FLU~~~~~~

The Great Dilemma

ERRATA

FLUORIDATION: The Great Dilemma (1978)

please correct the following errors:

p. xxvi, line 4: Yogoslavia to Yugoslavia

p. 241, line 1: pateints to patients

p. 356, Table 19-1, column 2, to read:

> *Fluoride*
> *from*
> *food*
> *(mg)*

p. 372, line 3 (line 1 of quotation) to
read: . . . in the drinking water

p. 421, line 14: bronchoscope to bronchoscopic

p. 421, line 17: fatility to fatality

p. 421, line 26: Moseby to Mosby

FLUORIDATION:
THE
GREAT
DILEMMA

by

GEORGE L. WALDBOTT, M.D.
WARREN, MICHIGAN

IN COLLABORATION WITH

ALBERT W. BURGSTAHLER, Ph.D.
The University of Kansas

and

H. LEWIS McKINNEY, Ph.D.
The University of Kansas

FOREWORD
by

ALTON OCHSNER, M.D.
Ochsner Medical Institutions
and
Tulane University School of Medicine

Coronado Press, Inc. Lawrence, Kansas

1978

ISBN 0–87291–097–0

Cover design by Robert Day

Set in 11 on thirteen point Press Roman and published in the United States of America by Coronado Press, Inc.
Box 3232
Lawrence, Kansas, 66044

AS EVERY past generation has had to disenthrall itself from an inheritance of truisms and stereotypes, so in our time we must move on from reassuring repetition of stale phrases to a new, difficult, but essential confrontation with reality.

For the great enemy of truth is very often not the lie – deliberate, contrived, and dishonest – but the myth, persistent, persuasive, and unrealistic. Too often we hold fast to the cliches of our forebears. We subject all facts to a prefabricated set of interpretations. We enjoy the comfort of opinion without the discomfort of thought.

President John F. Kennedy
Commencement Address,
 Yale University
June 11, 1962

CONTENTS

ILLUSTRATIONS

TABLES

FOREWORD

NO MEDICAL SUBJECT has aroused as much controversy as has fluoridation of community water supplies. According to many health authorities, fluoride supplied to children during the period of tooth development and maturation decreases the average incidence of dental caries. Various studies have compared the incidence of dental caries in twin cities using the same (or similar) water supplies, except that one is fluoridated and the other is not. The average incidence of dental caries among children in the fluoridated city appears to have been less. One disturbing fact, however, has been that in many cities with natural fluoridation, although the rate of tooth decay in the young population is frequently lower, premature dental deterioration occurs as the population ages and results in many edentulous individuals.

The tremendous emotionalism generated by the advocates for and those opposed to fluoridation is regrettable. If fluoride therapy could be proved never to be harmful, there would be no scientific argument against the fluoridation of the water supply, even though it has been apparently beneficial to a relatively small segment of the population, that is, those with developing teeth. In any event, health officials have assured us that fluoridation, at a concentration of about 1 part per million, is safe and effective for most persons subjected to its use.

The authors of *Fluoridation: The Great Dilemma* present a very comprehensive consideration of the subject of fluoride in its many applications, industrial and otherwise. They document the fact that there are many factors which influence the effect of fluoride on animals and humans, and there are many avenues by which fluoride can enter biological organisms.

Because of this, any consideration of total fluoride intake must take into account not only water supplies but also food, air, health of consumer, and many other factors including industrial pollution. Temperature of the air and physical activity are also critical, for vigorous persons in hot climates must replace large quantities of lost fluids. Should fluoride intake increase too much, sensitive persons will immediately react with bizarre, disabling symptoms. The authors authenticate many such cases. It is generally believed that most persons probably tolerate fluoride (less than 1-2 mg/day) fairly well during good health — but we really do not know.

Adverse susceptibility to small doses of fluoride is not unique, for it is well-known that many substances   such as drugs, antibiotics, and even foods — produce extreme sensitivity in patients. Moreover, there are individuals who have difficulty excreting excess amounts of fluoride because of kidney disease, thus promoting an abnormal accumulation of fluoride in the body.

Fluoridation: The Great Dilemma is a detailed, comprehensive survey of the fluoride question which presents both sides of the controversy with careful and extensive documentation. It is without doubt the most complete and authentic work on the highly emotional subject of fluoride and its use. A careful review of this splendid contribution is highly recommended for all persons interested in this important subject.

Alton Ochsner, M.D.
Department of Surgery,
Ochsner Medical Institutions
            and
Professor of Surgery, Emeritus,
Tulane University School of Medicine
New Orleans, Louisiana

ACKNOWLEDGMENTS

THIS BOOK owes a large debt to the innumerable contributions by many scientists, physicians, dental researchers, and lay persons throughout the world. Figures and photographs were contributed by A. V. Arma, G. Balazova, L. Capozzi, A. Y. Charnot, J. A. Csernyei, H. T. Dean, F. B. Exner, G. Fradà, J. Franke, K. Garber, L. Gisiger, S. S. Jolly, F. Marci, J. R. Marier, D. Milor, W. P. Murphy, G. Nalbone, A. E. Olson, F. Parlato, F. Pinet, O. Pribilla, M. O'Brien Rapaport, D. Rose, J. L. Shupe, M. Soriano, and S. P. S. Teotia.

For reading parts of the manuscript and offering helpful comments, special thanks are extended to Ernest E. Angino, Mrs. Arthur Case, N. Ray Hiner, S. L. Manocha, A. H. Mohamed, Lynn Nelson, Kevin Oliver, Dennis Quinn, Marjorie O'Brien Rapaport, Nell C. Taylor, H. Warner, John Yiamouyiannis, and Edward J. Zeller.

Photographic services were provided by E. Richard Marolf, The University of Kansas, Lawrence, Kansas, and Robert Shay, Hutzel Hospital, Detroit, Michigan.

Permission from the C. V. Mosby Co., St. Louis, Mo., to reproduce Figures 3-2, 4-3, 13-1, and 13-5 from *Health Effects of Environmental Pollutants* by G. L. Waldbott, 1973, is also warmly appreciated.

Ordinarily, publishers receive their accolades in the wings, but authors usually recognize the fundamental contributions made by these benefactors to knowledge. Professor John E. Longhurst, Ph.D., publisher of Coronado Press, and his son David have not only made publication of this book possible, they (and their staffs) have also extended themselves in every way on its behalf. They are gentlemen, creative scholars, and friends to those who wish to know.

NOTE ON REFERENCES

Periodical title abbreviations follow the BIOSIS List of Serials (BioSciences Information Service of Biological Abstracts, 2100 Arch Street, Philadelphia, Pa. 19103). Books are cited in full when first referred to and in abbreviated form thereafter.

INTRODUCTION

FLUORIDATION, a modern health procedure to counteract tooth decay, is part of our attempt to conquer disease and produce a better life for everyone. We all recognize that our health significantly affects the quality of our lives, and bright, sound teeth couched in a smiling face are perhaps the most visible manifestations of a happy state of being. Health officials have enthusiastically promised to maintain or even improve the condition of our teeth by fluoridating our water supplies.

Moreover, impressive benefits are not accompanied by any harmful side effects, except for a minimal amount of cosmetic mottling, so we are told. For about the last ten years, proponents have suggested that even this aesthetically offensive, permanent damage to teeth may really be desirable after all. Curiously, one fluoride toothpaste ad now claims that we do not get enough fluoride [protection] from fluoridated water alone, thus totally disregarding the problem of mottling.

We are also assured that all the dental benefits from fluoridation accrue with no effort on the consumer's part, that costs for the procedure are almost nothing, and that dental expenses will be tremendously reduced. Even politicians rarely promise quite so much to the public. That industries can concurrently dispose of an industrial waste product is still another less obtrusive benefit health officials rarely discuss.

Those of us concerned with the health of millions of persons heartily applauded fluoridation at first. We trusted health authorities, especially the United States Public Health Service (USPHS), to look after our best interests, and we sat back to await the Golden Age, when dentists would have more important duties than filling cavities. But over thirty years have passed, and the Millennium has not arrived: tooth decay is still a major disease ravaging civilization.

In English-speaking countries, supporters of fluoridation have been very successful in selling their dream, primarily because they have always emphasized the potential good to the exclusion of negative signs of danger in the scientific literature. For example, during an interview published on June 5, 1978, the Director of the National Institute of Dental Research stated:

> The National Cancer Institute, the National Heart, Lung, and Blood Institute, the Center for Disease Control, and population-study centers in Great Britain and Canada – all find that, *if you take into account population variations of age, sex, and race,* there's no difference in the cancer death rates between communities with or without fluoridated water.[1] [Emphasis added.]

On the basis of documented evidence, however, two scientists had already concluded in July 1977 that the excess cancer death rates in ten of the largest American cities "could *not* be ascribed to changes in the racial or sex compositions of the fluoridated and nonfluoridated populations." [Emphasis added.] Among persons 45 years of age or older, cancer death rates in the fluoridated cities have increased significantly compared to the nonfluoridated cities.[2]

On May 18, 1978, a USPHS scientist published analyses of mortality figures for 1969-1971 in 46 American cities having populations of 250,000 and over. *After* adjustments for differences in age, racial composition, and sex, he found a 4% *greater* cancer mortality rate in the 24 fluoridated cities than in the 22 nonfluoridated cities.[3] Two additional statistical manipulations of highly questionable merit[4] were necessary to swing the pendulum slightly in the opposite direction. Although the final verdict has not yet been rendered on this controversial subject, at the moment the evidence casts a suspicious shadow on the fluoridated cities, authoritative assurances notwithstanding.

Cancer is but one of a large assemblage of subjects connected with the fluoridation story. The overall adverse health effects many of us experience during everyday living – headaches, arthritis, colitis, (see Symptom List, pp. 392-393) – are of immediate and pressing interest to everyone, as are other potential problems. Pregnant mothers are naturally very sensitive about the health of their unborn children. Parents worry especially about their children's teeth; in fact, all of us feel strongly that depriving our children of the "birthright" of excellent teeth is a crime against humanity. With intelligent and effective health care programs, we hope that dental caries will eventually become only a bad memory. At the same time, we require that our general health not suffer at the expense of improved dental health: the human race is not expendable merely for the sake of our teeth.

Have we fallen into a disadvantageous risk-benefit situation with fluoridation? Has our daily fluoride burden exceeded a reasonable level? In 1939 Gerald J. Cox observed that the objective of fluoridation "is the optimum total amount of fluorine ingested per child *from all sources*."[5] [Emphasis added.] That amount has grown steadily from the 1940s until the present, when concern is widespread. In the State of Michigan, for example, the Governor recently launched an investigation of total fluoride intake. The study, although very incomplete, indicated an elevated intake from food.[6] A later publication by the National Research Council of Canada has emphasized fluoride intake from air, water, food, cigarettes, industrial exposure, Teflon cookware, etc.; the evidence demonstrates that total fluoride intake has clearly and undeniably grown well beyond prudent limits.[7]

Even the American Dental Association Council on Dental Therapeutics partially recognizes this problem: "Because differences of opinion exist on this matter, there is clear need for additional research to definitely establish the optimal dosage schedule for dietary supplementation."[8] Furthermore, the Health Services Administration of the U.S. Department of Health, Education, and Welfare has recently urged lowered fluoride supplementation, thus explicitly acknowledging the growing fluoride burden and its attendant dangers.[9]

The following book attempts the difficult task of revealing the truth about fluoridation. Standard claims are analyzed. Endorsements and sweeping generalizations about benefits are carefully examined. As expected, provocative questions have arisen: Is fluoridation really only a glowing promise that was never kept? Is it "a dental myth built out of misleading and unreliable statistics"?[10] Is it a revealing example of Man's best intentions degenerated into folly? Is it a dream turned into a nightmare?

Objective readers will be led irresistibly to the following

conclusion: what began as a triumphant march of the forces for public health — as a significant victory of science over disease — has ended as a nonscientific promotional effort where reason is subservient to methods abhorred by science, where unequivocal scientific facts have been ignored, and where scientists with adverse evidence have been denigrated and libeled.[11]

We assume that the laws of nature are universal and constant. Man, however, does not always understand nature's laws; his interpretations are imperfect, and today's wisdom is often merely tomorrow's folly. One of our foremost difficulties is that once we have become attached to certain views, we are extremely reluctant to give them up, even when the truth is known. For example, the Environmental Protection Agency (EPA) recently considered contaminant levels in drinking water, in accordance with the provisions of the Safe Drinking Water Act of 1974. Based on many explicit recommendations from the Department of Health, Education, and Welfare, Division of Dental Health,[12] with numerous citations to scientific publications, the EPA recommended that the maximum allowable fluoride level for drinking water be reduced from 2 times the "optimal" level to 1.5 times the "optimum."[13] By March 1975, however, DHEW dental officials did an abrupt about-face:

> We are convinced that to publish the lower maximum in these proposed regulations [as recommended by DHEW and accepted by EPA], when the basis for doing so is not well founded [sic], *would create unnecessary doubt on the safety of fluoridation and invite unwarranted attack by anti-fluoridationists.*[14] [Emphasis added.]

The scientific basis for lowering the levels was, on the contrary, very substantial, *as documented by DHEW scientists themselves.* On that point the evidence is uniquivocal. As the Environmental Defense Fund correctly concluded, the request for maintaining the old, outdated standard of 1962 arose from purely political considerations.[15] Science and truth took a back seat to entrenched policy on which reputations and careers were based. Adverse health effects were ignored.

Despite numerous denials of adverse effects caused by fluoridation, the elaborately documented harm remains as irrefutable testimony to the danger.[16] The tragic irony is that nonskeletal chronic fluoride toxicity more often than not is reversible if the following procedures are followed: switch to nonfluoridated water, consume only low-fluoride foods, and avoid fluoride from any other source. This is the path by which most persons intolerant to fluorides will recover their good health if they act soon enough. Refusing to perform such a simple experiment is hardly scientific or rational, especially since potable non-fluoridated water as consumed by humans presents no known health hazard in itself.

The history of science proves beyond question that few complex scientific questions are closed forever — "not debatable." Fluoridation most of all is not a closed subject: we all have much to learn and relearn about the effects of fluoride on life forms. The allegations that "there's no 'scientific controversy' over the safety of fluoridation" and that fluoridation is "safe, economical, and beneficial"[17] reveal a fundamental ignorance of the scientific literature, particularly the original sources. The evidence presented in the following book completely refutes such uninformed misrepresentations.

Is the so-called "fake controversy" over fluoridation "one of the major triumphs of quackery over science in our generation,"[17] or is fluoridation, scientifically speaking, far less effective than its public image suggests? Unquestionably, many of the arguments for fluoridation are superficially attractive and at first glance have persuaded many biologists and physicians. However, laborious examination of the scientific literature as well as first-hand experience with numerous cases of reversible nonskeletal chronic fluoride toxicity have compelled many scientists to abandon their early unwarranted support. If this work provides readers with an opportunity to reassess their own positions on the issue of fluoridation, the main goal of this book will have been achieved.

Recent political history has taught us many important lessons, not the least of which is that the public cannot be misled forever. Eventually, the truth will surface no matter how deeply it has been submerged. Fluoridation has been given trial runs all over the world, but it has not even begun to solve the problem of tooth decay. In fact, it has created a Pandora's box of its own. This glaring failure coupled with serious dangers to the health of millions of persons is widely recognized outside North America. Indeed, many nations have already abandoned water fluoridation.[18] Hungary, for example, discontinued fluoridation two years ago because of *deleterious effects,* according to Dr. Bozzay Jozsefne, Chief of the Chemical Section of the Municipal Water Works in Budpest. "She also stated that Yogoslavia had discontinued fluoridation recently."[19]

Throughout the world in the relatively few places that are still adding fluorides to their water supplies, the pillars of fluoridation are shaking. Will public health officials let this "health procedure" die a natural death, thereby salvaging a part of their tarnished reputations, or will the fight end as Lysenkoism ended in the USSR — in disgrace for hundreds of scientists — because USPHS scientists refuse to admit grave mistakes? These errors about fluoridation have caused pain to millions and death to many others. Surely, it is time for the curtain to fall on this human tragedy — The Great Dilemma.

REFERENCES

1. Interview, David B. Scott, Director, National Institute of Dental Research: From an Expert: Latest on Care of Your Teeth. U.S. News & World Report, June 5, 1978, pp. 81-82.

2. Yiamouyiannis, J., and Burk, D.: Fluoridation and Cancer. Age-Dependence of Cancer Mortality Related to Artificial Fluoridation. Fluoride, 10:102-123, 1977.

3. Erickson, J.D.: Mortality in Selected Cities with Fluoridated and Non-Fluoridated Water Supplies. N. Engl. J. Med., 298:1112-1116, 1978.

4. [Graham, J.R.] : H.E.W. Repackages Year-Old Study in an Attempt to Cover-Up Fluoridation-Cancer Link. Public Scrutiny, 1(7):14, Aug. 1, 1978: "As a matter of fact, the population density of fluorided cities *decreased* faster than the population density of the nonfluoridated cities, *a trend which would tend to increase the 10,000 figure* [of excess cancer deaths in the fluoridated cities] ." [Emphasis in original.]

5. Cox, G.J.: New Knowledge of Fluorine in Relation to Dental Caries. J. Am. Water Works Assoc., 31:1926-1930, 1939, at p. 1928.

6. The Department of Public Health and The Department of Agriculture, Michigan: Report on Fluoride Intake in Michigan. [July 1978], 26 pp., at pp. 9-11.

7. Rose, D., and Marier, J.R.: Environmental Fluoride 1977. National Research Council Canada, Report No. 16081, Ottawa, Ont., Can., [July 1978], 151 pp.; see esp. pp. 75-83.

8. Driscoll, W.S., and Horowitz, H.S. [Council on Dental Therapeutics] : A Discussion of Optimal Dosage for Dietary Fluoride Supplementation. J. Am. Dent. Assoc., 96:1050-1053, June 1978. See also Scholle, R.H.: Editorial:

Concern about Dietary Fluoride Supplementation. J. Am. Dent. Assoc., 96:1158, June 1978.

9. Fomon, S.J., and Wei, S.H.Y.: Prevention of Dental Caries, in Fomon, S.J., Ed.,: Nutritional Disorders of Children: Prevention, Screening and Followup. U.S. Department of Health, Education, and Welfare Publication No. (HSA) 76-5612, 1976. Cited in Trask, P.A.: Fluoride Dosage Update. J. Calif. Dent. Assoc., 6:50, March 1978, and Scholle, Ref. 8, above.

10. Douglas of Barloch, Lord: Blind Obstinacy: The Department of Health and Fluoridation. The National Pure Water Association [Great Britain], April 1978.

11. Consumers Union: Fluoridation: The Cancer Scare. Consumer Reports, 43(7):392-396, July 1978; Six Ways to Mislead the Public. Ibid., 43(8):480-482, August 1978. Libelous statements against opposing scientists have been rectified by public retractions. For example: Dismissal of suit: Waldbott v. Tossy, Travis. J. Mich. Dent. Assoc., 52:248, Sept. 1970; Apology [by R.D. Shortreed, M.D.], The Sarnia (Ontario) Observer, Tues., Jan. 5, 1971, p. 4; High Court of Justice: Queen's Bench Division. Fluoridation Dispute. Waldbott v. Sharp and Another. *Before* Mr. Justice Glyn-Jones. London Times, Nov. 24, 1961.

12. Greene, J.C.: Memo, Recommended Changes in Section 5.23, "Fluoride," PHS Drinking Water Standards, 1962 (8 references cited), Aug. 22, 1967; Memos on April 30, 1971 (W.B. Bock), Aug. 3, 1971 (G.R. Robeck), Aug. 24, 1971 (W.B. Bock), and June 4, 1973 (W.B. Bock). Copies in my possession.

13. Water Supply Division, Office of Water and Hazardous Materials, Environmental Protection Agency: Proposed Interim Primary Drinking Water Standards. Preliminary Draft, January 23, 1975; Environment Reporter, Current Developments, 5(42):1629, Feb. 14, 1975. EPA Schedules Four Public Hearings on Proposed Drinking Water Standards. Ibid., 5(47):1833, March 21, 1975: "In the only significant change from the later draft [discussed Feb. 28, 1975], EPA raised the proposed fluoride standard from one and one-half times the optimum level for dental purposes to two times the optimum after hearing that the lower limit would not be any better from a health standpoint and that many communities would find it difficult to meet."

14. Custard, C., Director, Office of Environmental Affairs, DHEW: Letter to Alvin L. Alm, EPA, March 7, 1975.

15. Environmental Defense Fund: Fluorides. Supplement C to the April 25, 1975, Comments of the Environmental Defense Fund on the Interim Primary Drinking Water Standards, May 16, 1975. Attachment, p. 13: "Thus, the recent arguments of DHEW ... do not contradict scientifically the evidence that maximum levels should be 1.5 times the optimum levels; rather, they seem to represent more a political decision than a scientific decision."

16. Spence, J.A., Ph.D.: Report to the MMWD [Marin Municipal Water District (California)] On the Health Effects of Fluoridation [April 1978], 3

pp. summary plus 16 pp. analysis and refs. to scientific literature. Cf. Lee, J.R., M.D. (Mill Valley, Calif.): Open Letter, Feb. 1975, and Report to the Marin Municipal Water District Board Concerning the Deliberations of the Citizens Committee on Fluoridation. April 1978. See also Hansen, K.: Effects of Fluoridated Water on Tissues of CSE Female Mice. Bios, 19(2):51-55, May 1978: "Histological observation revealed pathological changes in thyroid, kidney, liver, and spleen in mice receiving as little as 1 ppm fluoride [in their drinking water for ca. 26 weeks]."

17. Consumer Reports, Ref. 11, above, p. 482.

18. Status of Fluoridation in European Countries, Public Health Service, [Memo] FL-92, April 1977. Compare with State of the Nations Report. World-Wide Fluoridation Facts and Figures. 1st August, 1977. Anti-Fluoridation Association of Victoria, Melbourne, Australia. Cf. World-Wide Fluoridation Scorecard, National Fluroidation News, 23(3): 4, 1977, also p. 1 (Egypt declines fluoridation). Cf. Safe Water Coalition, Inc. [California]: Other Countries Reject Fluoridation. [1978].

19. Coalition for Pure Water, Allentown, Pa.: Memo re: Visit to Hungary [by E. Roth, June 1978]. June 27, 1978. Copy in my possession.

FLUORIDATION:

The Great Dilemma

CHAPTER 1

ENVIRONMENTAL DISEASES

UNTIL THE DAWN of our century, infectious diseases, not the medical profession, generally held the upper hand in the battle for life. Smallpox, diphtheria, typhoid, cholera, dysentery, tuberculosis, and anthrax sometimes decimated whole populations. Children succumbed in large numbers to scarlet fever, measles, and whooping cough, or else suffered long, drawn-out illness from these infections. Pneumonia was then one of the most dreaded diseases from which people rarely recovered, but any infectious disease could be terminal when no cure existed.

In the latter part of the 19th century, however, Robert Koch, Louis Pasteur, Joseph Lister, Paul Ehrlich, and others ushered in a new age in medicine. Particularly great moments occurred in 1882 when Koch identified the tiny rod-shaped bacillus that causes tuberculosis and in 1884 when Pasteur proved that man can be protected from the dreaded rabies virus by a vaccine to defend against the infecting organism, much as Edward Jenner had shown earlier in the case of smallpox. These and other similar developments laid the groundwork for an intensive drive against the numerous contagious diseases that had been ravaging mankind for thousands of years.

In rapid succession many new serums and vaccines were developed, and, by the middle of the 20th century, control of most infectious diseases was so effective that one modern author has optimistically claimed "we have healers so powerful that scarcely an illness remains beyond their power to control."[1] For instance, the genius and persevering industry of men such as Jonas Salk and Albert Sabin have led to the virtual eradication of the great crippler poliomyelitis. Not to be forgotten in this connection is the vital contribution of the U. S. Public Health Service, which provided extensive research support and nationwide distributional capabilities. Because vaccines, serums, and antibiotics – appropriately called miracle drugs – were prolonging human life, physicians in the 20th century could turn their attention to other health problems; for not all the scientific and technological advances of the past century benefited mankind.

The Industrial Revolution often meant pain as well as progress; it was indeed a two-edged sword. As the blue skies of former centuries gave way to industrial gray smoke and pollution, civilization seemed to be striking back at man, its creator. New, subtle maladies of unknown origin began to appear. The incidence of cancer rose alarmingly, and other degenerative ailments, especially arthritis, cardiovascular disease, and birth defects – these and many more afflictions – began to supplant infectious diseases, which man was learning to control. Man became his own enemy by poisoning not only the air he breathed and some of the medicines he took, but even the water and foods he consumed – indeed his entire environment. The slow, insidious manner in which the new afflictions crept up on man obscured the real causes of the problems and for a long time deceived physicians and other scientists.

Our medical literature now spotlights numerous health problems that were literally manufactured by man himself. Early in the Industrial Revolution physicians recognized the harmful effects of the fumes and dusts to which workers in many factories and mines were exposed. Only in recent years, however, has closer attention been given to the equally significant environmental dangers to people living near contaminating industrial operations.

INDUSTRIAL POLLUTANTS

In 1946 when H. L. Hardy and I. R. Tabershaw described delayed chemical pneumonitis in beryllium workers, they anticipated the discovery – by another group of scientists, three years later – of a serious "neighborhood disease" in the United States.[2] The latter group (six authors) reported the same characteristic beryllium-induced lesions in the lungs of 10 persons residing within ¾ mile of an Ohio beryllium plant, thereby indicating that the contamination had spread beyond the factory itself.[3] The slow development of these oftentimes fatal lesions, called granulomata, may not become apparent until some years after exposure to the poisonous agent. Additional studies on 26 persons residing within

1.7 to 6 miles downwind from a beryllium plant in Pennsylvania revealed the ability of this element to produce small-scale epidemics, reminiscent of those created by infectious diseases. When the work clothes of 100 employees at the plant were shaken out at the end of one work day, the dust in them contained about one-half microgram of beryllium per cubic meter — more than enough to trigger the diseases in the workers' families.[3]

Other industrial pollutants have also produced major outbreaks of chronic illness of unknown causes. In 1955, the Japanese physician F. Komatsu encountered a chronic disease among 357 of 1033 residents in the village of Kinasa, Nigano Prefecture, who were manufacturing floor mats.[4] During the winter months, the windows and crevices of the walls of their working areas were tightly sealed. Concentrations of carbon monoxide as high as 0.2 to 0.3% from open charcoal fires in the crowded rooms accounted, at first, for dizziness, fatigue, stiffness in shoulders, and headaches among the workers. As the disease progressed, the victims became short of breath and experienced tightness and pain in the chest. The carbon monoxide fumes had induced a specific kind of arteriosclerotic heart disease associated with high blood pressure, now referred to as "Shinshu myocardosis," in which the heart valves, particularly, were involved.

During the last decade, another Japanese physician, K. Tsuchiya, stumbled upon a new malady among the residents of the city of Toyama. This disorder was characterized by lumbago which gradually turned into bone pain so severe that the inhabitants called it "itai-itai byo" or "ouch-ouch disease."[5] Eventually their softened bones disintegrated even under slight pressure, thus giving rise to multiple fractures. In most cases, death was attributed to kidney failure that developed during the course of the disease. Extensive detective work ultimately identified the culprit as cadmium in rice and soybeans grown near a lead and zinc mining facility. Effluent water from the mine, combined with cadmium-laden fumes, had polluted the fields. Japanese health authorities eliminated the disease through strict pollution control measures. In the United States the late Henry Schroeder, a specialist in toxic trace metals, for many years emphasized the danger of cadmium, particularly its role in producing high blood pressure.[6] Pesticides, fertilizers, and water pipes are often the source of cadmium contamination of food and drinking water.

The searching minds and ingenuity of Japanese investigators have also penetrated the mystery of one of the most serious outbreaks of man-made poisoning of the industrial age – the widely publicized epidemic of mercury poisoning in the Minamata Bay of Japan. Between 1953 and 1960, 111 persons were disabled and 43 died.[7] A factory producing plastics from vinyl chloride and acetaldehyde was discharging its mercury wastes into the water; the wastes then accumulated in the fish consumed by the local population. A similar but less severe outbreak in 1965 killed 5 of 26 individuals stricken in the city of Niigata on the Japanese island of Honshu.[8] In the beginning, only general and vague symptoms were encountered: fatigue, marked weakness, irritability, numbness in arms and legs. Loss of hearing and vision, lack of muscle coordination, and progressive emaciation ensued. Tragically, permanent birth defects appeared in 19 babies, although, curiously, their mothers had expressed few or no complaints.

As a result of its volatility, mercury is dispersed for long distances from its original source. It settles to the bottom of lakes and rivers where bacteria convert the metal into the more toxic alkyl mercury derivatives. These in turn penetrate into plankton consumed by fish, which retain and further concentrate the poison during their lifetime. During the 1960s, widespread mercury poisoning also occurred in Sweden, where mercury-treated grain intended for seed purposes was unwittingly fed to domestic animals and resulted in severe contamination of meat and eggs.[9]

Another product of our industrial age – asbestos – has been the source of still more widespread environmental pollution. Asbestos is found almost everywhere – in homes, farms, factories, automobiles, planes, trains, ships, and missiles. It is widely used in roofing and siding, as insulation around air-ducts and water-pipes, in many electrical devices, and even in draperies and rugs. When sprayed on steel girders at construction sites or blown into spaces between walls, substantial amounts reach the lungs of non-workers, especially in metropolitan areas. In New York City, for example, minute asbestos fibers less than one micrometer in diameter were recovered in 1970 in the lungs of approximately two-thirds of 3,000 consecutive autopsied cases.[10] The presence of these fibers is often associated with scarring of lung tissue and other changes, especially the development of lung cancer. A malignant tumor involving the lining of the lungs and of the abdominal cavity, known as mesothelioma – a medical curiosity until two decades ago – is now being attributed to asbestos, even in persons who have had *no known exposure to asbestos.*[11] Most disconcerting is the extraordinary time lag – as much as 20 to 40 years – between the initial exposure to asbestos and the appearance of the malignancy. As though the harm from this airborne toxic agent was not enough, water supplies are also polluted with asbestos in effluents from iron mines that flow into rivers and lakes, including the Great Lakes. From such sources asbestos enters the water supplies of some communities, possibly in amounts sufficient to cause malignancies.

Another source of concern to our health authorities has been the upsurge – or perhaps the greater awareness – of chronic lead poisoning that has plagued mankind at least since the time of the Greek and Roman empires but has only recently received widespread attention by the medical profession. In ancient Rome, lead in pipes and in drinking and cooking vessels was a major source of excessive intake, especially for the upper classes.[12] Even today, lead water pipes (mainly in older plumbing) and soldered pipe joints pollute drinking water – especially "soft" and nonalkaline water. Perhaps still more hazardous, however, is the lead in automobile exhausts and smoke from burning trash and coal, since it settles on field crops, fruit, and vegetables. Thus, not only the air we breathe but also the food we eat may contain lead and account for an average daily uptake of about 0.3 mg,[13] about 10% of which is estimated to be stored in the body, especially in bones. Even more vexing and dangerous is the lead paint found in older homes, because small children often ingest paint from woodwork, plaster, floors, and furniture.

It is not surprising, therefore, that as many as 25% to 30% of American children have lead levels of more than 40 micrograms per 100 milliliters in their blood. This is enough to cause so-called "subclinical" lead poisoning, a disease which develops slowly and insidiously with symptoms common to many other kinds of chronic poisoning.[14] Patients become irritable, hyperactive, impulsive, restless, and clumsy; they look anemic and complain of pains and aches in muscles, of heartburn, nausea, and constipation – symptoms that ordinarily might not arouse serious concern. Low-grade lead poisoning may even induce abortions and stillbirths, since the levels of lead (and cadmium) in the bones of stillborn babies have been found to be 5 to 10 times higher than normal.[15] As the disease advances, the victims display visual and perceptual abnormalities, lethargy, loss of balance, epilepsy-like convulsions, and paralysis of the musculature of legs and arms—all manifestations of brain damage. Fortunately, modern techniques permit early detection of lead poisoning: (a) X-rays can disclose lead particles in the intestines; (b) laboratory tests can measure basophilic stippled red blood cells; (c) increased levels of delta-aminolevulinic acid in the urine indicate interference with the production of hemoglobin. Considerable progress has also been made in the treatment of lead poisoning by means of chelating agents that selectively remove lead, mercury, and other heavy metals from the body.

DIOXINS

Herbicides, fungicides, insecticides, and rodenticides also take their toll in illness and death. Among the highly toxic chemicals present in various sprays used as defoliants, the dioxins in 2,4,5-T (salts of 2,4,5-trichlorophenoxyacetic acid) and other polychlorinated phenol derivatives serve as tragic illustrations. (Dioxins are a class of persistent tricyclic by-products formed in the production of the trichlorophenol used to prepare 2,4,5-T and other chlorinated phenoxyacetic acid herbicides.) According to a recent report,[16] accidents during the manufacture of such compounds have caused acute dioxin poisoning of plant workers and even populations in Ludwigshafen, West Germany (1953), in The Netherlands (1963), and in Derbyshire, England (1968). In July 1976 a chemical explosion at a manufacturing plant in Seveso, Italy, released sufficient quantities of a dioxin (ca. 1.5-2 kg) to necessitate complete evacuation of large residential areas. Afterward, the dioxin was found in river water near Milan, in a sewage plant at Varedo, half-way between Milan and Seveso, and in the ground to a depth of 25 cm as far as 1 km (0.6 mile) from the plant.

In Vietnam, 2,4,5-T and related dioxin-contaminated defoliants were used extensively during 1961-1969. At least six different major toxic effects have been attributed to dioxins: (1) skin lesions, mainly "chloracne"; (2) eye disorders, including conjunctivitis, iritis, and corneal lesions; (3) gastrointestinal bleeding due to blood clotting abnormalities; (4) liver disease resembling viral hepatitis; (5) miscarriages and birth deformities; and (6) cancer. "Between 1956 and 1961 (the year in which spraying began), 159 cases of primary hepatic cancers were recorded among 5492 cancers [in the Hanoi area], while between 1962 and 1968, 791 primary hepatic cancers were observed of a total of 7911 [cancers]." This change represented an increase of over threefold in the proportion of primary cancer of the liver.[16]

SMOKING

Cigarette smoking produces some of the most serious and debilitating diseases arising from man's folly. The smoke itself contains not only nicotine, which affects capillary blood vessels, but also cancer-producing tars, such as benzo[a]pyrene. It also contains a higher concentration of carbon monoxide than a fume-laden garage or an automobile tunnel. Furthermore, a variety of other toxic agents are present in tobacco smoke, especially arsenic, lead (and related radioactive elements), cadmium, and fluoride – all of which are assimilated by the growing tobacco leaf from fertilizers and sprays. Even microscopic-sized particles of glass and asbestos derived from processing tobacco play a role in the kaleidoscope of toxic agents found in tobacco smoke.[17]

Although lung cancer and emphysema are the major part of the costly price of the smoking habit, smoking is one of the most common sources of myocardial infarction in the young, and it also contributes to gastric disturbances and decreases the birth weight of children of smoking mothers.[18] Likewise, tobacco smoke taxes the natural defense mechanism of the lungs, making them more susceptible to damage from airborne poisons such as asbestos, sulfur dioxide, and cadmium.[19]

Severe harm from smoking first made a vivid impression on me in 1953 when I realized that several of my patients and I suffered a common respiratory disease caused by smoking. The principal symptoms of this forerunner of emphysema are a chronically inflamed throat, chest pains, and a persistent irritating cough with asthma-like wheezing localized in the upper portion of the bronchial tree. After reflecting on my own condition, which was remarkably similar to that of many of my patients, and because I suspected a possible relationship to smoking, I decided to abandon cigarettes. To my pleasant surprise, the symptoms disappeared almost overnight. When I described this disease, which I designated Smoker's Respiratory Syndrome, in the *Journal of the American Medical Association*[20] —the first report of this kind in the medical literature—I observed that its most effective treatment was "complete elimination of smoking." Subsequently, hundreds of patients, many of whom had been suspected of having beginning lung cancer or what was mistakenly called "intrinsic asthma," have been cured of this chronic, debilitating ailment (and of emphysema in its early stage) simply by discontinuing smoking.

FLUOROCARBONS

Whereas the hazard of smoking is generally confined to a limited area such as a room or hall, other man-made air pollution may reach even beyond the lower regions of the earth's atmosphere. In the early 1930s the aerosol and refrigeration industries discovered what they believed were two ideal propellants and refrigerants: the gases dichlorodifluoromethane and trichloromonofluoromethane with the trade names Freon-12 and Freon-11. They revolutionized our economy because of their stability, apparent nontoxicity, and nonflammability; in 1973 their total U.S. production was about 830 million pounds. They were used in liquefied form in pressurized containers and released into the atmosphere whenever the product was propelled. Practically everything that can be sprayed has been packaged in aerosol containers, and today virtually every refrigeration plant utilizes Freons.

In 1970, J. E. Lovelock of the University of Reading, England, observed that these gases were present in the air over Western Ireland and in 1971 he discovered that one of them had pervaded the entire troposphere—the 6- to 10-mile-high layer of air that lies between the earth and the stratosphere. In 1973, two University of California scientists at Irvine, F. S. Rowland and M. J. Molina, discovered that once in the stratosphere, fluorocarbon molecules will dissociate and release chlorine atoms under the intense ultraviolet radiation of the sun. This process in turn then leads to a loss of ozone from the ozone layer that shields the earth from harmful ultraviolet solar radiation.[21] According to Lovelock's measurement, the total amount of Freon-11 in the troposphere was almost equal to the total amount ever manufactured. Researchers concluded that these gases are not removed from the atmosphere by rainfall, nor are they absorbed by the oceans, because they are so insoluble in water. Furthermore, they are not broken down rapidly by any other known mechanisms.[22] If manufacture of these gases were to continue at the 1972 worldwide rate of about one million tons a year, release of chlorine atoms and conversion of ozone to oxygen might appreciably diminish the earth's protective ozone layer or drastically alter it and disrupt, if not destroy, the biological systems of the earth.[23] The depletion of ozone would increase the solar radiation on earth, significantly affect the earth's climate, be detrimental to plant and animal cells, and induce skin cancer and genetic mutation in humans.

FOOD ADDITIVES

Air pollution from propellants, smoking, factories, and motor vehicles is but part of a larger picture, for we are also confronted with another man-made hazard in the form of food additives. I am referring to some 2500 items present in our daily diet ranging from chemical preservatives, dyes, bleaches, and the sequestering, drying, maturing, anti-caking, and anti-foaming agents, to extenders, emulsifiers, thickeners, plasticizers, artificial sweeteners and flavors, moisteners, fungicides, conditioners, hydrolyzers, antioxidants, and even to the antibiotics and hormones fed to the animals we eat.

The precise effects of these substances that are foreign to our bodies are often either unknown or unforeseen. For example, the administration of stilbestrol to chickens and cattle to stimulate growth was considered safe until gynecologists discovered that stilbestrol produced cancer in children whose mothers had taken it during pregnancy.[24] In light of a clear danger to health, intelligent consumers must wonder why stilbestrol is still used to fatten domestic animals in the U.S.A. even though the government has initiated strict regulations.

Another health threat associated with the advance of our civilization is derived from nitrites and their precursors, nitrates, which

are added as preservatives to many human and animal food substances, especially to processed meats for protection against deadly
botulism bacteria. Bacon in particular has long been linked with
this problem because of its high fat content and because it is fried
at a high temperature. In the stomach, under certain conditions,
especially when its acidity is high, nitrates are reduced to nitrites
that react with secondary amines to form highly toxic N-nitrosamines. Malignant tumors in the lungs, esophagus, and stomach
have been experimentally induced in animals by N-nitrosamines[25]
but in humans these poisonous agents have not, as yet, been conclusively linked with cancer. Since many other animal species are
subject to the same effect, however, complacency on this question
is unwarranted. Thus, government agencies are facing a grave
dilemma: in their attempt to protect consumers from serious
infections, they may thereby be inviting exposure to even greater
threats to health. The Food and Drug Administration, it is true,
has banned the use of many poisonous additives, but it is impossible to estimate how many others today are still shortening our
lifespan.

A PILL FOR EVERY ILL

Still another area of widespread assault upon our health is the
indiscriminate use of drugs. The desire of the public to have a "pill
for every ill" creates a vexing problem to a physician who must determine when a drug may be useful, or even lifesaving, and when it
may be destructive. In the past, drugs have all too frequently been
placed on the market before adequate testing, but even a generally
effective remedy can produce a tragedy. One of my own cases
illustrates this problem. In 1949 I published the first report of a
sudden fatal anaphylactic shock due to penicillin.[26] This tragedy
occurred to a 39-year old woman who collapsed and expired within minutes after her sister, a registered nurse, had injected the
drug. Many similar incidents are now on record. The unusual feature in this particular case was that the patient had experienced no
ill effects from previous treatments, which forces the conclusion
that during the three-week interval following her last injection, she
must have acquired the fatal sensitivity. That such sensitivity may

develop during a 2- to 3-week interval between one injection and the next is now well documented by animal experiments.

I had previously made extensive studies on sudden death from human anaphylactic shock that had been considered a curious laboratory phenomenon confined to animals.[27-34] After reviewing numerous hospital records involving sudden death from injections, I was able to demonstrate that nonprotein substances, such as local anesthetics, can cause the same manifestations of anaphylaxis as animal sera and can produce a generalized edema.[32] It is not uncommon that a drug as harmless as aspirin induces anaphylactic shock in highly sensitized patients, in spite of the fact that the victim may have been taking aspirin for years without apparent ill effects. In assessing such reactions from drugs, we must distinguish between hypersensitivity (or allergy) to a drug and intolerance to it.[35] In the case of aspirin, intolerance is characterized by hemorrhages in the stomach whereas allergy to aspirin results in such symptoms as hives, asthma, allergic nasal and sinus disease, or even shock — reactions that are not related to poisoning, and for which no excessive dose is required.

Nearly every drug can have grave side effects in persons who display intolerance to it. For example, in Europe phenacetin was used as a pain reliever for more than 50 years until 1961, when two Norwegian physicians, O. Nordenfeld and N. Ringertz, demonstrated that it had caused a fatal kidney disease in 27 men and 3 women, some of whom had been taking this medication regularly for as long as 20 years.[36]

Shortly after World War II, other deaths from kidney disease were attributed to a lithium compound prescribed as a salt-substitute for patients with heart disease. Nevertheless, lithium carbonate was approved in 1969 as a "mild, non-addictive sedative" for agitated mental patients by the Food and Drug Administration, and a researcher at the University of Texas has even suggested that it be added to water supplies.[37] He had found significantly lower admissions to mental hospitals from Texas towns where lithium levels in water were high. Nevertheless, lithium contributes to irreversible brain damage.[38]

For centuries, physicians used mercury in the treatment of syphilis. It was injected into the buttocks or routinely applied to the skin of the entire body. In the latter case, its high volatility accounted for absorption of toxic amounts through inhalation and frequently caused slowly developing, vague symptoms of kidney damage, which remained largely unnoticed. We shall never know how many deaths attributed to syphilis actually resulted from mercury poisoning.

One of the most vivid examples of our inability to recognize specific, long-term toxicities of drugs is the thalidomide tragedy during the 1960s that led to phocomelia—gross deformities of limbs of numerous infants here and abroad, after their mothers had used this tranquilizer during an early stage of pregnancy.[39] With the approval of the Food and Drug Administration, thalidomide had been made available for investigative purposes for six years to about 1200 physicians in the U.S.A. before its devastating effects became known.[40] It is certainly ironic that "about one third of American thalidomide babies were born to wives of physicians who had received free samples of the drug."[40]

Other helpless victims of inadequate testing of new medical procedures are the children blinded with retrolenticular fibroplasia due to routine administration required by health officials of concentrated oxygen to premature infants. Three to five weeks after delivery, the arteries and veins behind the lens of the eyes become congested, and an opaque mass develops in the retina and vitreous body of the eye. Finally, the vision is obscured by newly-formed scar tissue leading to complete blindness. It took eleven years before the cause of this disease was recognized and before health departments in the U.S.A. reversed their stand.[41]

Even the well-known poison arsenic was believed to be useful in minute doses for the treatment of certain skin diseases, especially psoriasis and bronchial asthma,[42] until it was determined that prolonged intake of arsenic caused dermatitis, nausea, abdominal pain, diarrhea, keratosis (scaling of hands and feet), and a tendency to fluid accumulation in the body. More recent discoveries indict it as carcinogenic to the skin, liver, and lungs,[43] particularly when released into the air by sprays and by combustion of coal, which contains an average of 16 micrograms of arsenic per gram.[44]

These are but a few examples of numerous man-made diseases that have littered the path of advances in technology, industrial development, and the medical sciences. It cannot be emphasized too strongly that in many of these instances, especially with air-

and water-borne pollutants, extremely minute amounts suffice to do the damage. These pollutants enter the body over long periods of time, causing diseases which begin slowly and unobtrusively, which are difficult to diagnose, and which therefore escape the attention of the healing profession.

In the following chapters, I shall discuss one of the most potent poisons in nature, one which has been inadequately assessed and often poorly understood, although countless articles have appeared in the medical literature clearly demonstrating its deleterious effects on human health. Few toxic agents are as widely distributed in the ecosystem – in air, in water, and in food – which affect as many organs of the human body and also damage plants and organisms – as is FLUORINE, an element that is now being widely added as inorganic fluorides to municipal water supplies at a concentration of 1 part of fluoride ion per million parts (ppm) of water for the prevention of tooth decay. This important question – whether fluoride is a poison or a panacea – has created one of the greatest dilemmas of the 20th century.[45]

REFERENCES

1. de Ropp, R.S.: The New Prometheans: Creative and Destructive Forces in Modern Science. Delacourte Press, New York, 1972, p. 56.

2. Hardy, H.L., and Tabershaw, I.R.: Delayed Chemical Pneumonitis Occurring in Workers Exposed to Beryllium Compounds. J. Ind. Hyg. Toxicol., 28: 197-211, 1946.

3. Eisenbud, M., Wanta, B.S., Duston, C., Steadman, L.T., Harris, W.B., and Wolf, B.S.: Non-Occupational Berylliosis. J. Ind. Hyg. Toxicol., 31:282-294, 1949.

4. Komatsu, F.: Shinshu Shinkinsho. Digest of Science Labour, 10:315-318, 1955.

5. Tsuchiya, K.: Causation of Ouch-Ouch Disease. Part II. Epidemiology and Evaluation. Keio J. Med., 18: 181-194, 195-211, 1969.

6. Schroeder, H.A.: Cadmium as a Factor in Hypertension. J. Chronic Dis., 18: 647-656, 1965.

7. Irukayama, K.: Paper No. 8, in Third International Conference Water Pollution Research, Washington, D.C., Water Pollution Control Federation, 1966.

8. Tsubaki, T., and Irukayama, K.: Minamata Disease: Methylmercury Poisoning in Minamata and Niigata, Japan. Elsevier, Amsterdam. New York and Oxford, 1977.

9. Westöö, G.: Mercury Compounds in Animal Foods. Nordic Conference on Mercury, Norforsk, Oct. 11, 1968. See articles in Environment (St. Louis), 13 (4): 2-33, May 1971.

10. Langer, A.M., Selikoff, I.J., and Sastre, A.: Chrysotile Asbestos in the Lungs of Persons in New York City. Arch. Environ. Health, 22:348-361, 1971.

11. Selikoff, I.J., Bader, R.A., Bader, M.E., Churg, J., and Hammond, E.C.: Editorial: Asbestosis and Neoplasia. Am. J. Med., 42:487-496, 1967.

12. Gilfillan, S.C.: Roman Culture and Dysgenic Lead Poisoning. Mankind Q., 5:131-160, 1965.

13. Editorial Note: Atmospheric Contamination with Lead. Ann. Intern. Med., 68:488, 1968.

14. Waldron, H.A.: The Blood Lead Level Threshold. Arch. Environ. Health, 29: 271-274, 1974.

15. Bryce-Smith, D., Deshpande, R.R., Hughes, J., and Waldron, H.A.: Lead and Cadmium Levels in Stillbirths. Lancet, 1:1159, 1977.

16. Laporte, J.-R.: Effect of Dioxin Exposure. Lancet, 1: 1049-1050, 1977; see also Crossland, J., and Shea, K.P.: The Hazards of Impurities. Environment (St. Louis), 15(5): 35-38, June 1973. For recent accounts of similar disasters from the pesticides Kepone (Hopewell, Va.) and Phosvel (Bayport, Tex.), see Sterret, F.S., and Boss, C.A.: Careless Kepone. Environment (St. Louis), 19(2): 30-37, March 1977; Shea, K.: Profile of a Deadly Pesticide, ibid., 19(1): 6-12, Jan./Feb. 1977.

17. For references to primary sources, see Waldbott, G.L.: Health Effects of Environmental Pollutants. The C. V. Mosby Co., St. Louis, 1973.

18. MacMahon, B., Alpert, M., and Salber, E.J.: Infant Weight and Parental Smoking Habits. Am. J. Epidemiol., 82: 247-261, 1965.

19. Selikoff, I.J., and Langer, A.M.: Inorganic Particles in Cigars and Cigar Smoke. Science, 174: 585-586, 1971.

20. Waldbott, G.L.: Smoker's Respiratory Syndrome. J. Am. Med. Assoc., 151: 1398-1400, 1953.

21. Molina, M.J., and Rowland, F.S.: Stratospheric Sink for Chlorofluoromethane: Chlorine Atomic-Catalysed Destruction of Ozone. Nature (Lond.), 249: 810-812, 1974.

22. Karim Ahmed, A.: Unshielding the Sun, Human Effects. Environment (St. Louis), 17(3): 6-14, April/May 1975.

23. Brodeur, P.: Annals of Chemistry. New Yorker, 51: 47-50, 55, 56, 58, April 7, 1975; cf. Jesson, J.P.: The Chlorofluorocarbon/Ozone Theory - A Scientific Status Report. Angew. Chem. Int. Ed. Engl., 16:513-519, 1977.

24. Greenwald, P., and Nasca, P.C.: Stilbestrol Exposure in Utero: Long Term Effect, in Congenital Defects: New Directions in Research, edited by D.T. Janerich, R.G. Salko, and I.H. Porter. Academic Press, New York and London, 1974, pp. 149-160.

25. Lijinsky, W.: Health Problems Associated with Nitrites and Nitrosamines. Ambio, 5: 67-72, 1976.

26. Waldbott, G.L.: Anaphylactic Death from Penicillin. J. Am. Med. Assoc., 139: 526-527, 1949; comment and reply, ibid., 140:125, 1949.

27. Waldbott, G.L.: The Prevention of Anaphylactic Shock. J. Am. Med. Assoc., 98: 446-449, 1932.

28. Waldbott, G.L.: So-called Thymic Death. V. Respiratory Sensitization to General and Local Anesthetics. Arch. Otolaryngol., 17: 549-553, 1933.

29. Waldbott, G.L.: So-Called Thymic Death. VI. The Pathologic Process in 34 Cases. Am. J. Dis. Child., 47: 41-60, 1934.

30. Waldbott, G.L.: Allergic Shock. III. From Substances Other Than Pollen and Serum. Ann. Intern. Med., 7: 1308-1318, 1934.

31. Waldbott, G.L., and Snell, A.D.: Pulmonary Lesions Resembling Pneumonia as the Result of Allergic Shock. J. Pediatr., 6: 229-233, 1935.

32. Waldbott, G.L.: Allergic Shock from Local and General Anesthetics. Anesth. Analg., 14: 199-204, 1935.

33. Waldbott, G.L., and Ascher, M.S.: The Role of Accidental Puncture of Veins in the Production of Allergic Shock. Ann. Intern. Med., 9: 1232-1239, 1936.

34. Waldbott, G.L., Ascher, M.S., and Rosenzweig, S.: Serial Studies of Blood, Sugar, Blood Pressure and White Blood Count in Allergic Shock. J. Allergy, 10: 220-225, 1939.

35. Waldbott, G.L., Blair, K.E., and McKeever, R.: Drug Tolerance in Asthma. Fatal Salicylate Poisoning from a Physiologic Dose. Ann. Allergy, 11: 199-203, 1953.

36. Nordenfeld, O. and Ringertz, N.: Phenacetin Takers Dead with Renal Failure. Acta Med. Scand. 170: 385, 1961.

37. Wells, B.G.: Adding Lithium to Drinking Water Keeps You Sane, Claims Scientist. National Enquirer, Jan. 23, 1972.

38. Cohen, W.J., and Cohen, N.H.: Lithium Carbonate, Haloperidol, and Irreversible Brain Damage. J. Am. Med. Assoc., 230: 1283-1287, 1974.

39. Curran, W.J.: Thalidomide Tragedy in Germany: The End of a Historic Medicolegal Trial. N. Engl. J. Med. 284: 481-482, 1971, and A.M.A.'s Drug Councils to Study Thalidomide. A.M.A. News, Aug. 8, 1962.

40. O'Brien, W.M.: Drug Testing: Is Time Running Out? Bull. At. Sci., 25-(1): 8-14, Jan. 1969.

41. Trevor-Roper, P.D.: The Eye and Its Disorders. 2nd ed. Blackwell Scientific Publications, Oxford, England, 1974, pp. 569-597.

42. Waldbott, G.L.: New Trends in the Treatment of Bronchial Asthma. Med. Clin. N. Am. (Nation-wide Number), 33: 411-425, 1949.

43. Hueper. W.C.: Environmental Carcinogenesis in Man and Animals. Ann. N.Y. Acad. Sci., 108: 963-1068, 1963.

44. Blot, W.J., and Fraumeni, J.F.: Arsenical Air Pollution and Lung Cancer, Lancet, 2: 142-144, 1975.

45. Cf. Gotzsche, Anne-Lise: The Fluoride Question: Panacea or Poison? Stein and Day, New York, 1975.

CHAPTER 2

FLUORINE AND ITS COMPOUNDS

HISTORICAL BACKGROUND

ONE OF THE EARLIEST references to the effects of fluorine in the environment is found in a passage written by the Roman poet Marcus Valerius Martialis (40-104 A.D.). Describing the distinctive teeth of Thais, a mistress of Alexander the Great, he observed:

> Thais has black teeth, Laecania has snow-white ones.
> Why? The latter's teeth were bought, the former has her own.[1]

The "black" or "mottled teeth" (Fig. 2.1, opposite), as we now call them, were probably common in the volcanic area of Italy where Martialis lived; they indicate the specific involvement of the fluoride ion (F$^-$), although nearly 2000 years passed before the cause of this dental abnormality was traced to fluoride. Because of the black horizontal lines especially prominent on the incisor teeth, which resemble inscriptions, contemporary Italians call them "denti scritti," – marked teeth – or teeth which have been inscribed.[2] They are also referred to as "denti di Chiaie," after the physician Stefano Chiaie, who described them in residents of Messina, Italy, where the drinking water that flowed through the lava beds had been contaminated with fluoride.[3] Another version identifies these teeth with Chiaia, a section of the city of Naples – also situated near a volcano – where this dental abnormality had been recorded by Benedetto Croce in 1892.[4]

As early as 1670, according to some authors, the Nürnberg glassworker Heinrich Schwanhardt made artistic etchings on glass with fumes evolved from the reaction of sulfuric acid with fluorspar.[5] The late chemist-historian J. R. Partington has questioned the validity of this traditional account, however, and states that

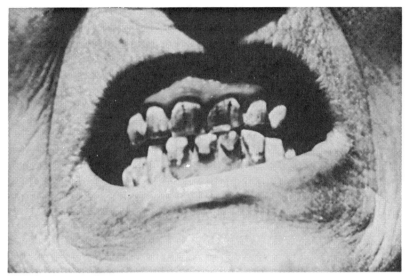

Fig. 2-1. "Black" teeth in a 56-year-old female residing in a high-fluoride-water (3-6 ppm) area of northern Sicily.
(Courtesy Prof. G. Fradà, Palermo, Italy.)

the first authenticated record of this reaction, which produces hydrofluoric acid or hydrogen fluoride (HF), dates from either the year 1720 or 1725.[6] A better understanding by chemists soon followed, and in 1771 the Swedish chemist Carl W. Scheele recognized in fluorspar the calcium salt of the new acid, which he called the "acid of fluorspar," or "fluoric" acid.[7]

In 1803 the Italian chemist Domenico Morichini made another significant discovery when he demonstrated the presence of the new element in a fossil tooth of an elephant disinterred near Rome. Two years later, in collaboration with L. G. Gay-Lussac, he showed that fluorine is also present in human teeth (1805).[5]

These discoveries gave rise to an interesting question originally posed in the last century: could the fluoride content of teeth and bones provide a clue regarding the age of a fossil?[8] It was suggested that calcium salts in bones attract fluoride from ground water and that the more fluoride thus stored, the older the fossil might be. The fluoride exchange method has recently found application in archaeology for ancient ivory.[9]

The term "fluorine" (French *le fluor*; Latin *fluere* – to flow) was originally used by the French physicist André-Marie Ampère in a letter dated August 25, 1812, to the British chemist Humphrey Davy.[10] The latter recognized that hydrofluoric acid contains a new element, a member of the halogen family, the other members being chlorine, bromine, iodine, and the radioactive element astitine. He called the element "fluorine," a name that refers to the ɥse of its calcium salt, fluorspar, as a flux in metallurgy.

Davy made numerous attempts to isolate the new element but failed because of its extraordinary reactivity. He observed that "liquid fluoric acid [HF] immediately destroys glass and all animal and vegetable substances, it acts on all bodies containing metallic oxides, and I know of no substances that are not rapidly dissolved or decomposed by it, except metals, charcoal, phosphorus, sulphur, and certain combinations of chlorine."[10] In his efforts to prepare fluorine either by electrolysis or by double decomposition reactions, he therefore used vessels of sulfur, carbon, gold, silver chloride, or platinum, but none appeared capable of resisting what he described as fluorine's "strong affinities and high decomposing agencies."[10]

Subsequently, other leading chemists of the 19th century, including Michael Faraday, Edmond Fremy, and George Gore, made further attempts to isolate fluorine but were as unsuccessful as Davy. In 1834 Faraday thought he had succeeded by electrolyzing fused fluorides, but he later realized that he had not. In 1855 Fremy reported that electrolysis of molten calcium fluoride liberated a gas at the anode which was so reactive that it could not be collected. In 1869 Gore described how he had momentarily obtained fluorine by electrolysis of anhydrous HF, but the gas immediately combined explosively with hydrogen from the cathode.[5,10]

Finally, on June 26, 1886, a major breakthrough occurred when Henri Moissan (Fig. 2.2, opposite) isolated the pale yellow, highly toxic and reactive gas by electrolyzing a cooled solution of potassium hydrogen fluoride in anhydrous hydrofluoric acid in an all-platinum apparatus.[5, 10] Moissan thereby solved what had been one of the most difficult chemical challenges of his time, an achievement recognized in 1905 by the award of a Nobel Prize.

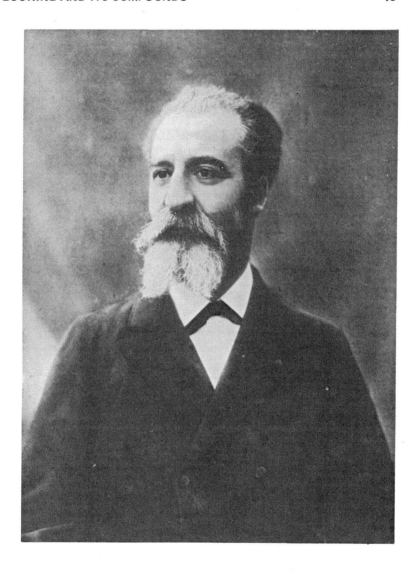

Fig. 2-2. Henri Moissan, 1852-1907. Professor of Chemistry at the École
Supérieure de Pharmacie and at the Sorbonne;
discoverer of elemental fluorine.
(From the frontpiece of his book
Le Fluor et ses Composés, Steinheil, Paris, 1900.)

Nevertheless, in the late 19th and early 20th centuries fluorine was generally regarded as a mere laboratory curiosity. Moissan himself had serious doubts that his discovery might ever be of practical use.[11] The decade of the 1920s, however, marked a new age in fluorine chemistry and many useful applications were discovered which have made the element indispensable to modern industry. Why have fluorine and its compounds become so important?

PROPERTIES OF FLUORINE

Widely distributed in nature, fluorine has been estimated to be the 13th most abundant element in the earth's crust (ca. 0.065% by weight).[12] Although trace amounts in uncombined form can be detected when certain radioactive fluorspars (e.g., from Wolsenberg, West Germany) are crushed, fluorine otherwise occurs only in combination with other elements. In the free state it is a pale yellow gas with a pungent, irritating odor. On cooling it condenses to a liquid boiling at -188°C., and on further cooling it freezes to a solid melting at -220°C.[12]

Elemental fluorine exists as a diatomic molecule with a remarkably low dissociation energy (38 kcal/mole). Consequently, it is highly reactive and has a strong tendency to combine with other elements to produce compounds called fluorides. As the most electronegative of all the elements, fluorine is the strongest oxidizing agent known. When liquid fluorine combines with hydrogen the reaction produces a temperature of 4700°C., which is even hotter than that obtained by burning atomic hydrogen in oxygen (4200°C.). Wood or rubber held in a stream of fluorine bursts into flames. Even asbestos, a fireproofing agent, reacts so vigorously with fluorine that it becomes incandescent. Another generally inert element, platinum, is also slowly attacked by fluorine.

This extreme reactivity makes fluorine very difficult to handle. Containers made of nickel, copper, or steel are attacked by it and become coated with a layer of nickel, copper, or iron fluoride, which then protects them from further corrosion. Curiously, Teflon, a plastic containing fluorine, is one of the most suitable materials for harnessing and shipping the compressed or liquefied gas.

SOURCES OF FLUORINE

The three most common sources of fluorine are the minerals fluorspar, or calcium fluoride (CaF_2), the aluminum compound cryolite (Na_3AlF_6), and apatite, a calcium phosphate complex of the formula $Ca_{10}X_2(PO_4)_6$, where X represents either fluoride, chloride, or hydroxide (OH^-) ions.

Fluorspar (CaF_2), often called fluorite, is a beautiful, transparent cube-shaped, glass-like crystal, with colors ranging from clear transparency to exquisite shades of green, blue, yellow, purple, brown, and blue-black (Fig. 2–3, below). It is found in veins of limestone and sandstone, mainly in Iceland, Mexico, England, Germany, and Newfoundland. In the United States, fluorspar is mined primarily near the border between Kentucky and Illinois, and in California, Montana, New Mexico, and Colorado.

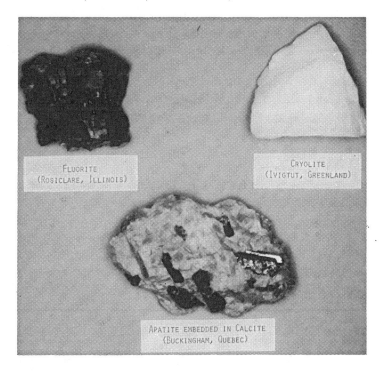

Fig. 2-3. Specimen samples of fluoride minerals; about ¼ actual size.
(Courtesy Mineralogy Collection,
University of Kansas Department of Geology.)

The usefulness of fluorspar has been known for centuries. In 1529 Georgius Agricola, who is often called the "father of metallurgy," referred to its value as a flux in smelting operations in his book *Bermannus*.[5,7] In Napoleonic times a variety of fluorite known as Blue John was exported from Devonshire, England, to France where it was worked into ornamental vases.[13] Today, the chemical industry is the largest consumer of fluorspar, particularly in manufacturing hydrofluoric acid. In steel production, it assists in the refining process because of its fluxing action to remove slag. Fluorspar is indispensable in making enamelware and in refining lead and antimony. Clear, colorless fluorite of optical quality is used in the manufacture of apochromatic lenses because of its low index of refraction and low dispersion of light.

Cryolite, sodium aluminum fluoride (Na_3AlF_6) (Fig. 2-3, above), the second industrially valuable fluoride compound found in nature, is (or at least was) mined mainly in Greenland, where it has been deposited through volcanic eruptions, but other large deposits occur in the Soviet Union, Spain, and Colorado. Since molten cryolite dissolves bauxite (aluminum oxide) and thereby facilitates the electrolytic reduction of Al^{+3} to the free metal, it is in great demand; indeed, natural sources are so heavily depleted that producers of aluminum now rely largely on synthetic cryolite made from fluorspar.[12]

Apatite, in the form of fluoroapatite, $Ca_{10}F_2(PO_4)_6$ (Fig. 2-3), another major natural source of fluorine, is found in vast coral deposits and volcanic rocks in Florida, Tennessee, and South Carolina, as well as in North Africa and the West Indies. Rich in phosphorus, apatite is mined primarily for the production of phosphate fertilizers and phosphoric acid, so vital to modern agriculture. In the conversion of fluoroapatite into superphosphate fertilizer by treatment with sulfuric acid, large amounts of hydrogen fluoride are evolved.

USES OF FLUORINE

Numerous other fluorine compounds have become extremely important during the past fifty years. Their uses range from automobile bearings that never need greasing to replacements for diseased or ruptured blood vessels in the human body; from clothing that resists stains to cancer drugs. The industrial application of fluorine seems endless (Table 2-1, below), and a glance at this new development is fascinating indeed.

Throughout the early part of the 20th century, fluorine compounds were by-products of industrial processes, such as the manufacture of aluminum and other metals, superphosphate fertilizers, and ceramics. Commercially, their only outlets were insecticides and rodenticides. With the development of new fluorine compounds, however, their usefulness increased remarkably during the 1940s when they began to be utilized as refrigerants, aerosols, lubricants, and plastics. Sodium fluoride and calcium fluoride were also added to many of the newer heat-resistant ceramics.

Simultaneously, the pharmaceutical industry discovered that fluorine reinforces the action of many molecules. The efficacy of a drug frequently depends on how soon the body metabolizes the molecule and terminates its action. By inserting fluorine at the weak point in the structure of a drug, chemists have made certain pharmaceuticals more resistant to breakdown in the body, thereby reinforcing their action. Some of the most popular fluorine-containing medications are: fluorosteroids (cortisone-like preparations) for the treatment of arthritis and allergic diseases; fluorouracil, which delays the growth of cancer of the prostate and bladder; and fluorine-containing antihistaminics, tranquilizers, anesthetics, and diuretics (which increase the flow of urine through the kidneys and thus counter the development of fluid accumulation).

Fluorine has also proved invaluable in the large-scale separation of the fissionable uranium isotope ^{235}U from stable ^{238}U for production of nuclear energy and weapons. Natural uranium is converted into volatile $^{235}UF_6$ and $^{238}UF_6$, which by virtue of their slight difference in molecular weight are separable by multistage diffusion.

The most widely used commercial fluorine products are hydrogen fluoride, hydrofluoric acid, and fluorocarbons. Hydrogen fluoride (HF), an easily liquified gas (boiling point 19.54°C), is so reactive that in water (as hydrofluoric acid) it dissolves every metal except extremely inert ones like gold and platinum. The U.S. production of HF, the most important of all industrial fluorine compounds, rose from about 150,000 tons in 1960 to nearly 400,000 tons only twelve years later. About 80% of the

Table 2-1

Commercial Uses of Some Inorganic Fluorides

SUBSTANCE	USES
Aluminum fluoride, AlF_3	Aluminum production (flux) Ceramics production (opacifier) Arc welding rods (coating)
Ammonium bifluoride, NH_4FHF	Glass (frosting) Brewery (sanitation) Special alloys (electrodeposition) Aluminum alloys (cleaning, polishing)
Antimony trifluoride, SbF_3	Organic fluorides (preparation)
Barium fluoride, BaF_2	Light metal industry Ceramic, enamel (ingredient)
Boron trifluoride, BF_3	Catalyst for alkylation, esterification, and polymerizations
Chlorine trifluoride, ClF_3	Rocket fuel Uranium production Oil drilling (chemical cutter) Chlorofluorocarbon lubricants (preparation)
Chromium trifluoride, CrF_3	Wool (treatment before dyeing)
Cryolite, Na_3AlF_6	Aluminum production (electrolyte) Steel (flux) Enamel, glass (opacifier)
Fluorine, F_2	Rocket fuel Uranium production Metal fluorides (preparation)
Fluoroboric acid, HBF_4 and its salts	Metals (cleaning, pickling) Electroplating
Fluorspar, CaF_2	Hydrogen fluoride (production) Steel production (flux) Glass, ceramics (opacifier)
Hydrofluorosilicic (also called hydrofluosilicic) acid, H_2SiF_6, and its salts e.g., sodium fluorosilicate, Na_2SiF_6	Electroplating Water (fluoridation) Wood (preservative) Concrete (hardening) Textile sours

Table 2-1 (cont'd)

SUBSTANCE	USES
	Metal casting (flux)
	Synthetic mica (production)
	Zirconium (extraction)
	Cements (acid resisting)
Hydrogen fluoride, HF	Organic fluorides (preparation)
	Aluminum (production)
	Uranium (production)
	Petroleum (alkylation)
	Inorganic fluorides (preparation)
Hydrofluoric acid (HF solution in water)	Glass (etching, frosting)
Lead fluoride, PbF_2	Pyrotechnics (flame colorant)
Magnesium fluoride, MgF_2	Optical industry
Perchloryl fluoride, $FClO_3$	Rocket fuel
	Gaseous dielectric
	Organic fluorides (preparation)
Potassium fluoride, KF	Organic fluorides (preparation)
Potassium fluorotitanate, K_2TiF_6	Titanium alloys (production)
Sodium fluoride, NaF	Insecticide, rodenticide
	Wood (preservative, fungicide)
	Water (fluoridation)
	Ceramics (production)
	Light metal (production, electrolyte)
Stannous fluoride, SnF_2	Toothpaste (additive)
Sulfur hexafluoride, SF_6	High-voltage equipment (dielectric)

1974 U.S. output went into the manufacture of aluminum and of fluorinated hydrocarbons.[14] Hydrogen fluoride and hydrofluoric acid are also used in manufacturing stainless steel, processing uranium, etching and frosting glass, and alkylating petroleum, as well as electroplating and cleaning copper and brass. Hydrofluoric acid is also useful in making filter paper and carbon electrodes and in galvanizing metals; it even has served as a sterilizer in breweries and distilleries.

Other fluorine-containing gases, known as refrigerants — Freon and Genetron — are carbon-fluorine compounds. Odorless, stable, noncorrosive, and nonflammable, they also comprise the bulk of aerosol sprays. When the ejection valve of a hand-sized fumigator is opened, the Freon begins to boil and discharges the contents of the container as a fine mist that remains suspended in the air for a long time. Until recently about 50% of the 800 million pounds of fluorocarbons produced annually in the U.S. were used in aerosols, more than 90% of which were toiletries such as hair-sprays and deodorants.[11] Widespread concern that use of fluorocarbons might deplete the ozone layer shielding the earth from harmful short-wavelength solar radiation has led manufacturers to turn elsewhere for ways to apply deodorants and many other substances.[15]

Another interesting group of carbon-fluorine compounds are the fluorocarbon plastics that are nonflammable, insoluble in most solvents, and stable to chemical attack. They also possess a high resistance to heat and are excellent dielectric materials. They are fabricated into special gaskets and packings, pump liners, tubing, pipe, wire, cablecoating, nonstaining cloth, and many other items.

The most important representative of this group is Teflon, which serves as a coating on rollers and cookware to prevent sticking because of its waxy surface with a low friction factor. Automobile manufacturers use Teflon for bearings in power-steering assemblies and for coating the sockets of ball joints that never require greasing or oiling. Teflon is also invaluable to the space industry as a lubricant in spacecraft because it is not affected by a vacuum, in contrast to oil which evaporates in the vacuum of outer space. Because of its durability and lack of toxicity, Teflon is also being used extensively in surgery to replace blood vessels and heart valves.

Thus fluorine and its compounds have emerged from virtual obscurity in their early history to a highly respected and extremely valuable position in modern industry. Their applications appear to be almost unlimited. Indeed, there are few chemicals with greater industrial potential than fluorides. On the other hand, this steadily growing expansion has subjected Man himself to intimate contact with these substances, and the full consequences of this exposure, particularly as related to his health, are not yet known. We must ask, therefore, has our knowledge about the biological effects of this all-important element and its compounds kept in step with the advances in industrial uses?

REFERENCES

1. Martialis, M.V.: The Epigrams of Martial, Bk. V, No. XLIII, ca. 89 A.D.

2. Eager, J.M.: Denti di Chiaie (Chiaie teeth). Public Health Rep., 16 (Part 2): 2576-2577, 1901; Dent. Cosmos, 43:300-301, 1902 (Reprinted in Mc-Clure, F.J., Ed.: Fluoride Drinking Waters. U.S. Department of Health, Education, and Welfare, Public Health Service, National Institute of Dental Research, Bethesda, Maryland, PHS Publication No. 825, 1962, p. 2).

3. Roholm, K.: Fluorine Intoxication. A Clinical-Hygienic Study with a Review of the Literature and Some Experimental Investigations. NYT Nordisk Forlag, Arnold Busck, Copenhagen, and H.K. Lewis and Co., London, 1937.

4. McClure, F.J.: Water Fluoridation: The Search and the Victory. U.S. Department of Health, Education, and Welfare, National Institutes of Health, National Institute of Dental Research, Bethesda, Maryland, 1970, p. 3.

5. Weeks, M.E., and Leicester, H.M.: Discovery of the Elements, 7th ed. Journal of Chemical Education, Easton, Pa., 1968, pp. 727ff.

6. Partington, J.R.: A History of Chemistry, Vol. 3. Macmillan, London, 1962, p. 213; and Historical and Industrial Discovery of the Elements. Chem. Ind. (Lond.), 60:109, 1941.

7. Mellor, J.W.: A Comprehensive Treatise on Inorganic and Theoretical Chemistry, Vol. 2. Longmans, Green, London, 1922, p. 3.

8. Middleton, J.: On Fluorine in Bones, Its Source and Its Application to the Determination of the Geological Age of Fossil Bones. Proc. Geol. Soc. Lond., 4:431- 433, 1844.

9. Baer, N.S., and Indictor, N.: Chemical Investigations of Ancient Near Eastern Archaeological Ivory Artifacts, in Curt W. Beck, Ed.: Archaeological Chemistry. Advances in Chemistry Series 138, American Chemical Society, Washington, D.C., 1974, pp. 236-245.

10. Cited in Ref. 7, above, pp. 4ff.

11. Portier, J.: Solid State Chemistry of Ionic Fluorides. Angew. Chem. Int. Ed. Engl., 15:475-486, 1976.

12. Kirk-Othmer Encyclopedia of Chemical Technology, Vol. 9, 2nd ed. Interscience, New York, London, and Sydney, 1966, pp. 506ff. Cf. Finger, G.C.: Fluorine Resources and Fluorine Utilization, in M. Stacey, J.C. Tatlow, and A.G. Sharpe, Eds.: Advances in Fluorine Chemistry, Vol. 2, Butterworths, Washington, D.C., 1961, pp. 35-54.

13. Friend, J.N.: The Historical and Industrial Discovery of the Elements. Part IV. The Halogens. Chem. Ind. (Lond.), 60:64-68, 1941.

14. Hydrofluoric Acid Makers Enjoy Good Times. Chem. Eng. News., 53(1): 8-9, Jan. 6, 1975.

15. Editorial: End of Aerosol Age. Science News, 107:396, 1975. Cf. National Research Council: Halocarbons. Effects on Stratospheric Ozone. National Academy of Sciences, Washington, D.C., 1976; also Ref. 23 in Ch. 1.

CHAPTER 3

SOURCES OF FLUORIDE INTAKE

IT IS FREQUENTLY thought that fluoride enters the human organism almost entirely through drinking water, although this assumption is far from the truth. In fact, because of its ubiquity in the environment, the fluoride in our bodies is derived from many different sources. The atmosphere, soil, water of rivers, lakes, wells, and oceans, rain, snow, drugs, and the food chain – all contribute significantly to the total intake of fluoride into the human body. These various sources of fluoride will now be examined in the light of the far-reaching man-made fluoride chain generated by modern industry and commerce (Fig. 4-1, opposite).[1]

AIR

In the United States the total inorganic fluoride emissions from major industrial and commercial operations are estimated to be between 120,000 and 155,000 tons per year (calculated as HF).[2] As seen in Table 3-1 (p. 30), the main sources are the combustion of coal (now greater and increasing), the processing of phosphates, and the manufacture of aluminum, steel, and ceramics (brick, tile, cement, glass, etc.), with lesser amounts from such activities as welding and the production of nonferrous metals. Other sources (not shown in the table) include the manufacture of high-octane gasoline and the production of hydrogen fluoride, fluorinated hydrocarbons, and other fluorides. Unfortunately, even assuming 90% containment with advances in pollution control equipment, "the estimated emissions of fluoride [worldwide] are expected to double between 1971 and 1980."[3]

The distribution of airborne fluorides depends on numerous factors, especially climatic and topographic conditions in the area involved (Table 3-2, page 31),[4] a fact which must be taken into

THE MAN-MADE FLUORIDE CHAIN

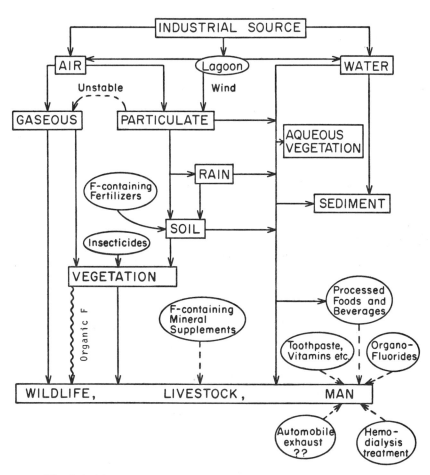

Fig. 3-1. Dispersion of commercial fluorides in the environment.
(From J. R. Marier and D. Rose: *Environmental Fluoride.*
National Research Council of Canada, Publication No. 12,226,
Ottawa, [1971], Appendix 6.)

account when interpreting the results of air-monitoring for fluoride. In areas of high industrial pollution, the heavy solids or particulates (such as sodium fluoride) are deposited in the immedi-

Table 3-1

**Estimated Total Atmospheric Inorganic Fluoride Emissions
from Major Industries in the United States, 1968[2]**

SOURCES	EMISSIONS TONS/YEAR
Steel industry	40,100
Ceramics industries	21,200
Phosphate fertilizer and processing industries	18,700
Aluminum industry	16,000
Combustion of coal	16,000
Nonferrous metal foundries	4,000
Welding operations	2,700

(See also V.A. Cecilioni, *Fluoride*, 7:164, 1974.)

ate vicinity of the emission, whereas gases are dispersed over wide areas. Mists or vapors form in the air when gaseous fluorides, mainly hydrogen fluoride and silicon tetrafluoride, are dissolved in fine water droplets.[5] In atmosphere thus polluted, the fluoride entering the human body from air and food may actually exceed the amounts consumed from fluoride in water, as demonstrated by the distribution of the major sources of fluoride intake near a fluoride-emitting aluminum factory in Czechoslovakia (Fig. 3–2, page 32).[6]

Ordinarily in large cities, one cubic meter of air averages less than 0.05 μg (microgram) or 0.0625 parts per billion (ppb) fluoride.[7] The highest level recorded by the National Air Sampling Network in 1966 and 1967 was 1.89 μg/m³ (2.4 ppb). These extremely small amounts, however, represent mean values subject to many variables and do not reflect conditions arising from sudden smoke episodes, especially in areas close to a factory.[7]

Near fluoride-emitting industries the amounts of airborne fluoride are significantly higher. For instance, investigators have found from 0.0 to 15.14 μg per cubic meter of air or up to 19.5 ppb near an Italian aluminum factory surrounded by high mountains.[8] At this concentration a person could inhale up to 0.3 milligram of fluoride per day. On the other hand, in the industrial Detroit-Windsor area – which is flat and where there are fewer concentrated sources of fluoride emission – atmospheric fluoride averages only 0.16 to 2.9 ppb according to the International Joint U.S.-Canadian Commission.[9]

Table 3-2

Climatic and Topographic Effects on Pollution by Airborne Fluorides[4]

INCREASE IN	TYPICAL EFFECT	POLLUTION CHANGE
Precipitation	Cleanses the air	Decrease
Humidity	Dissolves solids; forms mists	Increase
Wind velocity	Promotes dispersion to longer distances	Mixed
Wind from source	Enhances contamination	Increase
Temperature with height (inversion)	Retards dispersion	Increase
Barometric pressure	Reduces wind; retards dispersion	Increase
Height of source	Promotes dispersion	Decrease
Distance from source	Promotes dispersion	Decrease
Mountains, hills	Breaks force of winds; forms pockets	Increase
Valleys	Traps pollutants	Increase
Plains	Promotes dispersion	Decrease

SOIL

Since much of our food is derived from vegetation growing in contaminated areas, fluoride in soil can also be an important source of intake. Fluoride enters the soil through weathering of rocks, precipitation, and contaminated water, mainly from waste run-off and fertilizers. Generally, little fluoride is found in sandy soils where, dissolved in rainwater, it leaches into lower levels, in contrast to clay, which absorbs and retains fluoride. The range of fluoride in "normal" soils is between 100 and 300 ppm with higher levels at increasing depth; but sampling in the "high-fluoride" regions of Idaho and Tennessee has revealed concentrations up to 8,300 ppm. One of the highest fluoride levels in soil, 184,000 ppm,

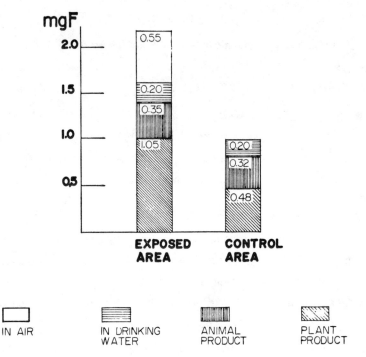

Fig. 3-2. Sources and daily fluoride intake of 6- to 14-year-old children
residing near an aluminum factory compared to children living in a
noncontaminated control area.
Fluoride content of drinking water 0.1-0.3 ppm in both areas.
(Courtesy Dr. G. Balazova and co-workers,
Research Institute for Hygiene, Bratislava, Czechoslovakia.)

was recorded in the wastes from a fluorspar mine in England.[10]
Fallout of particulate fluoride from the air and absorption of
gaseous fluoride in rain and snow account for considerable
accumulation in soil, and each year fluoride in phosphate
fertilizers can contribute up to 17 pounds of the halogen
per acre.[11]

WATER

The natural fluoride content of water in different areas varies according to the source of the water (surface or subterranean), the geological formation of the area, the amount of rainfall, and the quantity of water lost by evaporation. The majority of untreated wells throughout the United States ordinarily contain less than 0.5 ppm of fluoride. Springs in New England have some of the lowest fluoride levels in the country ranging from 0.02 to 0.1 ppm.[12] As a general rule, the fluoride content of wells depends on the rock strata as well as the depth of the well.

Spring water which flows through high-fluoride rock strata sometimes dissolves extraordinary amounts, as in Bruneau, Idaho, where the U.S. Public Health Service recorded 28 ppm in 1959, the highest level in communal well water in the country[13] (Table 3-3). In many communities of Western Texas, Arizona, Tennessee, Arkansas, and South Dakota, the fluoride in water supplies was formerly quite high. For example, in Bartlett, Texas (8 ppm),[14] and in Britton, South Dakota (6.7 ppm),[15] the concentration is now being reduced by defluoridation to approximately 1 ppm, in the former by means of activated alumina, in the latter by bone char.

Deep wells, mineral springs, and geysers contain unusually high fluoride levels. Striking examples are Old Faithful geyser in Yellowstone National Park, with as much as 40 ppm, and Vichy water, with 8 ppm. In other mineral waters concentrations range from 0.8 to 12.2 ppm[16] (Table 3-3, page 35).

Uncontaminated **surface water**, on the other hand, is generally low in fluoride, in the range of 0 to 0.2 ppm,[2] but rivers receiving effluents from factory wastes have much higher values. For instance, the U.S. Geological Survey of 1959 to 1961 reported as much as 46 ppm in the water of the Peace River in Florida, whereas prior to industrial contamination (ca. August 30, 1951) the fluoride level was about 1 ppm.[17] The effluent water of an aluminum factory in Bolzano, Italy, contained 14 to 35 ppm in 1971,[18] and near a fertilizer factory in Dunnville, Ontario, cistern water showed fluoride levels as high as 37.8 ppm on December 6, 1965.[19] The Rhine River, which is notorious for its pollution after its passage through the industrial Ruhr region, shows fluoride levels on the order of 0.25 to 0.45 ppm[20] compared to 0.13 to 0.16 ppm in the Mississippi River near Minneapolis–St. Paul.[21]

In **lake water** the highest natural fluoride value ever recorded is 2,800 ppm or 0.28%, in Lake Nakuru, located in a volcanic area of Kenya, East Africa,[24] but in the United States even higher concentrations have been reported – up to 5,150 ppm in so-called gypsum ponds, the collection pools for the effluent water from phosphate fertilizer factories.[25]

Oceans maintain a relatively constant fluoride level of about 1.3 ppm even at depths of 2500 meters or more.[31] Approximately half (47%) of the dissolved fluoride in the oceans occurs as MgF^+, 2% as CaF^+, and 51% as free, unbound F^-.[32] Although colorimetric assays indicate that the fluoride content and the F/Cl ratio in deep-lying waters in certain areas of the North Atlantic Ocean are slightly elevated,[27] more recent measurements by the ion-selective electrode method do not show any increase.[31] Fluoride levels as high as 8.72 ppm in the Persian Gulf and 3.36 ppm in the Mediterranean Sea have been reported,[28] but do not appear to have been confirmed.

Rainwater also contributes fluoride to the ocean as well as to the land and to fresh water because it absorbs the halogen from the atmosphere. Although the oceans serve as a "sink" for airborne and riverborne fluoride, there is evidence that they also release significant amounts of fluoride into the atmosphere, thus recycling it back to the land.[3] Over the mid-Atlantic Ocean up to 0.025 ppm fluoride was found in rainwater, but over other oceans the concentrations were lower.[27] On the other hand, measurement of fluoride in rainwater near polluting factories – for example, within 500 meters of a German phosphate fertilizer plant near Hamburg – has disclosed concentrations up to 10 ppm.[29] Snow also collects fluoride. Samples of snow falling in an urban environment contained 0.04 ppm ionized and 0.05 ppm total fluoride. In a heavy traffic area of Minneapolis–St. Paul ground snow had 0.45 ppm ionized fluoride and 3.27 ppm total fluoride.[21]

Daily Fluoride Intake from Water. In the past the water generally consumed by human life on earth contained only minute amounts of fluoride. With the advent of the Industrial Revolution, however, man has probed deeper into the earth for his water, and

Table 3-3

Fluoride Content of Water

	ppm
IN SURFACE WATER[2]	0.0-0.2
Near a fluorspar mine[10]	1.1-26.8
Cistern water near fertilizer factory (Ontario)[19]	37.8
After volcanic eruption in Iceland 1970[22]	4.0-70.0
(2 weeks later)	0.3-14.0
IN DEEP WELLS	
Old Faithful (Yellowstone National Park)	40.0
Bruneau, Idaho[13]	28.8
Bartlett, Texas[14]	8.0
Colorado Springs[13]	1.6-2.0
Near Detroit, Mich.[13]	1.0
Punjab, India[23]	0.2-40.0
IN LAKES	
Great Lakes	0.05-0.2
Lake Nakuru (Kenya)[24]	2800.
In "gypsum pond" (Florida)[25]	5150.
IN SNOW[21]	
Fresh falling	0.05
On streets with heavy traffic	1.62-3.27
Melting on street	2.41
IN RIVERS	
Most rivers in U.S.A.	$\leq$1.0
Rhine (Holland)[20]	0.25-0.45
Meuse (Belgium)[26]	$\leq$9.0
Peace River (Florida)[17]	46.0
Near aluminum factory (Bolzano, Italy)[18]	14.0-35.0
IN OCEANS	1.3
Near Newfoundland[27]	$\leq$1.4
Mediterranean[28]	3.36
Persian Gulf[28]	8.72

(Cont'd on page 36)

Table 3-3 (Cont'd)

Fluoride Content of Water

	ppm
IN RAINWATER	
Over ocean[27]	0.025
Near fertilizer factory[29]	≤10.
IN MINERAL SPRINGS	
Vichy (France)	8.0
Baden Baden (Germany)[30]	9.98
Bottled waters (Spain)[16]	0.8-12.2
ARTIFICIALLY FLUORIDATED	0.7-1.2
IN SEWAGE[21]	
Fluoridated	1.16-1.25
Nonfluoridated	0.38

has thus raised the fluoride content of much of the water which he consumes. Moreover, during the current century, industry has released substantial amounts of the halogen into the environment, thereby further raising the fluoride levels of our drinking water. In recent decades the final step has been the addition of specified amounts of fluoride to communal water supplies in the United States and in a number of other countries for the purpose of reducing tooth decay. In doing so, however, we have increased our total fluoride intake 2- to 10-fold above what we were consuming because many food items and beverages are now being processed and prepared with fluoridated water. In specific terms, when we drink water containing one part of fluoride per million parts (ppm) of water, we are consuming 1 mg of fluoride with each liter of water.

FOOD

Whereas individual fluoride intake from water and air can be roughly estimated, it is more difficult to determine the exact quantities of fluoride ingested in the food by any given population. The presence of fluoride depends upon numerous variables: where the food is produced; whether the edible portion is leaf, root, or fruit; whether the food is grown in a dry or wet season; the composition of the soil; the kind of fertilization and sprays employed; and the method by which the food is processed and prepared.[33]

From Plant Life. Virtually every food contains at least some fluoride.[33] Plants take it up from the soil and from the air. From the soil, fluoride is transmitted through fine hair rootlets into the stems, and some reaches the leaves. Plants absorb more fluoride from sandy than from clay soil and more from wet and acid soils than from dry and alkaline ones. Since phosphate fertilizers contain between one and three percent fluoride, fertilized tuber plants such as potatoes, beets, radishes, etc., assimilate more fluoride from the soil than from the atmosphere. The high fluoride content of artificially fertilized soil is also reflected in increased dietary intake. For example, a Japanese study has shown that in rural communities daily fluoride consumption rose from an average of 4.38 mg in 1958 to as much as 11.13 mg in 1965 because of the increase in the use of fluoride-containing phosphate fertilizer.[34]

The fluoride that a plant absorbs from the air is derived primarily from chimney smoke, volcanic eruptions, and insect sprays. It settles on leaves, permeates through the stomata of the leaf surface —fine pores between the cells—into the ribs of the leaves, and tends to damage the margins and tips of the leaf (Figs. 3–3 and 3-4, pages 38 and 39). A brown line usually sharply demarcates the "burned" from the healthy portion of the leaf and makes the effects of fluoride readily distinguishable from similar lesions, especially those due to airborne hydrochloric acid.[35]

Turgid (firm) plants are more susceptible to fluoride accumulation than are wilted ones. Fruit and leafy vegetables such as lettuce, cabbage, and celery are especially prone to deposition of airborne fluoride, mainly at their outside structures that contain more fluoride than their inner parts. Tea leaves accumulate more fluoride than any other edible plant. Recent analyses of 15 different kinds of dry tea leaves by Belgian scientists revealed from 50 to 125 ppm fluoride.[36] Scientists at the University of Minnesota found 52 to 144 ppm in five black teas and 336 ppm fluoride in one green tea; between 41% and 78% of this amount of fluoride could be extracted in the first infusion.[37] In general, six cups of an average brew of tea contain about 1 mg, which is approximate-

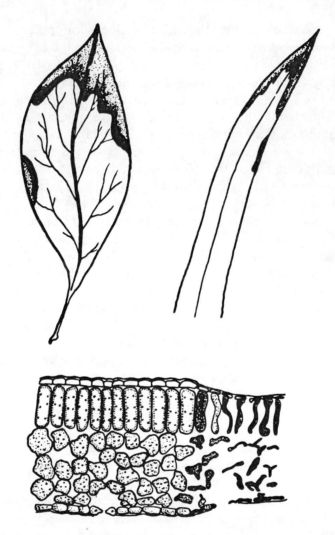

Fig. 3-3. Typical patterns of leaf margin and tip necrosis due to fluoride. Bottom cross section shows sharp demarcation between (healthy) left and fluorosed (right) structure.
(Courtesy Dr. K. Garber, State Institute for Applied Botany, Hamburg, Germany.)

ly the daily amount recommended for prevention of tooth decay in children.

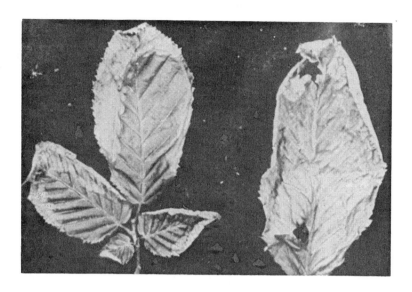

Fig. 3-4. Beech leaves injured by airborne fluoride.
(Courtesy Dr. L. Gisiger, Agricultural Chemistry Institute,
Liebefeld-Bern, Switzerland.)

From Animal Life. Among food derived from non-plant sources, seafood and fish are richest in fluoride.[38] The calcium in fish attracts fluoride from sea water, especially to their outer portions and to their bones. Extensive analyses of fluoride in food in Germany indicate levels of the order of 1.37 to 5.21 ppm in the flesh of fish, but the skin and bones contain 5 to 20 times more.[39]

Other animals also concentrate fluoride in bone, ligaments, and in skin. For example, food items made with bone meal, especially from older animals, can be a significant source of fluoride. Pablum, a popular infant food prepared from bone meal, formerly contained as much as 18 ppm. When this amount of fluoride was found to be excessive — it produced mottled teeth — manufacturers reduced the fluoride content of Pablum to between 1.33 and 2.12 ppm.[40] Strained chicken in baby foods averages between 1.51 and 3.14 ppm fluoride due to its accumulation in the skin of chickens (Table 3-4, page 41).[41] Gelatin, made from the skin and hides of animals, normally contains less than 10 ppm fluoride, but when

1-ppm fluoridated water is used in its preparation and final processing the fluoride content is increased to 29–34 ppm.[42] Even
more fluoride – up to 370 ppm – is present in fish-protein concentrate distributed to undernourished people throughout the world.
Because of the low solubility of fluoride in this form, however,
only a fraction of it is absorbed in the blood stream, and the
remainder is eliminated through the bowels.[43]

Wild animals such as deer and rabbits also accumulate fluoride
in their bones, especially in industrial areas, but predators generally
demonstrate higher levels than their prey.[44] In laboratory animals
fluoride storage is frequently excessive since their food contains
amounts on the order of 35 ppm.[45] Because little attention has
been paid to this fact in the past, data dealing with food intake in
animal experiments and their application to human diets are not
always reliable.

TOTAL FLUORIDE INTAKE

The calculation of the total amount of fluoride in our daily food
becomes even more complex when we consider the manner in
which food is processed and prepared.[46] When vegetables are
boiled in water containing fluoride, the fluoride becomes more
concentrated as the water boils off. Furthermore, protein and minerals in food absorb fluoride from water, even if the water is not
boiled away. This effect contrasts markedly to that of chlorine in
drinking water, which is lost during cooking through liberation of
oxygen and conversion into dilute hydrochloric acid. On the other
hand, if carbonated soft drinks are stored in metal cans over a
four-month period, their fluoride content drops by about 30%.[47]

In 1943, F. J. McClure, of the National Institute of Dental Research, USPHS, estimated that the diet of a typical adult American
contributed about 0.3 to 0.5 mg of fluoride per day to the total
daily fluoride ration,[48] and in 1971 a U.S. National Research
Council committee stated that 0.2 mg, "rarely as much as 1 mg,"
is the amount of fluoride present in our daily diet.[49] In 1966, however, scientists at the Canadian National Research Council had
already demonstrated that the total average daily fluoride intake
of food processed with artificially fluoridated water plus the
amount imbibed with drinking water has increased from the range

Table 3-4
Fluoride Content of Baby Foods[41]

	ppm
FRUITS	
Peaches	0.70-0.76
Pears	0.54-0.67
Apricots	0.86-1.17
Pineapple and pears	0.63
Apricots and applesauce	0.71
Applesauce	0.82
FRUIT JUICES	
Orange	0.33-0.36
Pineapple and grapefruit	0.58
Apple	0.68-2.15
Apple and cherry	1.17-2.38
MIXED CEREAL WITH APPLE AND BANANAS	0.69-1.05
VEGETABLES	
Green beans	0.40-0.58
Peas	0.59-1.20
Carrots	0.39-0.64
Beets	0.80
Creamed spinach	2.01
STRAINED MEATS	
Beef	0.29-0.34
Pork	0.20-0.41
Chicken	1.51-3.14
Ham	0.31
Veal	0.29
Lamb	0.32
Beef liver	0.41
Turkey	0.64
STRAINED MEAT COMBINATIONS	
Beef and noodles	0.84
Ham, vegetables, and bacon	0.87
Turkey, vegetables, and noodles	0.82
Ham and vegetables	0.49
Beef, noodles, and vegetables	0.39
Chicken and vegetables	0.63

of 1–1.5 mg to 2–5 mg.[50] More recently, analyses of typical hospital diets in 16 U.S. cities confirmed the increase of fluoride in the daily diet: about one mg per day from food *alone* in nonfluoridated communities and *more than twice as much* (1.7 to 3.4 mg) in fluoridated ones.[51]

Chemical additives – especially preservatives and insecticides – are additional sources of fluoride in food. A bone meal supplement to flour, for instance, adds about 1 mg to the daily diet.[52] Talcum used to polish rice and peas has been found to raise their fluoride content to 10–14 ppm;[40] a large-sized apple sprayed with an insecticide containing fluoride provides about 1 mg of fluoride.[53] Calcium and vitamin supplements prescribed by physicians for pregnant women may contribute further to fluoride intake, since some of these preparations are made from phosphate rock, from which naturally occurring fluoride has not been completely removed.

Moreover, certain dietary habits may augment our fluoride consumption, often without our knowledge or intent. For example, there is a case on record of nonfatal skeletal fluorosis (chronic fluoride poisoning) in a patient who obtained practically his whole daily intake of water from a mountain spring containing 7.5 ppm fluoride; he mistakenly thought that all spring water was especially conducive to good health.[54]

How such hidden sources of dietary fluoride add up to substantial amounts was further demonstrated in 1960 by two Toronto scientists.[52] They showed that the diet of Newfoundland residents, who are surrounded by the sea, consists largely of fish which provided an average of 0.74 mg fluoride per day. Typical of their English ancestry, they also consumed another 1 mg by drinking about six cups of tea per day, and an additional 1 mg was added to the total because of a fluoride-containing calcium supplement in bread!

A final example of how fluoride from multiple sources adds up is the case of a woman in England whose arthritis was related to her consumption of 6.3 to 9.3 mg fluoride per day from tea and water alone.[55] It is clear, therefore, that an unpredictable amount of fluoride ingested with food, imbibed in water, and inhaled from the air enters our bodies and that even to approximate our total daily consumption of fluoride, many variables must be taken into consideration.[56]

REFERENCES

1. Marier, J.R., and Rose, D.: Environmental Fluoride. National Research Council of Canada, Publication No. 12,226, Ottawa, [1971], Appendix 6. Cf. Oelschläger, W., and Waldbott, G.L.: Fluorides in the Environment. Fluoride, 7:220-222, 1974.

2. National Research Council Committee on Biologic Effects of Atmospheric Pollutants: Fluorides. National Academy of Sciences, Washington, D.C., 1971, Ch. 2. Cf. Groth, E. III: Fluoride Pollution. Environment (St. Louis), 17(3): 29-38, April/May 1975.

3. Dobbs, C.G.: Fluoride and the Environment. Fluoride, 7:123-135, 1974.

4. Waldbott, G.L.: Health Effects of Environmental Pollutants. 1973, Table 3-1, p. 33 (adapted).

5. Ref. 4, above, Chs. 1 and 3.

6. Balazova, G., Macuch, P., and Rippel, A.: Effects of Fluorine on the Living Organism. Fluoride, 2:33-36, 1969.

7. Yunghans, R.S., and McMullen, T.B.: Fluoride Concentrations Found in NASN Samples of Suspended Particles. Fluoride, 3:143-152, 1970.

8. Cavagna, G., and Bobbio, G.: Contributo allo studio delle caratteristiche chemico-fisiche e degli effetti biologici degli effluenti di una fabbrica di alluminio. Med. Lav., 61:69-101, 1970.

9. Report by the International Air Pollution Board for the International Joint Commission, St. Clair/Detroit. Ottawa, Canada, and Washington, D.C., Jan. 1971.

10. Johnson, M.S.: Natural Colonization and Reinstatement of Mineral Waste Containing Heavy Metals and Fluoride. Fluoride, 9:153-162, 1976.

11. Oelschläger, W.: Fluoride Uptake in Soil and Its Deposition. Fluoride, 4:80-84, 1971.

12. Cholak, J.: Fluorides, A Critical Review. I. The Occurrence of Fluoride in Air, Food, and Water. J. Occup. Med., 1:501-511, 1959.

13. Natural Fluoride Content of Communal Water Supplies in the United States. U.S. Department of Health, Education, and Welfare, Public Health Service, Bureau of State Services, Division of Dental Public Health, Public Health Service Publication No. 655. Washington, D.C., 1959.

14. Likins, R.C., McClure, F.J., and Steere, A.C.: Urinary Excretion of Fluoride Following Defluoridation of a Water Supply. Public Health Rep., 71:217-220, 1956. (Reprinted in Fluoride Drinking Waters, 1962, pp. 421-423.)

15. Horowitz, H.S., Stanley, B.H., and Driscoll, W.S.: Partial Defluoridation of a Community Water Supply and Dental Fluorosis. Public Health Rep., 87:451-455, 1972.

16. Mazarrasa, O., and Lazuen, J.A.: Fluoride in Spanish Bottled Waters. Fluoride, 9:201–203, 1976.

17. Johnson, L.: Memorandum to the Governing Board of the Peace River Valley Water Conservation and Drinking District, P.O. Box 448, Bartow, Florida, Nov. 1, 1961.

18. Waldbott, G.L., and Steinegger, S.: New Observations on 'Chizzola' Maculae. Proceedings of the 3rd International Clean Air Congress, Oct. 8–12, 1973, Düsseldorf, Federal Republic of Germany, Verein Deutscher Ingenieure, Düsseldorf, 1973, pp. A63-A67.

19. Report to W.C.B. Mills, Medical Officer of Health, Township of Sherbrooke, Ontario, by the Ontario Water Resources Commission Chemical Laboratories. Date of water sampling: Nov. 30–Dec. 6, 1965.

20. Jaarverslagen 1971-1974 van de Rijncommissie Waterleidingbedrijven (1971-1974 Annual Reports of the Rhine Commission of the Dutch Waterworks).

21. Singer, L., and Armstrong, W.D.: Fluoride in Treated Sewage and in Rain and Snow. Arch. Environ. Health, 32:21–23, 1977.

22. Georgsson, G., and Pétursson, G.: Fluorosis of Sheep Caused by the Hekla Eruption in 1970. Fluoride, 5:58-65, 1972.

23. Jolly, S.S., Prasad, S., Sharma, R., and Rai, B: Human Fluoride Intoxication in Punjab. Fluoride, 4: 64–79, 1971.

24. Williamson, M.M.: Endemic Dental Fluorosis in Kenya. A Preliminary Report. E. Afr. Med. J., 30:217-233, 1953.

25. Cross, F.L., Jr., and Ross, R.W.: High Fluoride Levels in a Citrus Grove Due to a Gypsum Pond Dyke Break. Fluoride, 3:27-30, 1970.

26. Verheyden, R., Van Craenenbrosck, V., and Meheus, J.: Verhoogd Fluoridegehalte Van Leidinwater Te Antwerpen Door Een Fluoridelozing in de Maas. Rev. Belge Med. Dent., 28:125-138, 1973.

27. Kester, D.R.: Fluoride Analysis in the Northwest Atlantic Ocean. U.S. Clearinghouse Fed. Sci. Tech. Inform., AD 1971, No. 723237.

28. Azar, H.A., Nucho, C.K., Bayyuk, S.I., and Bayyuk, W.B.: Skeletal Sclerosis Due to Chronic Fluoride Intoxication. Cases from an Endemic Area of Fluorosis in the Region of the Persian Gulf. Ann. Intern. Med., 55:193–200, 1961.

29. Garber, K.: Fluoride in Rainwater and Vegetation. Fluoride, 3:22–26, 1970.

30. Rub, K.: Resorption and Retention of Fluoride Present in Mineral Waters and Soft Drinks in Humans and Experimental Rats (Abstract). Fluoride, 3:41–42, 1970.

31. Wilson, T.R.S.: Salinity and the Major Elements of Sea Water, in J.P. Riley and G. Skirrow, Eds.: Chemical Oceanography, Vol. 1, 2nd ed. Academic Press, London, New York, and San Francisco, 1975, pp. 403-404.

32. Stumm, W., and Brauner, P.A., in Ref. 31, above, p. 213.

33. Waldbott, G.L.: Fluoride in Food. Am. J. Clin. Nutr., 12:455-462, 1963. Also see Ref. 40, below.

34. Okamura, T., and Matsuhisa, T.: The Fluorine Content in Favorite Foods of Japanese. Japn. J. Public Health, 14:41-47, 1967.

35. Hindawi, I.J.: Air Pollution Injury of Vegetation. U.S. Department of Health, Education, and Welfare, Public Health Service, National Air Pollution Control Administration, Raleigh, N.C., 1970.

36. Srebrnik-Friszman, S., and Van der Mijnsbrugge, F.: Teneur en Fluor de quelques thés prélevés sur le Marché Belge et de leurs Infusions. Arch. Belg. Med. Soc. Hyg. Med. Trav. Med. Leg., 33:551-556, 1976.

37. Singer, L., Armstrong, W.D., and Vatassery, G.T.: Fluoride in Commercial Tea and Related Plants. Econ. Bot., 21:285-187, 1967.

38. Nielson, F.H., and Sandstead, H.H.: Are Nickel, Vanadium, Silicon, Fluorine, and Tin Essential for Man? A Review. Am. J. Clin. Nutr., 27:515-520, 1974.

39. Oelschläger, W.: Fluoride in Food. Fluoride, 3:6-11, 1970.

40. Waldbott, G.L.: Fluoride in Food. Am. J. Clin. Nutr., 13:393, 1963.

41. Wiatrowski, E., Kramer, L., Osis, D., and Spencer, H.: Dietary Fluoride Intake of Infants. Pediatrics, 55:517-522, 1975. Cf. summary of report by D. R. Taves in Waldbott, G.L., and Yiamouyiannis, J.: AAAS Fluoride Symposium in Denver. Fluoride, 10:142, 1977, and Taves D.R.: Normal Fluoride Intake and Metabolism, in E. Johansen and D.R. Taves, Eds.: AAAS Symposium: Continuing Evaluation of the Use of Fluorides. Westview Press, Boulder, Colorado, in press, 1978.

42. Bartlet, J.C.: The Fluoride Content of Gelatin. Analyst, 86:200-201, 1961.

43. Zipkin, I., Zucas, S.M., and Stillings, B.R.: Biological Availability of the Fluoride in Fish Protein Concentrate in the Rat. J. Nutr., 100:293-299, 1970.

44. Kay, C.E.: Fluoride in Levels in Indigenous Animals and Plants Collected from Uncontaminated Ecosystems. Fluoride, 8:125-133, 1975.

45. Parsonson, I.M., Carter, P.D., and Cruickshanks, J.: Letter: Chronic Fluorosis in Laboratory Guinea Pigs. Aust. Vet. J., 51:362-363, 1975.

46. Martin, D.J.: The Evanston Dental Caries Study. VIII. Fluorine Content of Vegetables Cooked in Fluorine Containing Waters. J. Dent. Res., 3: 676-681, 1951.

47. Enno, A., Craig, G.G., and Knox, K.W.: Fluoride Content of Prepackaged Fruit Juices and Carbonated Soft Drinks. Med. J. Aust., 2:340-342, 1976.

48. McClure, F.J.: Ingestion of Fluorine and Dental Caries. Quantitative Relations Based on Food and Water Requirements of Children One to Twelve Years Old. Am. J. Dis. Child., 66:362-369, 1943. Also: Fluorine in Foods — Survey of Recent Data. Public Health Rep., 64:1061-1074, 1949. (Reprinted

in Fluoride Drinking Waters, 1962, pp. 283-294.

49. Ref. 2, above, p. 168.

50. Marier, J.R. and Rose, D.: The Fluoride Content of Some Foods and Beverages—A Brief Survey Using a Modified Zr-SPADNS Method. J. Food Sci., 31:941-946, 1966.

51. Kramer, L., Osis, D., Wiatrowski, E., and Spencer, H.: Dietary Fluoride in Different Areas in the United States. Am. J. Clin. Nutr., 27:590-594, 1974. For further references and discussion, see Marier, J.R.: Some Current Aspects of Environmental Fluoride. The Science of the Total Environment, 8:253-265, 1977.

52. Elliott, C.G., and Smith, M.D.: Dietary Fluoride Related to Fluoride Content of Teeth. J. Dent. Res., 39:93-98, 1960.

53. Smith, M.C., Lantz, E.M., and Smith, H.V.: Further Studies in Mottled Enamel. J. Am. Dent. Assoc., 22:817-829, 1935.

54. Odenthal, H., and Wieneke, H.L.: Chronische Fluorvergiftung und Osteomyelosklerose. Dtsch. Med. Wochenschr., 84:725-728, 1959.

55. Cook, H.A.: Fluoride Studies in a Patient with Arthritis. Lancet, 2:817, 1971, and Crippling Arthritis Related to Fluoride Intake (Case Report). Fluoride, 5:209-212, 1972.

56. Jerard, E., and Patrick, J.B.: The Summing of Fluoride Exposures. Int. J. Environ. Stud., 4:141-155, 1973. Cf. Rose, D., and Marier, J.R.: Environmental Fluoride 1977. National Research Council Canada, Report No. 16081 [July 1978].

CHAPTER 4

FLUORIDE IN THE BODY

WHAT HAPPENS to fluoride once it has entered the human body? To answer this question one of two methods is usually used: in one the total quantity of fluoride consumed over a given period from all food and drink is measured and compared with the amounts of fluoride eliminated through the kidneys and bowels. This approach, however, is only partially reliable because some fluoride leaves the body with sweat, saliva, and tears, all of which are difficult to collect. The procedure was first reported in 1891 by two German pharmacologists, J. Brandl and H. Tappeiner, who over the course of 21 months fed slightly more than 14 ounces (403 g) of sodium fluoride to a 28-pound dog.[1] During this period the dog excreted 81% of the fluoride through the kidneys and bowels. Of the fluoride detected in the dog when they then killed it, over 92% was present in the bones and cartilage. The rest, in decreasing amounts, was found in the skin, muscle, liver, teeth, and blood.

The second approach uses the radioactive tracer technique. Radioactive fluoride, ^{18}F, is imbibed with water or injected into a vein, and a Geiger counter then records the amount of radiation which emanates from ^{18}F as it passes through the body. Thus, it can be determined exactly where the radioactive fluoride localizes and how much is eliminated. In these experiments, all information must be obtained in about 8–10 hours because of the rapid disintegration of ^{18}F, which has a half-life of 1.87 hours as it decays (by loss of a positron) to ^{18}O, a stable isotope of oxygen. Radioactive tracer studies were first reported on rats in 1954,[2] on sheep in 1955,[3] on rats and mice in 1958,[4] and on humans in 1960.[5] Many similar studies have been carried out subsequently.

BALANCE STUDIES

In 1945 fluoride balance studies were described on five healthy young men for 28 test periods, each consisting of five eight-hour days. These findings indicated that more than 80% of the fluoride ingested in drinking water was being excreted in urine and perspiration.[6] Indeed, sweat is "an important avenue for the elimination of fluoride," the authors stated.

In a later investigation, the daily diet of nine male ambulatory patients, which averaged 4.4 mg fluoride, was supplemented by 9.1 mg of fluoride (as sodium fluoride).[7] Of the total daily amount of fluoride (13.5 mg) thus consumed, 3.6 mg was retained, amounting to 115 mg during the 32-day experimental period. During the 18 days following termination of the experiment, the total amount of excess fluoride excreted in the urine and feces was 9.8 mg, which means that only about 10% of the 115 mg of fluoride retained during the experiment was subsequently eliminated.

ABSORPTION INTO THE BLOOD

Under ordinary conditions fluoride is detectable in the blood stream by ^{18}F tracer within 10 minutes after ingestion and reaches a maximum concentration about 50 minutes later.[5] About 47.5% is absorbed through the upper bowels and 25.7% through the stomach wall within one hour by simple diffusion, no active transport mechanism being involved.[8] This "normal" course of the metabolic fate of fluoride, however, may be modified considerably by many factors. For instance, when accompanied by calcium, aluminum, magnesium, and phosphates present in food or water, fluoride is absorbed more slowly,[9,10] although increased intake of calcium and phosphorus has only a limited effect on the amount that is absorbed.[7] Similarly, simultaneous ingestion of fat considerably delays the emptying of the stomach,[11] but enhances fluoride absorption into the blood stream.[12]

When the stomach is unduly acid, as in persons with stomach ulcers, fluoride is more rapidly and more completely absorbed than in a less acid stomach. Once fluoride has reached the lower bowels, little absorption takes place because, in contrast to the acidity of the stomach, the bowel content is alkaline, and some fluoride, instead of entering the blood stream, leaves the body with the fecal material. When fluoride is swallowed with food, tablets, or salt, less of it reaches the blood stream than when taken in water or most other liquids. With milk, in which the calcium and protein tend to bind fluoride, the absorption is slower and less complete. In an experiment with rats, continuous feeding of fluoride caused greater retention in the body than interrupted feeding.[13]

In workers and in persons residing close to factories which emit fluoride, however, the respiratory tract is a major route of fluoride ingress. In its gaseous form – essentially hydrogen fluoride – the halogen readily enters the blood stream, mainly in the upper portion of the respiratory tract. The uptake of particulate fluoride compounds is governed mainly by the size of the particles: the larger ones settle in the nose, sinuses, and pharynx and are promptly removed from the body with mucus or swallowed.[14] Particles with a diameter of $0.5-5\mu$ will be impacted in the alveolar-capillary bed, the terminal areas of the lungs, where they are absorbed into the blood stream within minutes, especially if they are water soluble.[15]

In the blood stream between 80% and 90% of the fluoride is present in a "bound" or nondiffusable form.[16] Most of this fluoride appears to be attached by stable covalent bonds to organic molecules. The rest of the fluoride in blood is in a free, ionic form, the concentration of which reflects both the level of intake and the efficiency of excretion. The "normal" level of serum ionic fluoride, according to D.R. Taves of the University of Rochester, is 0.2-0.4 micromole/liter (μM) or 0.004-0.008 ppm "when the drinking water contains only traces of fluoride, and about 0.5-1 μmol (0.01-0.02) ppm in a community with fluoridated water."[17]

In the most extensive studies to date, H. Hanhijärvi reported somewhat higher serum ionic fluoride levels (but in a comparable ratio) in 2200 hospital patients in a nonfluoridated and a fluoridated community in Finland.[18] His data showed that ionized plasma fluoride increases with age, diabetes, and renal insufficiency but decreases slightly during pregnancy. Diseases of the liver and heart also reflected higher serum fluoride levels, especially in the fluoridated community (Table 4-1, page 50).[19]

The small "free" or dissociated fluoride ion easily penetrates the walls of tiny capillary blood vessels and thereby reaches the cells of various organs in the body, especially the bones. In these

Table 4-1

Mean Ionic Plasma Fluoride Levels of 2200 Patients in Two Finnish Hospitals[19]

| | Plasma Fluoride (µM) | |
Age (years) or Disease	Nonfluoridated Area	Fluoridated Area
Mean age 7	0.79	1.1
27	0.87	1.2
47	0.86	1.4
67	0.96	1.6
87	1.0	1.8
Mean	0.88	1.3
Diabetes (adults)	0.98-1.6	1.4-4.0
Liver diseases	0.95-1.4	2.3-3.5
Cardiovascular diseases	0.94-1.3	1.2-2.6
Collagen diseases	1.7	2.6

movements the fluoride ion concentration and the calcium and carbon dioxide levels in the blood, together with the composition of the tissue fluids, all play a role in determining how much and how fast fluoride reaches the tissues.

TISSUE STORAGE

In bones and teeth, fluoride becomes incorporated directly into the crystalline mineral phase, called hydroxyapatite, to form fluoroapatite. The cancellous part of long bones and the surface of the shaft incorporate fluoride more rapidly than does the cortex.[20] Developing bones and teeth take up more fluoride than do mature ones.[21] In the absence of kidney impairment adults therefore accumulate fluoride more slowly than children.

Although most of the body fluoride is stored in hard tissues— bones, teeth, and nails—we now know that the fluoride ion can penetrate into and be "stored" in virtually any tissue of the body, sometimes in rather substantial quantities. Much fluoride is found, for instance, in the aorta, the main artery of the heart[22] —even at relatively uncalcified sites—and in ligaments. Under certain conditions, significant amounts of fluoride can also accumulate in the skin, bowels, kidneys, liver, muscles, and other organs.[23] The highest level of fluoride stored in soft tissue organs, 8400 ppm, was found in the aortas of two middle-aged men.[24]

EXCRETION

The elimination of fluoride from the body—through kidneys and less through feces, sweat, saliva, tears, and milk—in general is unpredictable. During a person's growth, the clearance of fluoride through the kidneys increases, but after age 50 it begins to decline, an indication of greater storage. Of a given dose in adults, 37% to 48% is usually retained, but these values vary considerably.[25] Early in my fluoride studies I administered to several patients, as a test dose, 15 mg of sodium fluoride (6.8 mg of F^-), which is seven times the daily intake of fluoride recommended for prevention of tooth decay in children.[26] One patient eliminated in the urine as little as 3.6% in 24 hours, another as much as 99.5%.

Fluoride excretion in excess of intake may continue for a long time after large amounts of the halogen have been ingested. For instance, 27 months after the drinking water in Bartlett, Texas, was defluoridated from 8 ppm to about 1 ppm, the average fluoride concentration in urine specimens of 116 white males, age 7 to over 70, decreased from 6–8 ppm to about 2 ppm.[27] These values indicate that previously stored fluoride was metabolized and excreted in the urine.

Because there are wide variations among people in their retention and excretion of fluoride (Fig. 4-1, page 52), it is logical to conclude that there must also be great differences in the health effects of fluoride from person to person. Unfortunately, our knowledge about the behavior of fluoride in the human organism is still very imperfect. We do not know why some individuals respond so much differently to fluoride than do others. Are there predisposing—perhaps inherited—factors which explain the variations in retention of fluorine in some persons? What role do malnutrition, vitamin deficiencies, differences in food habits, functional impairment of certain organs, presence of disease, occupa-

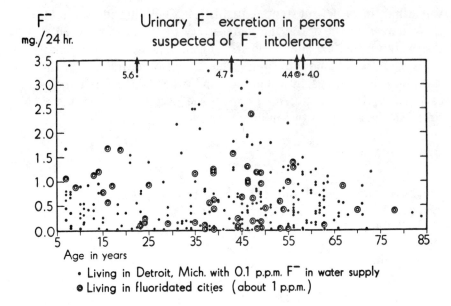

Fig. 4.1 Unpredictable variations in 24-hour urinary fluoride excretion by age among allergic persons living in fluoridated and nonfluoridated communities. (From G.L. Waldbott: Fluoride in Clinical Medicine. *Internat. Arch. Allergy Appl. Immunol.*, Suppl. 1 to Vol. 20, 1962.)

tional exposure, and socio-economic factors play in the action of fluoride in the body? These questions indicate clearly that there are important areas of research which still need answers. At the moment, we have scarcely begun to formulate the questions, much less to grope for answers. The area to which scientists have given most attention is the action of fluoride on teeth, specifically its value in preventing tooth decay, and even here our knowledge is still incomplete.

REFERENCES

1. Brandl, J. and Tappeiner, H.: Ueber die Ablagerung von Fluorverbindungen im Organismus nach Fütterung mit Fluornatrium. Z. Biol., 28:518-539, 1891.
2. Wallace-Durbin, P.: The Metabolism of Fluorine in the Rat Using F[18] as a Tracer. J. Dent. Res., 33:789-800, 1954.

3. Perkinson, J.D., Jr., Whitney, I.B., Monroe, R.A., Lotz, W.E., and Comar, C.L.: Metabolism of Fluorine 18 in Domestic Animals. Am. J. Physiol., 182:383-389, 1955.

4. Ericsson, Y., and Ullberg, S.: Autoradiographic Investigations of the Distribution of F^{18} in Mice and Rats. Acta Odontol. Scand., 16:363-374, 1958.

5. Carlson, C.H., Armstrong, W.D., and Singer, L.: Distribution and Excretion of Radiofluoride in the Human. Proc. Soc. Exp. Biol. Med., 104:235-239, 1960.

6. McClure, F.J., Mitchell, H.H., Hamilton, T.S., and Kinser, C.A.: Balances of Fluorine Ingested from Various Sources in Food and Water by Five Young Men. Excretion of Fluorine Through the Skin. J. Ind. Hyg. Toxicol., 27:159-170, 1945. (Reprinted in Fluoride Drinking Waters, 1962, pp. 377-384.)

7. Spencer, H., Kramer, L., Osis, D., and Wiatrowski, E.: Excretion of Retained Fluoride in Man. J. Appl. Physiol., 38:282-287, 1975.

8. Stookey, G.K., Dellinger, E.L., and Muhler, J.C.: *In vitro* Studies Concerning Fluoride Absorption. Proc. Soc. Exp. Biol. Med., 115:298-301, 1964.

9. Lawrenz, M., and Mitchell, H.H.: The Effect of Dietary Calcium and Phosphorus on the Assimilation of Dietary Fluorine. J. Nutr. 22:91-101, 1941.

10. Weddle, D.A., and Muhler, J.C.: The Effects of Inorganic Salts on Fluorine Storage in the Rat. J. Nutr., 54:437-444, 1954.

11. McGown, E.L., and Suttie, J.W.: Influence of Fat and Fluoride on Gastric Emptying of Rats. J. Nutr., 104:909-915, 1974.

12. McGown, E.L., Kolstad, D.L., and Suttie, J.W.: Effect of Dietary Fat on Fluoride Absorption and Tissue Fluoride Retention in Rats. J. Nutr., 106:575-579, 1976.

13. Lawrenz, M., Mitchell, H.H., and Ruth, W.A.: The Comparative Assimilation of Fluoride by Growing Rats During Continuous and Intermittent Dosage. J. Nutr., 20:383-390, 1940.

14. Task Group on Lung Dynamics (Bates, D.V., Fish, B.R., Hatch, T.F., Mercer, T.T., and Morrow, P.E.): Deposition and Retention Models for Internal Dosimetry of the Human Respiratory Tract. Health Phys., 12:173-207, 1966.

15. Collings, G.H., Jr., Fleming, R.B.L., May, R., and Bianconi, W.O.: Absorption and Excretion of Inhaled Fluorides: Further Observations. Arch. Ind. Hyg. Occup. Med., 6:368-373, 1952.

16. Taves, D.R.: Evidence That There Are Two Forms of Fluoride in Human Serum. Nature (Lond.), 217:1050, 1968.

17. Hodge, H.C., and Taves, D.R.: Chronic Toxic Effects [of Fluoride] on the Kidneys, in Fluorides and Human Health. World Health Organization Monograph Series No. 59, Geneva, 1970, p. 254.

18. Hanhijärvi H.: Comparison of Free Ionized Fluoride Concentrations of Plasma and Renal Clearance in Patients of Artificially Fluoridated and Non-Fluoridated Drinking Water Areas. Proc. Finn. Dent. Soc. 70: suppl. III, 1974.

19. Hanhijärvi, H.: Inorganic Plasma Fluoride Concentrations and Its Renal Excretion in Certain Physiological and Pathological Conditions in Man. Fluoride. 8:198-207, 1975.

20. Weidmann, S.M., and Weatherell, J.A.: The Uptake and Distribution of Fluorine in Bones. J. Pathol. Bacteriol., 78:243-255, 1959.

21. Savchuck, W.B., and Armstrong, W.D.: Metabolic Turnover of Fluoride in the Growing Skeleton. J. Dent. Res. 30:467-468, 1951; J. Biol. Chem., 193:575-585, 1951.

22. Waldbott, G.L.: Fluoride and Calcium Levels in the Aorta. Experientia (Basel), 22:835-837, 1966.

23. Waldbott, G.L.: Introduction to Symposium on the Non-Skeletal Phase of Chronic Fluorosis. Fluoride, 9:5-8, 1976.

24. Geever, E.F., McCann, H.G., McClure, F.J., Lee, W.A., and Schiffmann, E.: Fluoridated Water, Skeletal Structure, and Chemistry. Health Serv. Mental Health Admin. Health Rep., 86:820-828, 1971.

25. Largent, E.J., and Heyroth, F.F.: The Absorption and Excretion of Fluorides. III. Further Observations on Metabolism of Fluorides at High Levels of Intake. J. Ind. Hyg. Toxicol., 31:134-138, 1949.

26. Waldbott, G.L.: Comments on the Symposium "The Physiologic and Hygienic Aspects of the Absorption of Inorganic Fluorides." Arch. Environ. Health, 2:155-167, 1961.

27. Likins, R.C., McClure, F.J., and Steere, A.C.: Urinary Excretion of Fluoride Following Defluoridation of a Water Supply. Public Health Rep., 71: 217-220, 1956. (Reprinted in Fluoride Drinking Waters, 1962, pp. 421-423.)

CHAPTER 5

FLUORIDE AND THE TEETH

THE RAVAGES OF TOOTH DECAY

DENTAL CARIES – tooth decay – is evidently as old as civilization. Although skulls of prehistoric man from pre-neolithic times
prior to 12,000 B.C. show little evidence of carious teeth, ancient
Sumerians living in the period between 5000 B.C. and 3500 B.C.
at a comparatively high cultural level did have dental caries. In
Egypt decayed teeth have been found on skeletal remains of aristo-
crats who lived when the pyramids were being built, but Egyptians
of the lower classes, who were in the habit of eating coarse food,
rarely had cavities. Similar observations have been made in other
parts of the world, in Silesia for example, where at the end of the
stone age only 1.75% of the population had caries in permanent
teeth, as contrasted with 80% in modern times.[1]

It is now well established that consumption of sugar and other
refined carbohydrates associated with civilization has been primarily responsible for the recent dramatic increase in caries. Indeed, as
civilization has advanced the incidence of dental caries has risen
until it has literally soared during the current century. North
American Eskimos and Indians, Greenland Eskimos, and Siberian
tribes were nearly free of dental caries as long as their diet was re-
stricted to meat, fish, and berries. Skulls of 200 years ago found in
western parts of Greenland showed virtually no evidence of caries,
but access to ice-free harbors during the larger part of the year by
western Greenlanders brought higher carbohydrate consumption
and increased dental caries, which eventually affected nine out of
ten persons. In contrast, the people in eastern Greenland, who
were isolated from contact with civilization for nine months of the
year, were unaffected. For similar reasons – diminished sugar consumption and increased consumption of whole-grain products – the

incidence of caries in occupied Norway and Denmark fell dramatically during World War II compared to Sweden. During the period
of most severe rationing, the incidence of caries was lowest in children whose molar teeth were erupting.[2]

Although diet is of fundamental importance in the development
of tooth decay, other factors are clearly involved. Certain elements – especially calcium, phosphorus, magnesium, molybdenum,
vanadium, strontium and fluorine – seem to afford protection in
varying degrees against dental caries. A constitutional genetic background might also predispose one to tooth decay. For instance, in
1933 at a time when southern blacks were strictly segregated from
whites in Tennessee, 74% of the Caucasian population had tooth
decay compared with only 41% of blacks,[3] but here, too,
differences in the diet might have played an undertermined, yet
significant role.

Tooth decay begins shortly after eruption of the primary teeth
and in modern societies continues at an extraordinary rate up to
puberty. In 1940 one of the first large-scale epidemiological surveys made in the United States of an entire elementary school
population of 4,416 children age 6 to 15 years at Hagerstown,
Maryland, revealed that at age 6, 50% of the boys and 56% of the
girls were afflicted with tooth decay. This alarming rate rose to
95% and 96% by the time the children reached age 14.[4]

A 1974 U.S. survey of 7,514 youths aged 12 to 17 years revealed
an average of 6.2 decayed, missing, and filled (DMF) permanent
teeth per person, comprising 1.7 decayed, 0.7 missing, and 3.8
filled teeth.[5] At every given age, males had a lower DMF count
than females, and white youths had slightly higher DMF indexes
than black youths. No correlation of the indexes was found with
either family income or parents' education. White youths living in
the northeastern states had a higher DMF count than those living
elsewhere.

The enormous impact of the ravages of tooth decay can be better appreciated if we consider that during the 1960s the average
person in the United States required about three dental restorations per year because of dental caries with a peak of slightly over
four at ages 15 to 24.[6] Another survey estimated that of the 91
million adults who still had their natural teeth, about 855 million
teeth were missing, 127 million had unfilled carious lesions, and

637 million had been filled.[7] In terms of cost, the American people paid $1.25 billion for fillings in 1965; five years later, in 1970, the total expenditure on dental disease had increased to more than $4 billion.

When a tooth is decayed, more is involved than a painful, swollen cheek, or an ugly-looking mouth. Many chronic diseases, especially the rheumatoid kind of arthritis and subacute bacterial endocarditis, can arise from cavities acting as portals through which bacteria and their toxins are transported by the blood stream and lymph channels. Kidney disease and diabetes may be precipitated, or at least aggravated, by dental caries. Even allergic reactions, in the form of chronic hives, are often traced to a decayed tooth. In my own practice, I vividly recall the case of a 40-year-old man with septicemia and daily spiking (i.e., rising) temperatures which progressed in spite of extensive antibiotic treatment. The extraction of an abscessed, decayed tooth brought a prompt change in the clinical picture and undoubtedly prevented a fatal outcome.

Such serious and numerous health problems have led dentists to renew their war on tooth decay. Among approaches they have explored are: improved oral hygiene, protective topical treatments, surface and fissure sealants, frequent use of dental floss, consumption of detergent foods (now questioned), restriction of refined carbohydrates, and better nutrition. The addition of chemical elements to food and water has also been recommended, and beginning in the late 1930s, scientists and public health dentists have advocated the addition of fluorides to drinking water. The prevailing view on caries prevention by fluoride is clearly summarized by L.M. Dalderup: "In the caries susceptible stages [ages] especially a sufficient supply of fluoride is extremely important for improving the caries resistance of the dentition."[8]

Early in the 1950s, the U.S. Public Health Service endorsed this view and began to promote fluoridation vigorously. Luther Terry, a former Surgeon General of the PHS, has described this measure as one of the "four horsemen of public health," comparable to "the pasteurization of milk, the purification of water, [and] immunization against disease."[9] Many other organizations here and abroad share this view. In 1975 the Council on Foods and Nutrition of the American Medical Association renewed its recommendation of fluoridation as a "desirable and safe health measure for total populations and urge[d] all communities to adopt the necessary measures."[10] The two fundamental issues pertaining to this health measure – its efficacy and safety – nevertheless require further consideration.

MECHANISM OF DENTAL CARIES

A tooth consists essentially of an outer layer called the enamel, a substance harder than any other part of the body, and an interior, less calcified, bone-like part called dentin (Fig. 5–1, below). It

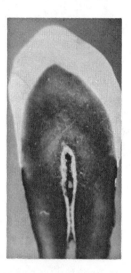

Fig. 5-1. Ninhydrin-stained section of a healthy premolar tooth showing the enamel (white), dentin (dark), and pulp chamber (center). This tooth-section has been demineralized by a neutral solution of phosphatase having a F/Mg ratio comparable to that present in carious lesions.
(Courtesy J. A. Csernyei, Milan, Italy: Fluoride and the Endogenous Theory of Dental Caries. *Fluoride,* 2:116-119, 1969.)

is held in the jaw by cementum, and in its center is a canal, the so-called pulp chamber, which houses the nerves, lymph, and blood vessels that supply the necessary nutrients during formation and development.

The enamel is formed by a group of cells called ameloblasts, one on top of the other in the form of tube-like structures similar to a stack of drinking straws. Inside these tubes, insoluble, inorganic salts containing mainly calcium and phosphorus and lesser quantities of many other elements accumulate. Eventually this process leads to calcification of the enamel through formation of hydroxyapatite, $Ca_{10}(OH)_2(PO_4)_6$.

Once the tooth is formed the enamel is relatively nonviable in contrast to the cells of bones that are constantly undergoing active metabolic changes and are capable of repair. After growth and calcification of the tooth are complete, the intake of chemicals, including fluoride, is almost entirely limited to the surfaces, particularly to the portion of the cementum lining the root canal which carries the blood vessel.

Several theories explaining the mechanism of tooth decay have been proposed. Toward the end of the 19th century, W.D. Miller, a German dentist, developed the so-called "chemico-parasitic" theory which maintains that caries consist of two stages: decalcification of enamel, followed by dissolution of the softened residue.[11] When Miller incubated bread, meat, and sugar for 48 hours, he produced enough acid to decalcify the dentin. Enamel attacked by an acid in the test tube loses calcium and phosphate ions which are then found in the solution.

In the mouth the decalcification of the enamel is brought about mainly by the action of the lactic acid bacillus *(Lactobacillus acidophilus)* that induces fermentation of carbohydrates. R. W. Bunting, former Dean of the University of Michigan Dental School, demonstrated the significant role of this microorganism when he found it universally absent in persons immune to caries, but abundant where caries were rampant.[12] The lactic acid formed by the bacillus can be partially neutralized by the alkaline property of saliva; however, sufficient amounts usually remain in the mouth to encourage formation of dental plaque, a gelatinous chemical-bacterial film that adheres to the tooth surface and often appears to be involved in the beginning of the decay process. Generally, plaque is formed at fissures and pits of the enamel surface or at adjoining surfaces of teeth, where food particles collect.

Defects in the enamel structure, inherited or environmentally-induced nutritional deficiencies, childhood diseases, exposure to toxic elements, such as selenium or strong acids, inadequate dental hygiene (lack of brushing and cleaning), and, particularly, a diet rich in refined carbohydrates and deficient in vital minerals — especially calcium, magnesium, and phosphorus — predispose the tooth to attacks by acid. Once the carious pits and fissures are created, they retain bacteria-laden fermentable matter that makes the defective faults more susceptible to further attack and to infection. When decay penetrates into the dentin, which is softer and less mineralized than the enamel, the process advances more rapidly, infects the pulp, and leads to abscess formation. (On the other hand, a view based on nutritional deficiency states that "dental caries originates with demineralization of an area of dentine and then proceeds to the enamel surface where cavity formation begins."[13])

A different kind of fermentation is brought about by oxidation of sugar to oxalic acid through the activity of another organism called *Leptothrix buccalis*. This type of fermentation forms a brittle, straw-colored tartar around the necks of teeth. The presence of this tartar is held by some dental researchers to counter the cariogenic effect of the lactobacillus.[14] A predominantly protein diet promotes formation of oxalic acid, in contrast to certain carbohydrate-rich foods that favor fermentation to lactic acid.

Another explanation of the mechanism of dental caries, quite different from Miller's theory, was proposed in 1929 by C. F. Bödecker, an American dentist. He suggested that decay originates in the organic, protein-containing matrix that constitutes about 0.6% of the tooth, not in the inorganic mineral components. This so-called proteolytic (protein-dissolving) theory postulates that the organic portion of the tooth, mainly the enamel lamellae and the sheaths of the enamel rods, are dissolved by microorganisms that invade the organic pathways and destroy them.[15]

In 1955, A. Schatz, co-discoverer with S. Waksman of streptomycin, developed the proteolysis idea further and introduced the "proteolysis-chelation theory," which explains the decay process under both acid and alkaline conditions.[16] Chelation is a process through which a metal cation* such as lead is complexed or "clawed" (Greek χηλή, claw) tightly to a bifunctional reagent to form a cyclic-structured species. Schatz postulates that, through enzymatic and bacterial attack on the organic constituents of enamel, chelating agents are formed from either constituents of enamel, food, or saliva. These agents then combine (chelate) with the calcium in the mineral phase of the enamel, thereby producing dental caries.

----

*A cation (pronounced "cat'-eye-on") is a positively charged particle or ion.

ACTION OF FLUORIDE ON TEETH

In view of these different explanations of the origin of tooth decay, how can we explain the decay-preventive action of fluoride? We know that fluoride accumulates in both the dentin and enamel of the teeth prior to eruption. Its uptake is more rapid during formation and development of the tooth than after it is fully formed. There is evidence that in the tooth the hydroxyl (OH) group of the apatite crystal is replaced by fluoride at the crystal surface. This exchange of ions enlarges the apatite crystal,[17] and as its size increases the enamel becomes less soluble and more resistant to decay. This process takes place mainly on the inner surface of the tooth, at the pulp chamber to which fluoride is carried by the blood stream. After the tooth is fully developed, the outer surface and the enamel-dentin border show the greatest deposition of fluoride.[18]

Other theories maintain that fluoride reduces the amount of dental plaque, which usually contains high concentrations of the halogen (6.4 to 179 ppm),[19] or that optimal fluoride intake during tooth formation produces a more rounded tooth with more tightly closed fissures that would be expected to be more self-cleaning[20] (cf. Fig. 5–2, page 62). Some authors believe that fluoride may inactivate the co-enzyme portion of the enolase system, thus preventing the degradation of carbohydrates[3] and particularly their accumulation in the plaque, which in turn encourages acid production beyond the time of eating when sugar is available. Others ascribe to fluoride a reduction in the amount of *Lactobacillus acidophilus* in the saliva, thereby inhibiting formation of cariogenic lactic acid in the mouth.[7] G. N. Jenkins summarizes the anti-caries action of fluoride as "a unique combination of properties all of which may play some part. The question is not which theory is right, but what is the relative importance of the various effects which F⁻ seems able to exert?"[20]

MOTTLED TEETH AND CARIES

In 1931 three different groups of scientists announced their discovery of the primary cause of the widely occurring endemic tooth defect known as dental mottling: fluoride in the drinking

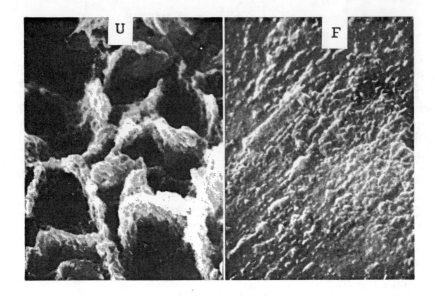

Fig. 5-2. Surface of tooth (magnification x 7,000) brushed twice daily for 12 days with fluoridated toothpaste (right) compared to untreated surface (left); both after immersion for 3 hours in lactic acid (pH 4). (Courtesy L. Capozzi and F. Marci, University of Rome: Observations with a "Scanning" Electron Microscope on Dental Enamel Treated with Fluorides.
Fluoride, 4:58-63, 1971.)

water of children. This extraordinary finding was reported independently by M. C. Smith and her colleagues at the University of Arizona Agricultural Experiment Station, Tucson;[21] H. V. Churchill at the Aluminum Company of America Research Laboratories, Pittsburgh, Pa.;[22] and H. Velu at phosphate mines in Morocco and Tunisia.[23] Shortly afterward the apparent decay-preventive action of fluoride in drinking water was investigated and brought to the attention of the dental profession.

Mottled teeth had been alluded to in medical literature as early as 1771 when John Hunter discussed a condition of dark spots underlying the intact enamel surface of otherwise sound teeth.[24] Later, in 1878, L. P. Meredith vividly described this dental "atrophy" in which "white, yellow, or brown spots of various sizes and irregular shapes may exist on the outer surfaces of teeth."[25] In 1901 J.M. Eager, a U.S. health officer stationed in Naples, wrote about similar defective teeth of Italian emigrants.[26] In the United States, however, mottled teeth did not become well known to the dental profession until 1916, when G.V. Black and F.S. McKay published their detailed observations with full-color illustrations.[27] Like Eager before them, they suspected that something in the drinking water was responsible for mottling, but they were unable to determine what it was.

Black and McKay were surprised by one particular aspect of their investigation: "This mottled condition in itself does not seem to increase the susceptibility of the teeth to decay, which is perhaps contrary to what might be expected."[27] In Bauxite, Arkansas, for example, where the fluoride content of the drinking water was as high as 13.7 ppm, and where *every* child born and raised there before 1928 had mottled teeth, 27% of these children were caries free as compared with 15% of the children born there after 1928 when a low-fluoride (≤ 0.2 ppm) source of water was introduced.[28]

After the discovery that fluoride was the cause of mottled enamel, extensive epidemiological investigations of the relation between the fluoride content of drinking water and the amount of mottling and dental caries were undertaken, especially by H. Trendley Dean of the U.S. Public Health Service, who was the first Director of the National Institute of Dental Research until his retirement in 1953. In his studies Dean correlated the occurrence of mottling or "dental fluorosis," as he labeled it, with the fluoride content of water supplies in 345 U.S. communities, located mostly in Texas, Colorado, South Dakota, Iowa, and Arizona.[29] (Figs. 5–3 and 5–4, pages 64 and 65). He also refined his investigations with a survey of 5824 white children 12 to 14 years old in 22 cities in 10 states and related both the incidence and severity of dental fluorosis to the concentration of fluoride in the drinking water[30] (Figs. 5–5 through 5–9, pages 66-70). By assigning a numerical weighting to each classification of mottled enamel according to its severity (see Chapter 12, below), he was able to determine a "community index" or weighted average of dental fluorosis in each community.[29,30]

In their surveys, Dean and his colleagues also reported a distinctly lower incidence of dental caries, particularly among 12- to 14-year-old children, in areas of endemic dental fluorosis. In South Dakota, for example, the amount of tooth decay in 8148 white

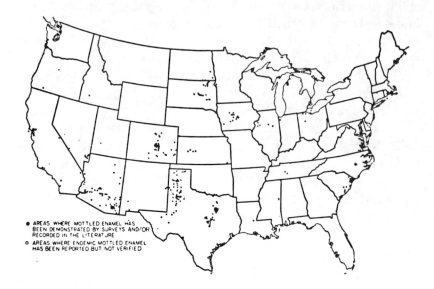

Fig. 5-3. Geographical distribution of mottled enamel in the United States (1936). (From H. Trendley Dean: Chronic Endemic Dental Fluorosis (Mottled Enamel). *J. Am. Med. Assoc.*, 107:1269-1272, 1936; reprinted in **F. J.** McClure, Ed.: *Fluoride Drinking Waters,* 1962, pp. 45-49.)

children 12 to 14 years of age "was inversely proportional to the prevalence of mottled enamel."[31] In other words, as mottling increased, the presence of caries decreased. More dental decay was also observed among American Indian children in the Pacific Northwest than among those living in the southwestern part of the United States, where mottling was widespread.[32] In a major study involving 7257 white children from ages 12 to 14 years in 21 cities in Colorado, Illinois, Indiana, and Ohio, Dean reported that the incidence of caries in communities with 0.9–1.4 ppm fluoride in the drinking water was only about one third that in the cities with 0.4 ppm or less.[31]

Meanwhile, other USPHS researchers devised the so-called DMF index—the number of decayed, missing, and filled permanent teeth per child (or 100 children)—in order to establish a quantitative measure of the incidence of dental caries in a given locality. A survey by this method in Hagerstown, Maryland, became a model for numerous other studies designed to measure the relationship of

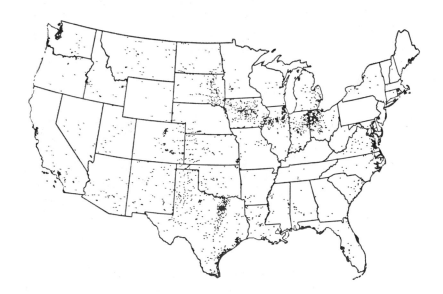

Fig. 5-4. Communities in the United States having 0.7 ppm or more natural fluoride in at least one water supply source (ca. 1955). Note correspondence with areas of endemic mottling in Fig. 5-3 (opposite). From U.S. Public Health Service Publication No. 655, Washington, D.C., 1959, p. IX.)

tooth decay to various environmental and other factors, especially fluoride in the drinking water.[33]

An obvious extension of Dean's findings was the idea of artificially raising the fluoride content of low-fluoride water supplies to levels sufficient to achieve a significant reduction in tooth decay without causing an undesirable increase in dental fluorosis. As early as 1938 Dean had written of "the possibility of partially controlling dental caries through the domestic water supply."[34] But it remained for G. J. Cox, a biochemist at the Dental School of the University of Pittsburgh, to be the first to make an actual proposal of "fluoridization" as "a means of very materially reducing the incidence of dental caries by a procedure that is applicable to whole communities. Furthermore, the prophylaxis could be applied in such a way that the individual would be hard put to escape the treatment. . . ."[35,36]

But what concentrations of fluoride in drinking water would yield the best results for caries control with the least amount of

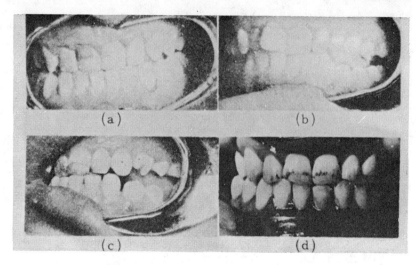

Fig. 5-5. Examples of "very mild" dental fluorosis. In this classification up to 25% of the surfaces of the two most affected teeth show mottling. Permanent yellow or brown staining not obvious in the teeth of the children (a), (b), and (c), is quite evident in the teeth of the adult (d). A 10% incidence of "very mild" fluorosis is not uncommon in communities with 1 ppm fluoride in the water supply. Even with only 0.5–0.6 ppm fluoride incidences of 3.5% (Elgin, Ill.) and 6.2% (Pueblo, Col.) have been reported.[30] (Courtesy F. B. Exner, M.D.; from his fluoridation testimony presented to the Ontario Investigating Committee, May 11, 1960, Plate XII.)

mottling? Dean's surveys revealed a steep acceleration in the incidence of dental fluorosis where the fluoride level of the water rose above 1 ppm, but only a minimal increase at concentrations between 0.1 and 1.0 ppm. In temperate climates a fluoride concentration of about 1 ppm was therefore adopted as optimal for the prevention of dental caries.[37] In communities with natural fluoride in the water in excess of 2 ppm, *removal* of fluoride to reduce the concentration to a level near 1 ppm was recommended.[38] Unfortunately, even at a concentration exceeding 1.4–1.6 ppm, according to an authoritative dental fluoride researcher,

the first signs of more serious dental fluorosis appear: some of the teeth of a few members of the population then show circumscribed spots, coloured

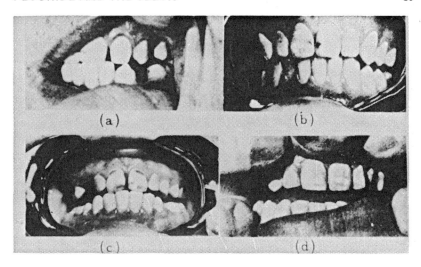

Fig. 5-6. Examples of "mild" dental fluorosis identified as "typical" by H. T. Dean and F. S. McKay. In this classification up to 50% of the surfaces of the two most affected teeth exhibit mottling, occasionally with brown staining, especially in adulthood. A 3.1% incidence of this degree of fluorosis has been reported in Joliet, Illinois, with 1.3 ppm fluoride in the drinking water.[30] A 6% incidence was found in Chandler, Arizona, with 0.8 ppm fluoride and a warmer climate (D. J. Galagan and G. G. Lamson, Jr.: Climate and Endemic Dental Fluorosis. *Public Health Rep.*, 68:497-508, 1953; reprinted in F. J. McClure, Ed.: *Fluoride Drinking Waters*, 1962, pp. 74-82.) (Courtesy F. B. Exner, *loc. cit.*, Plate IX.)

light-yellow to brownish. When the fluoride content exceeds 2.0 ppm, then brownish spots, varying from small to large in size, *can be seen on numerous teeth in the great majority of the members of the exposed community.*[39] [Emphasis added. See Figs. 5-6, 5-7, and 5-8.]

FLUORIDATION TRIALS

Newburgh. The cities of Newburgh, New York; Grand Rapids, Michigan; Brantford, Ontario; Evanston, Illinois; Southbury, Connecticut; Sheboygan, Wisconsin; Marshall, Texas; Ottawa, Kansas; and Lewiston, Idaho, were selected for the original experimental studies to add fluorides to municipal water supplies, and a 10- to 15-year plan was scheduled to begin in 1945 for the first three of

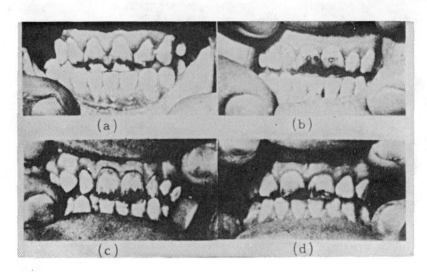

Fig. 5-7. Examples of "mild" dental fluorosis, tending toward "moderate" in which all teeth are affected. Brown staining seen here is not always present; often the tooth is a nearly uniform, opaque ("eggshell") white. In Elmhurst, Illinois, with 1.8 ppm fluoride in the drinking water, an incidence of 1.25% "moderate" fluorosis has been reported.[30] In Tucson and Chandler, Arizona, with only 0.7-0.8 ppm fluoride in the water, respectively, a 2% incidence was recorded (Galagan and Lamson, *loc. cit.* in Fig. 5-6).
(Courtesy F. B. Exner, M.D., *loc. cit.*, Plate XI.)

the above cities. Kingston, New York, with 0.05 ppm fluoride in the water, was selected as the control city for Newburgh. Located about 35 miles apart on the Hudson River, the two cities had 1940 populations of 31,956 and 28,817, respectively. Fluoridation of the Newburgh water supply began in May 1945. Initial dental examinations were made on all elementary grade school children aged 6 to 12 in both cities, and the information obtained was assembled according to an established classification of caries-free teeth, untreated caries, filled, missing, and unerupted teeth.[40]

In the baseline examinations (prior to the study) the DMF rate was approximately 20 DMF teeth per hundred teeth in both Newburgh and Kingston; in the former, the DMF rate of permanent molars was approximately 58 per hundred erupted teeth in each city. Thereafter, annual clinical dental examinations were made in Newburgh in each of the years 1944 through 1955

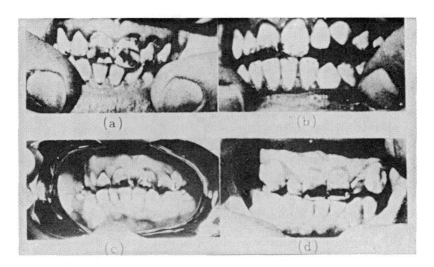

Fig. 5–8. Examples of "moderate" dental fluorosis cited as "typical" by H. T. Dean. In this classification some pitting and brown staining are common. This degree of mottling (in a temperate climate) is generally found only where the water contains at least 2 ppm fluoride; in Colorado Springs (2.5–2.6 ppm) an incidence of 8.9% was recorded.[30]
(Courtesy F. B. Exner, M.D., *loc. cit.,* Plate V.)

and in Kingston from 1945 through 1955. Roentgenograms (X-rays) were included in the examinations for the years 1949 to 1950, 1953 to 1954, and 1954 to 1955. All dental examinations in Newburgh and the first series in Kingston were made by the same examiner, S.B. Finn. In the subsequent examinations in Kingston the same technique was used by two dental hygienists trained by Finn. The study also included extensive pediatric examinations with measurements of height, weight, X-rays of the right hand and both knees, estimation of bone age, and various laboratory tests. such as urine analyses, hemoglobin levels, and total blood counts in order to detect any possible side effects from fluoridation.

Dental findings after three years of fluoridation in Newburgh were announced in October 1949 at the 77th Annual Meeting of the American Public Health Association. The investigators reported a marked downward trend in the DMF rate in Newburgh from 21.3 to 14.8 per hundred permanent teeth.[41] These figures indicated an increase of 6.5/100 sound permanent teeth in Newburgh,

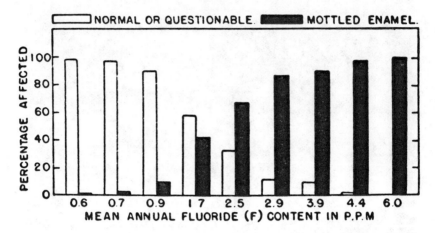

Fig. 5-9. Graphical presentation of the "quantitative relation" between the natural fluoride content of drinking water and the amount of mottled enamel. (From H. Trendley Dean: Chronic Endemic Dental Fluorosis (Mottled Enamel). *J. Am. Med. Assoc.,* 107:1269-1272, 1936; reprinted in F.J. McClure, Ed.: *Fluoride Drinking Waters,* 1962, pp. 45–49.)

or a 31% reduction in decay. Among the first permanent molars, which account for most of the caries in children, the rate in Newburgh was 48.0 DMF per hundred such teeth, whereas in Kingston it was 58.7, or a difference of 10.7 DMF teeth per hundred first permanent molars (18% decrease). The greatest benefits were reported for the younger age groups. Ten years after the start of fluoridation, the reports claimed 58% less decay in the permanent teeth of the 6- to 9-year-old children in Newburgh than in Kingston.[42]

Grand Rapids. In the 15th year of fluoridation in Grand Rapids, dental caries in lifelong resident children aged 12 to 14 years was found to be 50% to 63% less than in 1944-1945 and 48% to 50% less in children ages 15 to 16 years.[43] In this report the statistical validity of these differences and possible effects of examiner variability were given special attention, and the probability of the findings being due to chance was claimed to be less than one in 2,500,000. Four of the 1031 continuously resident children showed "mild" dental fluorosis, and about 10% of the entire study group had mottling which was classified as "questionable" or "very mild."

Other Cities. In Brantford, after 15 years of fluoridation, the overall DMF rate of continuously resident children aged 5 to 16 was reportedly reduced by 54%, while the reduction in decayed, extracted, or filled deciduous teeth was 42%, compared to levels in 1944-1945.[44] In 1963 the 16- and 17-year-old children in Brantford had a DMF count per child that was less than half (4.74 vs. 10.44) that of the low-fluoride (≤ 0.1 ppm) control city of Sarnia.[44] In Evanston, which began fluoridating in February 1947, no significant reduction in caries of the deciduous teeth apparently occurred until after 6 to 8 years of fluoridation.[45] After lifetime exposure to fluoridated water, however, children aged 12 to 14 had 57% to 48% fewer DMF teeth,[46] but the rates were not so low as those of the nearby comparison city of Aurora, Illinois, with 1.2 ppm natural fluoride in the water. In Evanston, on the other hand, dental examinations included X-ray films, whereas in Aurora no roentgenograms were taken.

For the most part findings similar to those summarized above have been reported from various other pilot studies of fluoridation both in the U.S. and in other countries. These investigations have led many scientists to conclude that fluoride in drinking water at a concentration of about 1 ppm produces a significant reduction in the incidence of dental caries – not to mention a parallel reduction in dental costs as well.[47] One author, in fact, claims that "for each dollar expended on fluoridation, about thirty-five dollars' worth of dental caries is prevented."[48]

Despite these promising results, the shadow of mottled enamel and the narrow latitude between the desirable and the toxic concentration of fluoride in water have been sources of constant concern to dental researchers. Indeed, the practicing dentist who wishes to explain the benefits of fluoridation to a mother, is confronted with a dilemma. Being more concerned with the acquisition of the technical skills required in his practice than with the critical examination of the intricate and involved scientific literature on fluoridation, he must rely upon the many reports of dental researchers telling him that fluoride makes teeth more resistant to decay. At the same time, he also encounters fluorosed teeth that can become discolored and difficult to repair. He may also wonder whether there might be other, perhaps less obvious, side effects from the practice of adding to drinking water a chemical known almost solely as a toxic agent before 1940.

This dilemma was well expressed by F. R. Moulton, who stated in his resumé on dental fluorosis in a 1942 monograph of the American Association for the Advancement of Science:

> A peculiarity of fluorine is that, so far as is known at present, its ingestion from natural sources by people living under sanitary conditions produces sensible biological effects only upon the teeth—*apparently* beneficial ones if in quantities that are somewhat below well-determined limits, and *certainly* tragically harmful ones if well-known limits are exceeded.[49] [Italics in the original.]

The dentist's dilemma is shared to an even greater extent by the physician, who constantly encounters in his practice unpleasant side effects from many medications. He knows that if a dangerous chemical is added to public waters, his patients cannot escape its effect. Yet, if reputable authorities tell him that no adverse medical problems can arise, he will, *ipso facto*, attribute any illness caused by fluoridated water to a multitude of other factors. We now need to examine the medical effects of fluoride.

REFERENCES

1. Dalderup, L.M.: Nutrition and Caries. World Rev. Nutr. Diet., 7:72-137, 1967.

2. Toverud, G., in National Research Council Publication 225: Review of the Literature of Dental Caries. National Academy of Sciences, Washington, D.C., 1952.

3. Shafer, W.G., Hine, M.K., and Levi, B.M.: A Textbook of Oral Pathology. W.B. Saunders, Philadelphia, 1974, p. 406.

4. Knutson, J.W., Klein, H., and Palmer, C.E.: Dental Needs of Grade School Children of Hagerstown, Maryland. J. Am. Dent. Assoc., 27:579-588, 1940.

5. Kelly, J.E.: Decayed, Missing and Filled Teeth Among Youths 12-17 Years. National Center for Health Statistics, Rockville, Md., 1974.

6. Report of Bureau of Economic Research and Statistics. American Dental Association, Chicago, 1965.

7. Young, W.O., and Striffler, D.E.: The Dentist, His Practice, and His Community. W.B. Saunders, Philadelphia, 1969, p. 184. Cf. Ref. 48, below.

8. Dalderup (in Ref. 1, above), p. 125.

9. McClure, F.J.: Water Fluoridation: The Search and the Victory. 1970, p. viii.

10. Fletcher, D.C.: Editorial: Revised Statement on Fluoridation. J. Am. Med. Assoc, 231:1167, 1975.

11. For citations to W.D. Miller, see Dalderup (in Ref. 1, above), p. 74.

12. Bunting, R.W., Mickerson, G., and Hard, D.G.: Further Studies of the Relationship of Bacillus Acidophilus to Dental Caries. Dent. Cosmos, 68:931-942, 1926.

13. Csernyei, J.A.: Fluoride and the Endogenous Theory of Dental Caries. Fluoride, 2:116-119, 1969.

14. Dillon, C.: Fluorosis and Dental Caries. Carlton Press, New York, 1969, p. 140.

15. Bödecker, C.F., and Bödecker, H.C.W.: The Bacterial Destruction of Dental Enamel. J. Dent. Res., 9:37-53, 1929.

16. Martin, J.J., Schatz, A., and Karlson, K.E.: Proteolysis-Chelation: A New Theory of Dental Caries. J. New Jersey State Dent. Soc., 27:7-8, 1955.

17. Posner, A.S., Eanes, E.D., Harper, R.A., and Zipkin, I.: X-ray Diffraction Analysis of the Effect of Fluoride on Human Bone Apatite. Arch. Oral Biol., 8:549-570, 1963.

18. Wörner, H.: Die Härte menschlichen Dentins in Abhängigkeit vom Calcium-, Phosphor- und Fluorgehalt. Dtsch. Zahnaerztl. Z., 29:58-62, 1974.

19. Hardwick, J.L., and Leach, S.A.: The Fluoride Content of the Dental Plaque. Arch. Oral Biol., Suppl. Vol. 8 (Proc. 9th Cong. European Organization for Research on Fluorine and Dental Caries Prevention, June 1962): 151-158, 1963.

20. Jenkins, G.N.: Mechanism of Action of Fluoride in Reducing Dental Caries. Fluoride, 2:236-240, 1969.

21. Smith, M.C., Lantz, E.M., and Smith, H.V.: The Cause of Mottled Enamel, A Defect of Human Teeth. Tech. Bull. No. 32, Univ. Ariz. Coll. Agric., Agric. Exp. Sta., Tucson, June 10, 1931, and Science, 74:244, 1931.

22. Churchill, H.V.: The Occurrence of Fluorides in Some Waters of the United States. J. Am. Water Works Assoc., 23:1399-1403, 1931; Ind. Eng. Chem., 23:996-998, 1931. (First announced in Ind. Eng. Chem., News Ed., 9:105, April 10, 1931.)

23. Velu, H.: Dystrophie dentaire des Mammifères des zones phosphatées (darmous) et fluorose chronique. C.R. Séances Soc. Biol. Ses. Fil., 108:750-752, 1931.

24. Hunter, J.: A Practical Treatise on the Diseases of the Teeth. Part II. American Society of Dental Surgeons, London, 1771, p. 2. (Reprinted in American Library of Dental Science, New York, 1839.)

25. Meredith, L.P.: The Teeth and How to Save Them. 2nd ed. William Tegg, London, 1878, p. 152.

26. Eager, J.M.: Denti di Chiaie (Chiaie teeth). Public Health Rep., 16(2): 2576-2577, 1901; Dent. Cosmos, 44:300-301, 1902. (Reprinted in Fluoride Drinking Waters, 1962, p. 2.)

27. Black, G.V., and McKay, F.S.: Mottled Teeth: An Endemic Developmental Imperfection of the Enamel of the Teeth, Heretofore Unknown in the Literature of Dentistry. Dent. Cosmos, 58:129-156; 477-484; 627-624; 781-792; 894-904, 1916.

28. Dean, H.T., Jay, P., Arnold, F.A., Jr., and Elvove, E.: Domestic Water and Dental Caries. I. A Dental Caries Study, Including L. Acidophilus Estimations, of a Population Severely Affected by Mottled Enamel and Which for the Past 12 Years Has Used a Fluoride-Free Water. Public Health Rep., 56: 365-381, 1941. (Reprinted in Fluoride Drinking Waters, 1962, pp. 101-109.)

29. Dean, H.T.: Chronic Endemic Dental Fluorosis (Mottled Enamel), in S. M. Gordon, Ed.: Dental Science and Dental Art. Lea and Febiger, Philadelphia, 1938, Ch. 12.

30. Dean, H.T.: The Investigation of Physiological Effects by the Epidemiological Method, in F.R. Moulton, Ed.: Fluorine and Dental Health, Am. Assoc. Adv. Sci., Washington, D.C., 1942, pp. 23-31.

31. Dean, H.T.: Epidemiological Studies in the United States, in F.R. Moulton, Ed.: Dental Caries and Fluorine. Am. Assoc. Adv. Sci., Washington, D.C., 1946, pp. 5-31.

32. Klein, H., and Palmer, C.E.: Dental Caries in American Indian Children. Public Health Rep., 50:1719-1729, 1935.

33. Klein, H., Palmer, C.E., and Knutson, J.W.: Studies on Dental Caries. I. Dental Status and Dental Needs of Elementary School Children. Public Health Rep., 53:751-765, 1938.

34. Dean, H.T.: Endemic Fluorosis and Its Relation to Dental Caries. Public Health Rep., 53:1443-1452, 1938. (Reprinted in Fluoride Drinking Waters, 1962, pp. 85-89.)

35. Cox, G.J.: New Knowledge of Fluorine in Relation to Dental Caries. J. Am. Water Works Assoc., 31:1926-1930, 1939.

36. Hodge, H.C., and Smith, F.A. in J.H. Simons, Ed.: Fluorine Chemistry, Vol. 4. Academic Press, New York and London, 1965, p. 514.

37. Hodge, H.C.: The Concentration of Fluorides in Drinking Water to Give the Point of Minimum Caries with Maximum Safety. J. Am. Dent. Assoc., 40:436-439, 1950. Using Dean's data, A.A. Hirsch (Chem. Eng. News, 32:4890, Oct. 8, 1956) has calculated that 0.75 ppm rather than 1.0 ppm is the optimum level for obtaining the best balance between decreased caries and the minimization of dental fluorosis.

38. USPHS Drinking Water Standards. 1961 Revision. Public Health Rep., 76:782, 1961.

39. Adler, P.: Fluorides and Dental Health, in Fluorides and Human Health. 1970, pp. 323-324.

40. McClure (in Ref. 9, above), pp. 123-124.

41. Ast, D.B., Finn, S.B., McCaffery, I., Schlesinger, E.R., Overton, D.E.,

and Chase, H.: The Newburgh-Kingston Caries-Fluorine Study. I. Dental Findings After Three Years of Water Fluoridation. Am. J. Public Health, 40: 716-724, 1950.

42. Ast, D.B., Smith, D.J., Wachs, B., and Cantwell, K.T.: Newburgh-Kingston Caries-Fluorine Study. XIV. Combined Clinical and Roentgenographic Dental Findings after Ten Years of Fluoride Experience. J. Am. Dent. Assoc., 52:314-325, 1956.

43. Arnold, F.A., Jr., Likins, R.C., Russell, A.L., and Scott, D.B.: Fifteenth Year of the Grand Rapids Fluoridation Study. J. Am. Dent. Assoc., 65:780-785, 1962.

44. Brown, H.K., and Poplove, M.: Brantford-Sarnia-Stratford Caries Study: Final Survey. J. Can. Dent. Assoc., 31:505-511, 1965.

45. Hill, I.N., Blayney, J.R., and Wolf, W.: The Evanston Dental Caries Study. XV. The Caries Experience Rates of Two Groups of Evanston Children After Exposure to Fluoridated Water. J. Dent. Res., 36:208-219, 1957.

46. Blayney, J.R., and Hill, I.N.: Fluorine and Dental Caries. J. Am. Dent. Assoc., 74(2):233-302, Jan. 1967.

47. For example, see Cross, C.O.: The Economics of Fluoridation. J. Southern Calif. Dent. Assoc., 36:499-500, Dec. 1968; Doherty, N. and Powell, E.: Effects of Age and Years of Experience on the Economic Benefits of Fluoridation. J. Dent. Res., 53:912-914, 1974.

48. Goldhaber, P.: The Teeth and Gums, in H. Wechsler, J. Gurin, and G.F. Cahill, Jr., Eds.: The Horizons of Health. Harvard University Press, Cambridge, Mass., and London, 1977, p. 290.

49. Moulton (in Ref. 30, above), Foreword.

CHAPTER 6

AN ESSENTIAL NUTRIENT?

ONCE IT BECAME widely accepted that fluoride hardens teeth and aids in preventing tooth decay, the question arose whether or not trace amounts might be necessary to maintain human health and life. This consideration, of course, represented an abrupt about-face: before the relationship between mottled teeth and fluoride in drinking water was established, certainly even afterward, fluoride was universally regarded as a toxic agent comparable in action to arsenic and lead.[1] Even Cox, the originator of the idea of fluoridation, had stated: "Fluorides are among the most toxic of substances."[2]

Several other chemical elements, however, do have such a dual, indeed a paradoxical function. A striking example is selenium, a member of the sulfur group, which is present in grain and vegetables. In minute concentrations—less than 1 ppm in forage and water—selenium is a required nutrient in domestic animals and probably in humans as well. Without selenium sheep and lambs develop "white muscle disease" with wasting of musculature, retardation of growth, infertility, and impairment of vision.[3] On the other hand, if humans consume food that contains more than ten times the normal amount, selenium causes chronic poisoning—general malaise, dizziness, excessive perspiration at first, and later a liver ailment associated with ascites.*

Similarly, the metal cobalt—found mainly in fish, cocoa beans, and molasses—is an essential building block of vitamin B_{12} involved in the synthesis of hemoglobin, the vital carrier of oxygen in the blood. As little as 0.0434 microgram of cobalt contained in one microgram of vitamin B_{12} suffices to prevent pernicious anemia.

---

*Ascites — hydroperitoneum; an accumulation of serious fluid in the peritoneal cavity.

Yet, when concentrations on the order of 150 ppm are ingested in the diet, the thyroid gland enlarges, congestive heart failure occurs, and, eventually, death can result. Moreover, when cobalt pollutes the atmosphere, minute amounts suffice to induce severe asthmatic attacks.

Other essential elements toxic in amounts larger than nutritional requirements are magnesium, manganese, and zinc, all of which are necessary constituents of many vital enzymes.[4] Too much iodine is toxic, but in small amounts it is indispensable for the function of the thyroid gland; although iron is necessary for the formation of hemoglobin, in large amounts it is also poisonous. A crucial question is: does fluorine (as a fluoride ion) share such a paradoxical property with other trace elements?

To explore this possibility, we must first establish whether the addition of fluoride to the diet contributes significantly to growth and good health and whether lack of it, in an otherwise adequate diet, leads to deficiency symptoms.[5] A recent statement reflects the position of many health authorities: "Fluoride is now considered to be an essential nutrient in man; this has been difficult to establish, however, because it is virtually impossible to prepare a fluoride-free diet for man or animals."[6]

LABORATORY STUDIES

Indeed, researchers on this subject have been confronted with the almost impossible task of obtaining a diet entirely free of fluoride to serve as a "nonfluoride" control. In 1953, McClendon and Gershon-Cohen fed 18 rats, for two months, a diet consisting exclusively of corn and sunflower seeds grown by culture in rainwater that was virtually free of fluoride (0.002–0.004 ppm).[7] These "low-fluoride" animals were reported to be smaller in size and to have more dental caries than a control group of 18 rats fed a standard laboratory diet and drinking water to which 20 ppm fluoride had been added.

On the other hand, in 1957 Maurer and Day of the University of Indiana succeeded in producing a diet nutritionally adequate in vitamins and minerals but so low in fluoride that it contained less than 0.007 ppm.[8] It was sugar-free and not conducive to impaction of food or formation of caries in the fissures of teeth. Rats maintained for three generations on this diet, but receiving 2 ppm of fluoride in their drinking water, did not show significant improvement in health or weight gain over their control counterparts that were kept on the same diet with redistilled, fluoride-free water. The authors concluded that "under the rigorous experimental conditions employed fluorine is not a dietary essential" for rats. The same probably holds true for most other animals.

In still other experiments, scientists at the University of Arizona, Tucson, reached the same conclusion.[9] They fed a "minimal fluofluoride" (0.005 ppm) diet of greenhouse sorghum and soybeans to one group of weanling rats for 10 weeks, while the same diet with the addition of 2 ppm fluoride was fed to another group of the same size. A third group of 9 weanling rats was fed a field-grown sorghum and soybean diet containing 2.67 ppm fluoride. During the 10-week period no significant differences in final body weight or weight gain were observed, although the second group weighed slightly less (av. 251.4 g) than the first (av. 267.8 g), which in turn was slightly lighter than the third (av. 277.7 g). No appreciable differences in alkaline or acid phosphatases, lactic dehydrogenase, or glutamic-oxalacetic and glutamic-pyruvic transaminases were seen; these results indicated no impairment of heart, kidney, or liver function in the low-fluoride group. On the other hand, the activity of isocitric dehydrogenase was significantly higher (by 21.7%) in the serum of the low-fluoride group, which suggests that fluoride is *not* essential; indeed, it is clearly deleterious for certain functions of the body.

Other experiments investigating essentiality of fluoride, with contrary results, were carried out on 344 rats fed a "fluoride-free" ("occasionally as low as 0.04 ppm"), highly-purified amino acid diet.[10] This diet by itself, however, produced deficiency symptoms such as scraggly fur, loss of hair, seborrhea, and a disturbance in the pigmentation of the tooth enamel. The addition of 2.5 ppm fluoride to the diet produced a 31% increase in the growth of the animals during a four-week period. However, weight gain *per se* has no necessary connection with a healthy organism, since fluoride is known to cause water retention and thus an increase in body weight. Furthermore, the diet in this study differs so radically from a "normal" diet that fluoride effects in it simply cannot be extrapolated to a normal one.

Another study claiming a beneficial effect of supplemental fluoride was reported in 1972 by scientists at the University of Minnesota.[11] These workers found that female mice receiving a low-fluoride (0.1–0.2 ppm) diet and fluoride-free (deionized) water demonstrated a significant delay in the birth of the first litter produced by the second generation and a progressive impairment in reproductive capacity, whereas mice on the same low-fluoride diet supplemented by 50 ppm fluoride in their drinking water delivered a normal number of offspring. Normal reproductive capacity was subsequently restored to the infertile females when 50 ppm fluoride was added to their drinking water. The authors believed, therefore, that fluoride is required for maintaining fertility in mice.

In a related study, pregnant mice were fed a low-fluoride (0.1–0.3 ppm) diet.[12] Although offspring of these animals had reduced iron levels in their blood (anemia) five days after birth, 60 days later there was no significant difference between them and the offspring of fluoride-supplemented mice. Of course, any iron deficiency in this diet would be offset by high-fluoride (50 ppm) intake, which would increase membrane transport of iron.

This interpretation is supported by S. Tao and J. W. Suttie, who concluded that the basal diet used by the Minnesota group was only "marginally sufficient in iron."[13] Tao and Suttie supplemented the iron-adequate diet of their mice with 2 ppm and 100 ppm fluoride and found *no* difference between the control and experimental mice in growth rate, reproductive ability, litter size, weight of pups, or incidence of stillbirths over three generations. The authors concluded: "Although fluoride may yet be shown to be essential for some physiological processes, sound evidence for a claim of essentiality of fluoride for reproduction is still lacking."[13]

A diet deficient in calcium also leads to serious impairment of growth and development and shortens the life span of quail unless the diet is supplemented by large amounts (up to 750 ppm) of fluoride.[14] Still another study indicates that under certain circumstances fluoride can prevent symptoms of magnesium deficiency in mice,[15] although exactly contrary findings have been reported in rats and dogs.[16] Therefore, in certain animal species, an insufficiency of calcium, magnesium, or iron in a purified or other special diet may produce deficiency symptoms that can be partially neutralized by fluoride supplementation. The results of such experiments, however, cannot be extrapolated to humans eating normal diets. They also do *not* prove that fluoride is in any way essential for the maintenance of good health in man.

FLUORIDE IN TEETH

Whether or not fluoride is required for the normal development of healthy teeth and bones also is relevant to the question of essentiality. Should the normal development of teeth be dependent upon the presence of fluoride, it would be reasonable to expect that a healthy nondecayed tooth would contain more fluoride than a decayed one; furthermore, teeth that received little or no fluoride should exhibit more decay than those of persons in whom fluoride intake has been adequate.

In 1938 Armstrong and Brekhus assayed the fluoride content of teeth and found more fluoride in the enamel of healthy teeth than in that of decayed teeth.[17] In 1948 McClure found no significant difference in the fluoride content of enamel of sound and carious teeth with the same history of exposure to fluoride.[18] A few years later, however, he agreed with the findings of Armstrong,[19] although other scientists—among them Ockerse of South Africa in 1943,[20] Restarski of the U.S. Navy,[21] Pincus of Melbourne, Australia,[22] and Bang in a survey in Alaska[23] —have found no difference in the fluoride content of enamel of sound and carious teeth among those who had been exposed to the same amount of fluoride throughout their lives.

In 1963 Armstrong himself re-examined his 1938 results and arrived at a new conclusion: "No difference in fluoride content of enamel of sound teeth from that of sound enamel of carious teeth was found in the same decade of life."[24] He realized that the sound teeth with a high fluoride content encountered in his 1938 report were those of older persons, and that more fluoride had been stored in their teeth because of their age.

Other studies since 1963 have confirmed that enamel fluoride increases with greater intake of fluoride as well as with age, but there is still no general agreement as to how reliably elevated enamel fluoride correlates with decreased tooth decay. A 1975 pilot study of 12- to 16-year-old subjects, for example, showed that while some correlation may exist in a group, at any given enamel fluoride level, "there is great individual variability in caries experience, including some rather high caries scores even in optimal [water] fluoride areas."[25] Likewise, from their data on 14-year-old children, Danish investigators in 1977 concluded that "it is not possible to demonstrate a relationship between surface enamel fluoride and caries status in the individual."[26]

FLUORIDE IN BONES

The action of fluoride on bones is similar to that on teeth. When incorporated into the apatite crystal, the main building block of bones, fluoride increases the crystallinity and size of the crystal and produces greater density of the skeleton.[27] However, the process of this new bone formation is also associated with bone resorption, and the newly-formed bone is not healthy; in particular, it tends to fracture easily.[28] These effects may be related to a reduction of citrate and magnesium in fluorotic bones.[29] Furthermore, the apposition of new bone substance is erratic; calcifications may appear anywhere at the periosteum (fibrous membrane covering the bone), on ligaments, or in the capsule surrounding joints. The newly formed bone can cause functional damage to joints (arthritis) and grotesque bony protrusions that encroach on nerves and induce a variety of symptoms ranging from numbness and pains to actual paralysis. Fluoride may even contribute to calcification of arteries.[30]

The treatment of osteoporosis with large doses of fluoride (up to 200 mg per day) has provided an excellent opportunity for studying these changes as well as the nonskeletal effects of long-term fluoride intake. C. Rich, who originated this treatment in 1961, believed that the increase in calcification and formation of new bone substance would be conducive to prevention of bone softening and spontaneous fractures. Five years later, however, he warned that such side effects as gastric pain and osteoarthritis as well as visual disturbances may occur from such large doses.[31] Two English clinicians encountered a case of retinitis in a patient treated with 20 mg of sodium fluoride three times a day for six weeks.[32] Previously undetected abnormal, "giant" cells have also been discovered in the bone marrow of patients undergoing mega-fluoride treatment.[33] Furthermore, there are several reports of increased bone softening, spontaneous fractures, and excess loss of vital calcium resulting from administration of fluoride.[34,35] As a consequence, many medical centers in the U.S. and abroad have abandoned this treatment for osteoporosis.

*

Neither laboratory studies on animals nor data on human teeth and bones, therefore, have provided conclusive evidence that fluoride is *essential* for life. No specific biochemical pathway requirement or essential metabolic role for fluoride has yet been discovered in any mammals, including man. The fact that fluoride affects and is incorporated in the mineralization of bones and teeth does not demonstrate its indispensability. Although lead, mercury, and cadmium share this property, this fact does not make them essential nutrients.

In any event, whether or not minute amounts of fluoride are absolutely required to maintain human vital functions is almost completely irrelevant, for it is impossible to avoid at least some fluoride in the diet, even in unfluoridated communities. As McClure has observed:

> Numerous attempts have been made to obtain proof of an indispensable requirement for fluoride but this proof is still lacking. The ubiquitous occurrence of fluoride in nature has made it virtually impossible to prepare a diet which is entirely free of fluoride. It seems evident, however, that *if* fluoride is essential for life *its daily requirement is extremely small.*[36] [Emphasis added.]

REFERENCES

1. DeEds, F.: Fluorine in Relation to Bone and Tooth Development. J. Am. Dent. Assoc., 23:568-574, 1936.

2. Cox, G.J.: New Knowledge of Fluorine in Relation to Dental Caries. J. Am. Water Works Assoc., 31:1926-1930, 1939.

3. Waldbott, G.L.: Health Effects of Environmental Pollutants. 1973, p. 171.

4. Underwood, E.J.: Trace Elements in Human and Animal Nutrition. 3rd ed., Academic Press, New York and London, 1971.

5. NRC Committee on Biologic Effects of Pollutants: Fluorides. 1971, p. 66.

6. Wisconsin Division of Health: What Today's Literature Tells About Fluoridation. Fluoridation News, Combined Issue, Vols. 11 and 12, July 1974-June 1975, p. 2. From Am. Med. Assoc. Report: Efficacy and Safety of Fluoridation, Sept. 1975, point 6.

7. McClendon, J.F., and Gershon-Cohen, J.: Trace Element Deficiencies. Water-Culture Crops Designed to Study Deficiencies in Animals. J. Agric. Food Chem., 1:464-466, 1953.

8. Maurer, R.L., and Day, H.G.: The Non-Essentiality of Fluorine in Nutrition. J. Nutr., 62:561-573, 1957.

9. Doberenz, A.R., Kurnick, A.A., Kurtz, E.B. Kemmerer A.R., and Reid, B.L.: Minimal Fluoride Diet and Effects on Rats. Fed. Proc., 22:554, 1963; and Effect of a Minimal Fluoride Diet on Rats. Proc. Soc. Exp. Biol. Med., 117:689-693, 1964.

10. Schwarz, K., and Milne, D.B.: Fluorine Requirement for Growth in the Rat. Bioinorg. Chem., 1:331-338, 1972.

11. Messer, H.H., Armstrong, W.D., and Singer, L.: Fertility Impairment in Mice on a Low Fluoride Intake. Science, 177:893-894, 1972.

12. Messer, H.H., Wong, K., Wegner, M., Singer, L., and Armstrong, W.D.: Effect of Reduced Fluoride Intake by Mice on Haematocrit Values. Nat. New Biol., 240:218-219, 1972.

13. Tao, S., and Suttie, J.W.: Evidence for a Lack of an Effect of Dietary Fluoride Level on Reproduction in Mice. J. Nutr., 106:1115-1122, 1976.

14. Chan, M.M., Rucker, R.B., and Riggins, R.S.: The Relationship of Fluoride to Bone Strength and Related Biochemical Properties. Fluoride, 8:163-173, 1975.

15. Hamura, Y.: Prevention by Fluoride of Magnesium Deficiency Defects such as Growth Inhibition, Renal Abnormalities, Hyperuremia, and Hyperphosphatemia in KK Mice. J. Nutr., 102:419-425., 1972.

16. Chiemchaisri, Y., and Phillips, P.H.: Effect of Dietary Fluoride Upon the Magnesium Calcinosis Syndrome. J. Nutr., 81:307-311, 1963.

17. Armstrong, W.D., and Brekhus, P.J.: Possible Relationship Between the Fluorine Content of Enamel and Resistance to Dental Caries. J. Dent. Res., 17:393-399, 1938.

18. McClure, F.J.: Fluorine in Dentin and Enamel of Sound and Carious Human Teeth. J. Dent. Res. 27:287-298, 1948. (Reprinted in Fluoride Drinking Waters, 1962, pp. 384-389.)

19. McClure, F.J., and Likens, R.C.: Fluorine in Human Teeth Studied in Relation to Fluorine in the Drinking Water. J. Dent. Res., 30:172-176, 1951.

(Reprinted in Fluoride Drinking Waters, 1962, pp. 392-394.)

20. Ockerse, T.: The Chemical Composition of Enamel and Dentin in High and Low Caries Areas in South Africa. J. Dent. Res., 22:441-446, 1943.

21. Restarski, J.S.: Incidence of Dental Caries Among Pure Blooded Samoans. U.S. Nav. Med. Bull., 41:1713-1714, 1943.

22. Pincus, P.: Fluoride and Dental Caries. Aust. J. Dent., 56:185-187, 1952.

23. Bang, G.: Developmental Microstructure and Fluorine Content of Alaskan Eskimo Tooth Samples. J. Am. Dent. Assoc., 63:67-75, 1961.

24. Armstrong, W.D., and Singer, L.: Fluoride Contents of Enamel of Sound and Carious Human Teeth: A Reinvestigation. J. Dent. Res., 42:133-136, 1963.

25. DePaola, P.F., Brudevold, F., Aasenden, R., Moreno, E.C., Englander, H., Bakhos, Y., Bookstein, F., and Warram, J.: A Pilot Study of the Relationship Between Caries Experience and Surface Enamel Fluoride in Man. Arch. Oral Biol. 20:859-864, 1975.

26. Richards, A., Joost Larsen, M., Fejerskov, O., and Thylstrup, A.: Fluoride Content of Buccal Surface Enamel and Its Relation to Dental Caries in Children. Arch. Oral Biol., 22:425-428, 1977.

27. Zipkin, I., Posner, A.S., and Eanes, E.D.: The Effect of Fluoride on the X-Ray Diffraction Pattern of the Apatite of Human Bone. Preliminary Notes. Biochim. Biophys. Acta, 59:255-258, 1962. Cf. Posner, A.S.: Crystal Chemistry of Bone Mineral. Physiol. Rev., 49:760-792, 1969.

28. Rockert, H.: X-Ray Absorption and X-Ray Fluorescence Microanalyses of Mineralized Tissue of Rats Which Have Ingested Fluoridated Water. Acta. Pathol. Microbiol. Scand., 59:32-38, 1963.

29. Singer, L., Armstrong, W.D., Zipkin, I., and Frazier, P.D.: Chemical Composition and Structure of Fluorotic Bone. Clin. Orthop. Relat. Res., 99:301-312, 1974.

30. Waldbott, G.L.: Fluoride and Calcium Levels in the Aorta. Experientia (Basel), 22:835-837, 1966.

31. Rich, C.: Osteoporosis and Fluoride Therapy. J. Am. Med. Assoc., 196:149, 1966.

32. Geall, M.G., and Beilin, L.J.: Sodium Fluoride and Optic Neuritis. Br. Med. J. 2:355-356, 1964.

33. Duffey, P.H., Tretbar, H.C., and Jarkowski, T.L.: Giant Cells in Bone Marrows of Patients on High-Dose Fluoride Treatment. Ann. Intern. Med., 75:745-747, 1971.

34. Henrikson, P.A., Lutwak, L., Krook, L., Kallfelz, F., Sheffy, B.E., Skogerboe, R., Belanger, L.F., Marier, J.R., Romanus, B., and Hirsch, C.: Fluoride and Nutritional Osteoporosis. Fluoride, 3:204-207, 1970.

35. Inkovaara, J., Heikinheimo, R., Jarvinen, K., Kasurinen, U., Hanhijarvi,

H., and Iisalo, E.: Prophylactic Fluoride Treatment and Aged Bones. Br. Med. J., 3:73-74, 1975. For comment, see Jowsey, J., and Riggs, B.L.: ibid., 3:766, 1975; and reply by Inkovaara, J., and Heikinheimo, R.: ibid., 4:758, 1975.

36. McClure, F.J.: Water Fluoridation: The Search and the Victory. 1970, pp. 191-193. For the same view, see Ref. 5 above, p. 67.

CHAPTER 7

ACUTE FLUORIDE TOXICITY

THE ACUTE TOXIC effects of single large doses of a chemical can often greatly help in assessing the long-term, *chronic* effects of that substance. Indeed, the symptomatologies may bear striking similarities, although cases of acute toxicity are obviously much more dramatic and easier to observe. Chronic toxicity, on the other hand, probably is more widely experienced throughout the world, and its symptoms are frequently masked by other health problems. Recognizing acute toxic effects can therefore provide a key to understanding and treating chronic toxicity.

In general, the toxicity of fluoride compounds is determined by whether they are organic or inorganic. In organic fluorides, the fluorine atom forms a tight covalent (non-ionic) bond with a carbon atom. The more strongly the two atoms are linked together, the more inert and, as a rule, the less poisonous is the molecule. In many organic compounds, therefore, the fluorine atom *per se* contributes less to the toxicity than does the remainder of the molecule.

ORGANIC FLUORIDES

Some of the most toxic of all organic compounds are fluoroacetates, salts of fluoroacetic acid (compound 1080), which are used as exterminators of rodents and predatory mammals. They also occur in several poisonous plants, such as the notorious gifblaar *(Dichapetalum toxicarium)*, which has often been responsible for cattle deaths in Africa. As little as 1.0 mg of this "delayed convulsant" can kill a 22–pound dog.[1] After first swallowing the poison, the dog appears to be in perfect health; 8 to 10 hours later, it develops fatal convulsions attributable to blockage of the citric acid cycle by conversion of the intact fluoroacetate moiety into fluorocitrate.[2]

On the other end of the organo-fluoride toxicity scale is the polymer Teflon, a substance so stable and innocuous that it can be used to replace blood vessels and can remain in the human organism for years without causing any known harm. If heated to about 300°C., however, Teflon breaks down and gives off perfluoroisobutene, an extremely poisonous gas. In one instance, a burning cigarette laid on some Teflon became contaminated with enough toxic decomposition products to kill the person smoking the cigarette.[3] Freon, a fluorocarbon used as a refrigerant, is believed to be inert, although its use as a propellant in sprays in conjunction with adrenalin-like substances may cause irregularity of the heart.[4] Fluorinated anesthetics are generally considered safe, but methoxyflurane (Penthrane) is metabolized to high blood levels of inorganic fluoride, sometimes leading to excessive urine flow and even lethal renal failure.[5]

INORGANIC FLUORIDES

In his classical treatise on fluoride intoxication, Kaj Roholm (Fig. 7-1, page 89) divided inorganic fluorine compounds into three categories according to their toxicity. As shown in Table 7-1 (next page), first and foremost in toxicity are the fluoride gases: hydrogen fluoride (HF) and silicon tetrafluoride (SiF_4). Then follow, in order of decreasing toxicity, aqueous solutions of HF and hydrofluorosilicic acid (H_2SiF_6) and the more readily soluble fluoride and fluorosilicate salts.

Fluoride compounds that are relatively insoluble in water, such as cryolite and calcium fluoride, are much less poisonous in the solid form. In aqueous *solution* – necessarily very dilute because of its low solubility – the toxicity of calcium fluoride is comparable to that of sodium fluoride (at the same concentration).

The amounts of these fluorides that are required to cause illness or death vary considerably and depend not only on the particular fluoride compound but also on a person's state of health and nutrition, where the fluoride enters the body (skin, lungs, stomach), and other factors such as the acidity and content of the stomach.

Table 7-1

Comparative Toxicity of Inorganic Fluorides[6]

Extremely Toxic

Hydrogen fluoride (anhydrous)	HF
Silicon tetrafluoride	SiF_4
Hydrofluoric acid (aqueous)	HF
Hydrofluorosilicic acid	H_2SiF_6

Very Toxic

Easily soluble fluorides and fluorosilicates

Sodium fluoride	NaF
Potassium fluoride	KF
Ammonium fluoride	NH_4F
Sodium fluorosilicate	Na_2SiF_6
Potassium fluorosilicate	K_2SiF_6
Ammonium fluorosilicate	$(NH_4)_2SiF_6$

Moderately Toxic

Poorly soluble (almost insoluble) fluorides

Cryolite	Na_3AlF_6
Calcium fluoride	CaF_2

Table 7-2

Lethal Dose of Fluorides in Adult Guinea Pigs[7]

Compound	Oral (mg/kg)	Subcutaneous (mg/kg)
NaF	250	400
CaF_2	>5,000	>5,000
AlF_3	600	3,000
HF (aqueous)	80	100
H_2SiF_6	200	250
Na_2SiF_6	250	500
$Al_2(SiF_6)_3$	5,000	4,000

Table 7-2 shows the acute toxicity of the most important fluoride salts to guinea pigs, expressed in milligrams per kilogram of body weight. It also demonstrates the difference in the lethal dose following oral and subcutaneous administration.

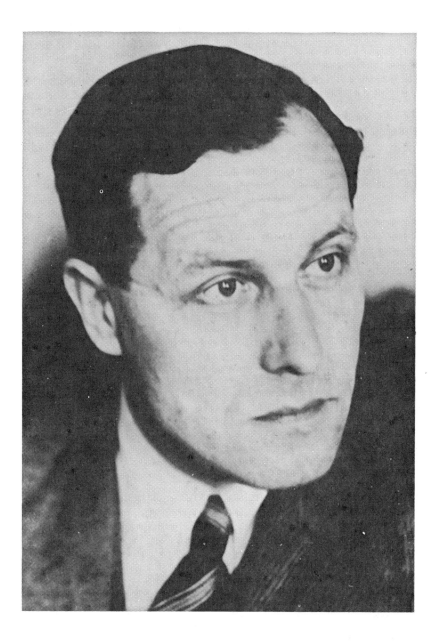

Fig. 7-1. Prof. Dr. Med. Kaj Roholm, 1902-1948.
Deputy City Health Officer of Copenhagen; author of the first
and most comprehensive monograph on fluorine toxicity.

For sodium fluoride (NaF) the lethal toxic dose in man, if the patient is left untreated, is 2.5 to 5 grams.[8] Even larger doses may not be fatal if adequate medical aid is administered quickly. For instance, in 1971 a 25-year-old male recovered following ingestion of 120 grams of roach powder containing 97% NaF that he had taken in a suicide attempt. Immediate medical attention – including lavage of the stomach and intravenous injections of calcium and magnesium combined with treatment to counter cardiac failure – saved his life.[9]

SYMPTOMATOLOGY

More than 300 cases of acute fluoride intoxication have been recorded in which a single massive dose of fluoride was either ingested – by intent or by accident – inhaled, or entered the body through the skin. Usually fluoride poisoning results from mistaking sodium fluoride for sugar, cornstarch, baking powder, epsom salt, or powdered milk.[10] Other instances represent intentional poisoning for suicidal or homicidal purposes. The symptoms in such attempts are similar to those of many other kinds of acute poisoning and involve mainly vomiting, cramps in the abdomen, diarrhea, and, depending on the severity of the case, varying degrees of shock (see Table 7-3, opposite).[11]

Because of the highly corrosive nature of the hydrofluoric acid formed through the reaction of the fluoride compound with the hydrochloric acid of the stomach (Fig. 7-2, page 92), the material that is vomited usually contains considerable amounts of blood. After several hours, if the victim survives, characteristic neurological symptoms appear: numbness in arms and legs, pain in and fibrillation of muscles, and convulsions.[10] Hives over the entire body indicate an existing allergy to fluoride. In one case the calcium level of the blood dropped to as low as 2.6 milligram per cent (normal about 10 milligram per cent), thus accounting for muscle spasms and general convulsions.[12] Heart failure may be the disastrous end of the clinical picture.[9]

When fluoride is inhaled – usually as silicofluoride or hydrogen fluoride – the respiratory tract is the primary target for fluoride toxicity and normally results in nasal irritation, nose bleed, spasmodic cough, a tendency to upper respiratory infection, shortness

Table 7-3

**Roholm's Classification of Symptoms in 34 Cases
of Acute Fatal Fluoride Poisoning[11]**

Symptoms	No. of Cases
Vomiting	31
Pains in abdomen	17
Diarrhea	13
Convulsions, spasms	11
General weakness, muscular weakness, collapse	8
Dyspnea	7
Pains and paresthesias in extremities	6
Paresis, paralysis	5
Difficulties with speech, inarticulation	5
Thirst	5
Perspiration	5
Weak pulse	5
Change in facial color	5
Nausea	4
Unconsciousness	4
Salivation	3
Impaired swallowing	3
Motor restlessness	2
High temperature	2
Dizziness, headache, hiccup, urticaria; cold shivers, choking sensation, pupil contraction, uncoordinated eye movements; pains in sacral region; low temperature	1

of breath and wheezing, and, in extreme cases, pulmonary edema (flooding of the lungs). These respiratory conditions are found in fluoride workers and also in residents near fluoride-emitting factories and will be discussed further in Chapter 10.

ACCIDENTS INVOLVING FLUORIDE

Of historical interest is the fact that several pioneer investigators died from the effect of inhaling small quantities of hydrogen fluoride – for example, the 32–year–old P. Louyet of Brussels,[13] whose attempts at isolating fluorine formed the groundwork for the

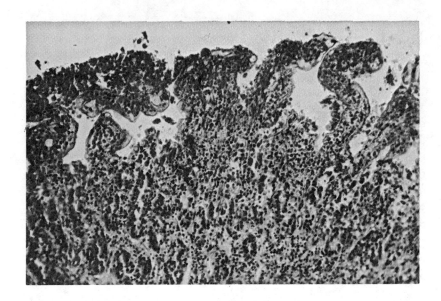

Fig. 7-2. Gastric mucosa in acute fluoride poisoning of a 42-year-old female (homicide). Note cellular infiltration with loss of surface epithelium (upper left) and obliteration of normal glands (upper right).
(From G.L. Waldbott: Acute Fluoride Intoxication. *Acta. Med. Scand.,* 174, Suppl. 400, 1963; courtesy Dr. A.V. Arma, St. Luke's Hospital, Kansas City, Missouri.)

ultimate success of Moissan (Chapter 2 above, pages 18–20). Hydrogen fluoride (HF) burns also result from industrial exposure. In such cases the fluoride ion penetrates the skin tightly bound to the hydrogen ion (undissociated HF) and forms hydrofluoric acid on contact with the body fluids. This acid causes extremely severe pain and ulceration resembling heat burns. Mishaps of this kind occur in factories to workers who are careless about protecting themselves adequately with suitable clothing, masks, and gloves. Although these data do not deal with poisoning from fluoridated water, they cannot be disregarded because accidents sometimes happen in handling and in feeding fluoride into municipal water supplies and through breakdown of equipment. For instance, in 1952, in Coeur d'Alene, Idaho, a waterworks employee, J.R.S., age 32, developed repeated episodes of acute fluoride poisoning, affecting his liver and causing hepatitis. He later recovered when he changed his job.[14]

At least two examples of mass poisoning from mechanical difficulties with artificial fluoridation have occurred: one in 1965 in Szolnok, Hungary,[15] and the other in 1974 in Stanly County, North Carolina.[16] In the Hungarian incident about 80 individuals (at a restaurant and a school) became seriously ill within minutes after drinking soda water or an orangeade made with the soda water. Everyone afflicted was nauseated and then vomited violently, followed by immediate, spontaneous recovery. The contaminated soda water contained 300 to 900 ppm fluoride, which had apparently collected in a temporarily unused supply pipe to the bottling plant. In the North Carolina episode, fluoridation equipment at a rural school pumped excess fluoride into the water. "All 213 individuals experienced nausea, and all 201 children (age 6-12) and 7 of the 12 adults vomited" shortly after drinking orange juice made from an uncontaminated concentrate diluted with the tap water. Analysis indicated that the reconstituted beverage contained 270 ppm fluoride.

Of graver consequence was the fate of Mr. W.B.D., age 49, of Highland Park, Michigan (fluoridated since 1952), who had been under my care because of marked intolerance to fluoridated water. By using distilled, fluoride-free water for drinking and cooking, he had remained free of symptoms for three years. On October 2, 1962, he was found dead in bed. For several months prior to his demise he had been using a water filter that was supposed to eliminate all fluoride from the tap water. A subsequent check of the filter by a Detroit water engineer indicated that some of the fluoride removed by the filter had accidentally contaminated the water. At autopsy Mr. W.B.D. showed no evidence of a cardiac or cerebral infarct, the two common causes of sudden death; *but his stomach was completely disintegrated, as is often the case in acute fluoride intoxication.* This finding, plus the fact that the patient had previously displayed an extraordinary intolerance to fluoride, very likely accounted for his death by a single large dose of the halogen. When such incidents as this occur, physicians are rarely able to recognize their causal relationship to fluoride. It is not surprising, therefore, that after 25 years of fluoridation, the medical literature appears to contain no examples of similar cases.

ACUTE POISONING FROM AIRBORNE FLUORIDES

A different kind of acute poisoning is encountered in the environs of fluoride-emitting factories when sudden outbursts of poisonous smoke clouds are ejected from the chimneys. In Chapter 10 I will relate how patients have been stricken during such smoke episodes with acute pulmonary ailments, mainly cough, shortness of breath and wheezing followed by fever and a pneumonia-like condition. Others who consume fluoride-contaminated food, mostly vegetables and fruit grown near the factory, develop acute gastrointestinal symptoms resembling ordinary food poisoning.

Massive outpouring of smoke pollution from factories may also involve large segments of populations rather than individual persons. This is especially true when the clouds of smoke fail to disperse because of unusual weather or environmental conditions. Only recently have scientists recognized that fluoride was the principal culprit in the two major air pollution disasters, one in the Belgian Meuse Valley in 1930, and the other in Donora, Pennsylvania, in 1948. Sixty persons lost their lives in the Meuse Valley calamity and an unknown number, perhaps several thousands, contracted upper respiratory diseases such as asthma and emphysema. In Donora, the death toll was 20 persons.

After examining both episodes, commissions of health scientists were unable to determine what was responsible for the pollution. The Donora committee thought the level of exposure to fluoride was not excessive.[17] Nevertheless, an independent study for the Borough of Donora by the chemist Phillip Sadtler showed 12 to 25 times more fluoride in the blood of victims than in normal blood.[18] Furthermore, he recorded other damage typical of fluoride toxicity to vegetation and domestic animals, as well as extensive mottling of children's teeth. He thus proved beyond question that the area had been subject to severe exposure to fluoride, and he regarded the 1948 episode as but an acute phase of a long-term exposure. Similarly, a group of scientists independent of industry and government examined the evidence of the Meuse Valley disaster and concluded, after extensive studies, that the most noxious ingredient of the killing smoke was fluorosilicate emitted from fertilizer and zinc factories in the area.[19]

There is good reason to believe that fluoride compounds also played a major role in the two London fog disasters of 1952 and 1956 in which the death count was several thousand in excess of normal. At first, investigators believed that sulfur dioxide fumes from London's coal-burning fireplaces accounted for widespread pulmonary involvement of the deceased persons. We now know that sulfur dioxide fumes are generally less harmful than airborne fluorides, since sulfur dioxide reacts with moist air and eventually yields relatively nontoxic salts of sulfuric acid that rarely reach the terminal portions of the bronchial tree and the lung tissue proper.[20,21] Furthermore, recent research demonstrates that fumes from burning coal can contain as much as 1440 ppm of fluoride.[22] In view of the widespread use of soft coal in London at that time and the extent and duration of the smoke stagnation, sufficient fluoride was undoubtedly produced to cause considerable damage to the lungs of the victims.

Acute fluoride poisoning occurs under widely differing circumstances ranging from accidental ingestion to inhalation of airborne fluoride. Various symptoms are: severe gastrointestinal distress, including nausea, vomiting, diarrhea, and cramps; fibrillation or convulsions of muscles; neurological disturbances; extreme weakness; paresthesias; skin irritations; respiratory complications; heart disorders, to name only some of the main effects. The same symptoms, usually with diminished intensity, are found in chronic fluoride poisoning, which will now be discussed.

REFERENCES

1. Bredemann, G.: Biochemie und Physiologie des Fluors und der industriellen Fluor-Rauchschäden. Academie-Verlag, Berlin, 1951, p. 40. Cf. Egyed, M.N.: Clinical, Pathological, Diagnostic and Therapeutic Aspects of Fluoroacetate Research in Animals. Fluoride, 6:215-224, 1973.

2. Peters, R.A.: Keynote and Historical Perspective of Organic Fluorides in Plants. Fluoride, 6:189-194, 1973. Cf. Buffa, P., Guarriero-Bobyleva, V., and Costa-Tiozzo, R.: Metabolic Effects of Fluoroacetate Poisoning in Animals. Ibid., 6:224-245, 1973.

3. Mack, G.L.: Letter to the Editor. J. Can. Med. Assoc., 85:995, 1961.

4. Taylor, G.J., IV, and Harris, W.S.: Cardiac Toxicity of Aerosol Propellants. J. Am. Med. Assoc., 214:81-85, 1970.

5. Taves, D.R., Fry, B.W., Freeman, R.B., and Gillies, A.J.: Toxicity Following Methoxyflurane Anesthesia. II. Fluoride Concentrations in Nephrotoxicity. J. Am. Med. Assoc., 214:91-95, 1970.

6. Roholm, K.: Fluorine Intoxication: A Clinical-Hygienic Study. 1937, p. 264.

7. Simonin, P., and Pierron A.: Toxicité brute des derivés fluorés. C.R.Séances Soc. Biol. Fil., 124:133-134, 1937.

8. Caruso, F.S., Maynard, E.A., and DiStefano, V.: Pharmacology of Sodium Fluoride, in F.A. Smith, Ed.: Pharmacology of Fluorides, in Handbook of Experimental Pharmacology, Vo. XX/2. Springer-Verlag, Berlin, 1970, pp. 144-165.

9. Abukurah, A.R., Moser, A.M., Jr., Baird, C.L., Randall, R.E., Jr., Setter, J.G., and Blanke, R.V.: Acute Sodium Fluoride Poisoning. J. Am. Med. Assoc., 222:816-817, 1972.

10. Waldbott, G.L.: Acute Fluoride Intoxication. Acta Med. Scand., 174, Suppl. 400, 1963.

11. Roholm (in Ref. 6, above), p. 27.

12. Rabinowitch, J.M.: Acute Fluoride Poisoning. J. Can. Med. Assoc. 52: 345-349, 1945.

13. Weeks, M.E., and Leicester, H.M.: Discovery of the Elements, 7th ed. 1968, p. 735.

14. Editorial: Liver Damage in Chronic Fluoride Intoxication, in Fluoride, 2:140-141, 1969. Cf. Nesin, B.C. in Panel Discussion on Experience in Applying Fluorides. J. Am. Water Works Assoc., 49:1252, 1957.

15. Horvath, I., Palicska, J., and Hanny, I.: Szikvízzel terjedő tömeges fluormérgezés [Mass Intoxication with Fluoride in Soda Water]. Orvosi Hetilap, 108:306-307, 1967.

16. Clarke, R., Welch, J., Leiby, G., Cobb, W.Y., and MacCormack, J.N.: Acute Fluoride Poisoning. Morbid. Mortal. Weekly Rep., Communicable Disease Control Center, USPHS, Atlanta, Ga., 23:199, 1974.

17. Schrenk, H.H., Heimann, H., Clayton, G.D., Gafafer, W.M., and Wexler, M.: Air Pollution in Donora, Pennsylvania. Epidemiology of the Unusual Smog Episode of October, 1948. Preliminary Report. U.S. Public Health Bull. No. 306, 1949.

18. [Re. P. Sadtler] Fluorine Gases in Atmosphere as Industrial Waste Blamed for Death and Chronic Poisoning of Donora and Webster, Pennsylvania Inhabitants. Chem. Eng. News, 26:3692, 1948.

19. Roholm, K.: The Fog Disaster in the Meuse Valley: A Fluorine Intoxication. J. Ind. Hyg. Toxicol., 19:126-137, 1937. (Abstracted in Fluoride, 2: 62-70, 1969.)

20. Amdur, M.O.: The Physiological Response of Guinea Pigs to Atmospheric Pollutants. Int. J. Air Pollution, 1:170-183, 1959.

21. Waldbott. G.L.: Health Effects of Environmental Pollutants. 1973, p. 83.

22. Dassler, H.G., Börtitz, S., and Auermann, E.: Untersuchungen über Fluor-Immissionen aus Braunkohlen-Kraftwerken. Z. Gesamte Hyg. Grenzgeb., 19:568-570, 1973.

CHAPTER 8

CHRONIC FLUORIDE TOXICITY

AS EARLY AS 1933, F. DeEds, one of the pioneers in fluoride research, perceived the difficulties doctors experience in recognizing chronic fluoride intoxication:

> There is usually a gradual transition from a condition of normality to one of protracted abnormality. Frequently there is no sharp line of demarcation of symptoms as in acute poisoning, and this fact in itself often makes it difficult to associate a pathological condition with the fundamental causes. . . . Chronic intoxications are of greater importance to the public health than are acute toxicities, but in comparison little is known about chronic intoxications as to scope, significance, and ultimate tissue and functional changes.[1]

In chronic fluoride poisoning there are obviously differences between the effects of the minute amounts of fluoride that are being added to drinking water at the concentration of 1 ppm and the effects of larger amounts encountered in water naturally, in food, and occasionally in air. Numerous reports in the medical literature describe chronic fluorosis due to "high-fluoride" drinking water — mostly in the range of 1.5 to 10 ppm — and to protracted exposure to fluoride dust and fumes among workers in mining, smelting, and chemical industries.

DENTAL AND SKELETAL FLUOROSIS

Although changes in teeth and bones are the two most conspicuous signs of chronic fluorosis, neither is an obligatory feature of the disease. Mottling of teeth — a disturbance of the enamel-building cells (ameloblasts) associated with a decrease in cementing substance — develops exclusively from fluoride intake during the first 10 to 12 years of life when the permanent teeth are being

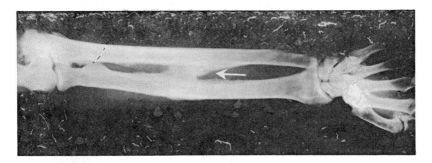

Fig. 8-1. X-Ray showing fluorotic calcification (arrow) in forearm of a 65-year-old North African male residing in Tolga (2.5 ppm F) in the Sahara. (Courtesy Prof. F. Pinet, Lyon, France.)

formed. Changes in the skeleton consist mainly of increased bone density, of abnormal apposition of bone substance, and of calcifications in ligaments and joints (Figs. 8-1 to 8-4). Ten to twenty years of continuous intake of excessive amounts of fluoride are usually required before these effects become detectable by X-rays. Most observations on skeletal fluorosis have been made in endemic "fluoride belts" in India where concentrations of fluoride in drinking water are generally higher than 1 ppm (Tables 8-1 and

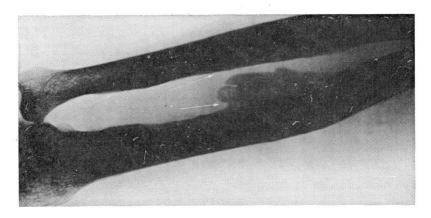

Fig. 8-2. X-Ray showing typical skeletal fluorosis in forearm from 3-6 ppm fluoride in drinking water in Sicily. Note new grotesque ossification of membrane between radius and ulna. Arrows point to newly developed bone substance. (Courtesy Prof. G. Fradà, Palermo, Italy.)

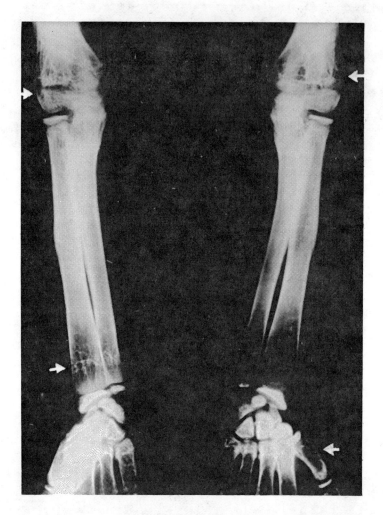

Fig. 8-3. X-Ray showing fluorosis in forearms of Indian patient with hyperparathyroidism involving both erosion (arrows) and thickening of bones.
(Courtesy Prof. S.P.S. Teotia, Meerut, India.)

8-2 below, page 103), in volcanic areas of Italy,[2] in North Africa,[3]
and in Arabia.[4,5] In the United States "natural fluoride" areas include western Texas,[6,7] parts of Arizona,[8] and portions of South
Dakota.[9] In the Indian province of Punjab (fluoride content of
water 0.2–40.0 ppm, mostly 2–5 ppm), S. S. Jolly has reported

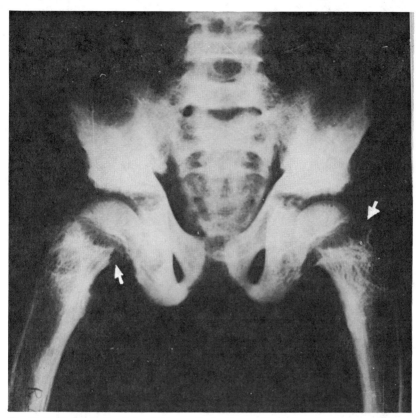

Fig. 8-4. X-Ray of pelvis of fluorotic Indian patient showing increased bone density with irregular erosions (arrows) in the femoral neck and metaphyses indicative of hyperparathyroidism secondary to fluorosis.
(Courtesy Prof. S.P.S. Teotia, Meerut, India.)

1320 radiologically demonstrable cases. Of these, 309 were without symptoms, 742 had rheumatic arthritic complaints, 144 exhibited crippling deformities (Fig. 8-5, next page), and 125 showed serious neurological complications.[10] In general, the incidence of skeletal fluorosis correlates with the fluoride concentration in drinking water (Table 8-1 below, page 103).[11] Other factors, however, such as magnesium hardness, account for differences between communities as shown in Table 8-2 below, page 103. It should be noted that in a community with only 0.7 ppm fluoride

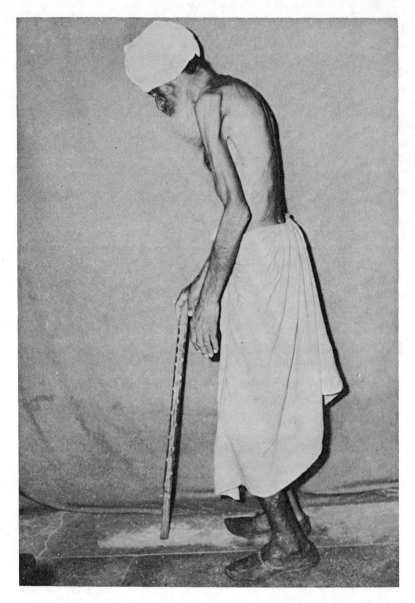

Fig. 8-5. Example of advanced skeletal fluorosis in Punjab, India, showing
crippling effect of rigid, "poker-back" spine.
(Courtesy Prof. S. S. Jolly, Patiala, India.)

Table 8-1

Radiological Study of Males Over Age 21 in Ten Villages of India[11]

VILLAGE	Water F⁻ in ppm	Number of Cases Evaluated	% Skeletal Fluorosis[a]
Mandi Baretta	0.73	70	2.9 (2)
Kooriwara	2.25	30	40.0 (12)
Gurney Kalan	2.45	67	19.4 (13)
Ganza Dhanaula	4.2	38	26.3 (10)
Baja Khana	5.09	98	46.9 (46)
Rajia	5.2	180	52.2 (94)
Village Baretta	5.49	71	29.6 (21)
Rorki	7.02	59	52.5 (31)
Saideke	8.2	38	52.6 (20)
Khara	9.4	131	80.9 (106)

[a] Numbers in parentheses indicate number of cases.

Table 8-2

Incidence of Skeletal Fluorosis in Adult Males in Villages of India with Different Levels of Fluoride in Water[11]

VILLAGE[a]	Mean F⁻ Content of Water (ppm)	Mean Mg⁺⁺ Hardness (ppm)	% Skeletal Fluorosis in Adult Males
Kooriwara	2.25	112	40.0
Gurney Kalan	2.45	169	19.4
Baja Khana	5.09	93.6	46.9
Village Baretta	5.49	179.5	29.6
Rajia	5.20	83.0	52.2
Village Baretta	5.49	179.5	29.6
Kooriwara	2.25	112	40.0
Village Baretta	5.49	179.5	29.6

[a] Note that in each pair the villages in italics with the lower incidences of skeletal fluorosis have higher magnesium hardness levels in the drinking water, even though the fluoride content is greater than in the villages with the higher incidences.

in water, the so-called optimal concentration in that warm climate, 2 of 70 males examined by Jolly showed skeletal changes. That children are not immune to skeletal fluorosis has also been demonstrated in India, where examples of the disease in children aged 5 to 15 have been found.[12]

SOFT TISSUE ORGANS

Teeth and bones are not the only parts of the body affected by fluoride. Large doses of fluoride – or persistent intake of small amounts extending over a number of years – can adversely influence many other organs as well. This fact was clearly recognized as early as 1937 by Roholm when he described as a part of chronic fluoride poisoning a variety of non-skeletal symptoms in workers exposed to cryolite dust.[13] The most important manifestations were gastrointestinal, neuromuscular, and cardiovascular symptoms, as well as allergic skin lesions (Table 8–3, opposite). These features have been subsequently confirmed by other clinicians in studies on skeletal fluorosis (see Chapter 10), but evidence dealing with the nonskeletal phase of the disease is often ignored or minimized in the medical literature.

FATALITIES

Because many organs can be involved in chronic fluoride poisoning, various causes are likely to be responsible for its fatal outcome. To date, only a few deaths have been reported, mainly in endemic regions in India,[14–17] and in industrial workers, afflicted with skeletal fluorosis.[13,18] Except for skeletal damage and its consequences such as injury to the spinal cord and peripheral nerves, no other characteristic changes have been identified at autopsy that would permit one to establish the specific pathological diagnosis "death from fluorosis." Therefore, should a disease of the kidneys, liver, or brain, or a terminal pneumonia be found at autopsy – as is the case in many other kinds of chronic poisoning – it would be difficult to attribute incontrovertibly such changes to fluoride without extensive studies, including analysis of many organs for fluoride.

In the United States a number of fatalities have been recorded for which fluoride must be considered either the primary or an

Table 8-3

Symptoms in 68 Cases of Chronic Industrial Fluorosis[13]

SYSTEM (SYMPTOMS)	NO.	% INCIDENCE
GASTRIC		
Lack of appetite, cardialgia, nausea, vomiting	55	80.9
INTESTINAL		
Disposition to diarrhea, constipation	23	33.8
MUSCULO-SKELETAL		
Feeling of stiffness, indefinite or localized rheumatic pains	24	35.3
NEUROLOGICAL		
Tiredness, sleepiness, indisposition, headache, giddiness	15	22.1
DERMATOLOGICAL		
Rash	8	11.8
RESPIRATORY-CIRCULATORY		
Shortness of breath, palpitation, cough, expectoration	35	51.5

important contributing cause. In 1943, a 22-year-old Texas soldier died with advanced bone changes and complete destruction of both kidneys.[6] For 19 years he had been drinking water that contained fluoride naturally at a concentration ranging from 1.2 –*not* 12 parts per million as frequently incorrectly cited – to 5.7 parts per million. Although the patient had sustained a minor injury to the right kidney at age 15, the damage to one kidney should not have led to destruction of both kidneys without long-term ingestion of fluoride. Indeed, one of the authors of this famous report specifically reiterated this view.[19] That fluoride can cause kidney damage has also been shown in connection with fluoride released in the body during methoxyflurane anesthesia[20] and more recently by Kaushik in endemic fluorosis.[21] Moreover, a study of the effects of fluoride on the kidneys of monkeys has demonstrated deleterious renal changes from even such a small amount as 1 ppm fluoride in the drinking water.[22]

The death of a 64-year-old Texan is another important fluoride-related case.[7] For 20 years his kidney disease and constant thirst (polydipsia) had caused him to consume excess water—up to 2.5 gallons a day—containing 2.2–3.5 ppm fluoride naturally as well as considerable amounts of tea. In all probability, both sources were responsible for poisoning. The patient finally succumbed to terminal pneumonia. At autopsy his bones contained as much as 6100 ppm fluoride. The high fluoride content of his liver (61 ppm) undoubtedly contributed to his demise.

In a third case artificially fluoridated water must be implicated. A premature male infant expired 16 hours after birth with extensive calcifications on the entire aorta and of arteries in the pelvis and extremities. The cause of this unusually rare disease was not established by the physician who reported the case in the *Journal of the American Medical Association* in 1964.[23] My subsequent inquiry, however, revealed the fact that neither parent had drunk an excessive amount of water nor had they ingested excess fluoride from food. They had lived about four years in Ames, Iowa, where the water is artifically fluoridated. In view of the absence of any other known cause of death in this heretofore insufficiently explored case, and because a significantly high incidence of arterial calcification has been well documented as a manifestation of fluorosis,[24] a causal relation of this child's illness with the mother's consumption of fluoride in drinking water during her pregnancy must be seriously considered. This interpretation is further supported by the unusually high fluoride content of the baby's aorta —59.3 ppm—which was analyzed at my request.[24] Normal aorta values in children with healthy kidneys are below 1 ppm.

Other cases of unexplained death are undoubtedly related to fluoridated water. For instance, in 1955, in Lubbock, Texas (at that time 4.4 ppm in water naturally), after I had presented a paper on skeletal fluorosis before the local medical society, I was shown the X-rays of a deceased 20-year-old man with advanced skeletal changes typical of fluorosis, whose illness and death had baffled his physicians. It was impossible for me to obtain complete clinical data on this case, but it appears that general cachexia (gradual wasting away) accounted for a slowly progressing deterioration of his health. This condition is characteristic of the terminal stages of chronic skeletal fluorosis.

NARROW MARGIN OF SAFETY

With the realization that crippling bone changes and even fatalities have occurred from drinking water containing fluoride at levels not much different from that designated as optimal, and that many organs might become involved in fluorosis, advocates of fluoridation have been faced with a serious dilemma. They are confronted with the question of whether the daily consumption of relatively small quantities of fluoride might constitute a greater risk than heretofore assumed. Might not water fluoridation jeopardize the health of some individuals who are unusually sensitive to fluoride either because of an inherited intolerance or because of an existing disease such as a kidney ailment, diabetes, or an allergy? In other words, could the toxic action of fluoride outweigh the supposed benefit to teeth?

Certainly the latitude of safety between a toxic dose of fluoride and a safe one is narrow or sometimes nonexistent. H.C. Hodge, whose credentials as a toxicologist are most impressive, recommends in general at least a 100-fold margin of safety in the dietary use of a potentially toxic agent.[25] Referring to toxicity studies in experimental animals and their relevance to humans, he points out that there should be a tenfold safety factor for species variability, i.e. for extrapolation from the animal experiment to human conditions, and another tenfold allowance for individual susceptibility of one person compared to another. In light of the extremely narrow safety factor associated with the above-cited fatalities, the twofold safety factor advocated by the U.S. Public Health Service for water fluoridation is obviously at great odds with that proposed by Hodge, who astutely observed in his article:

> It is virtually impossible in most instances to discover toxic effects in the human consumer by standard epidemiological procedures. Only when there is some devastating and tragic outcome, for example the deaths from agranulocytosis in the early use of chloramphenicol (and, more recently, thalidomide), will a danger be identified and the use of the compound appropriately limited. Reliability in guaranteeing that no human will be injured can only be achieved by making the tolerance values reliable.[25]

Others who support fluoridation have partially acknowledged this dilemma when they concede that in warm climates, where people drink more water, the 1-ppm concentration of fluoride is too high. They readily admit that: "Adding fluoride to communal water supplies will inevitably expose large sections of the population to higher levels of the element than they have hitherto been accustomed."[26] They also know that fluoridation requires that assessments "be made not only of its effectiveness as a weapon against dental decay, but also of possible hazards of increased fluoride ingestion and absorption."[26]

Do increased levels of fluoride intake resulting from artificial fluoridation produce detectable harm to health even before there are perceptible changes in the bones and teeth? In other words, are there *preskeletal* symptoms connected with chronic fluorosis? This question -- of vital importance to every one of the millions of persons now drinking fluoridated water and consuming products made with it - will be explored in the following chapters.

REFERENCES

1. DeEds, F.: Chronic Fluorine Intoxication. A Review. Medicine (Baltimore), 12:1-50, 1933 (at pp. 19-20).

2. Waldbott, G.L.: Comments on the Symposium "The Physiologic and Hygienic Aspects of the Absorption of Inorganic Fluorides." Arch. Environ. Health, 2:155-167, 1961.

3. Pinet, F., Pinet, A., Barrière, J., Bouché, B., and Bouché, M.M.: Les osteopathies fluorées endemiques d'origine hydrique 40 observations d'ostéoses condensantes du Souf (Sud-Algérien). Ann. Radiol., 4:589-612, 1961.

4. Azar, H.A., Nucho, C.K., Bayyuk, S.I., and Bayyuk, W.B.: Skeletal Sclerosis Due to Chronic Fluoride Intoxication. Cases from an Endemic Region of the Persian Gulf. Ann. Intern. Med., 55:193-200, 1961.

5. Kumar, S.P., and Harper, R.A.K.: Fluorosis in Aden. Br. J. Radiol., 36:497-502, 1963.

6. Linsman, J.F., and McMurray, C.A.: Fluoride Osteosclerosis from Drinking Water. Radiology, 40:474-484, 1943; correction of misprint, ibid., 41:497, 1943.

7. Sauerbrunn, B.J.L., Ryan, C.M., and Shaw, J.F.: Chronic Fluoride Intoxication with Fluorotic Radiculomyelopathy. Ann. Intern. Med., 63:1074-1078, 1965.

8. Morris, J.W.: Skeletal Fluorosis Among Indians of the American Southwest. Am. J. Roentgenol. Radium Ther. Nucl. Med., 94:608-615, 1965.

9. Gilbaugh, J.H., Jr., and Thompson, G.J.: Fluoride Osteosclerosis Simu-

lating Carcinoma of the Prostate with Widespread Bony Metastasis: A Case Report. J. Urol., 96:944-946, 1966.

10. Jolly, S.S., Prasad, S., Sharma, R., and Rai, B.: Human Fluoride Intoxication in Punjab. Fluoride, 4:64-79, 1971.

11. Jolly, S.S., Prasad, S., Sharma, R., and Chander, R.: Endemic Fluorosis in Punjab. I. Skeletal Aspect. Fluoride, 6:4-18, 1973.

12. Teotia, M., and Teotia, S.P.S.: Further Observations on Endemic Fluoride-Induced Osteopathies in Children. Fluoride, 6:143-151, 1973.

13. Roholm, K.: Fluorine Intoxication. A Clinical-Hygienic Study. 1937, p. 138.

14. Teotia, S.P.S., Teotia, M., Burns, R.R., and Heels, S.: Circulating Plasma Immun[o]reactive Parathyroid Hormone Levels (IPTH) in Endemic Skeletal Fluorosis with Secondary Hyperparathyroidism. Fluoride, 7:200-208, 1974.

15. Chawla, S., Kanwar, K., Bagga, O.P., and Anand, D.: Radiological Changes in Endemic Fluorosis. J. Assoc. Phys. India., 12:221-228, 1964.

16. Singh, A., Jolly, S.S., Bansal, B.C., and Mathur, C.C.: Endemic Fluorosis. Epidemiological, Clinical and Biochemical Study of Chronic Fluorine Intoxication in Punjab (India). Medicine (Baltimore), 42:229-246, 1963; addendum, ibid., 44:97, 1965.

17. Lyth, O.: Endemic Fluorosis in Kweichow, China. Lancet, 1:233-235, 1946.

18. Franke, J., Rath, F., Runge, H., Fengler, F., Auermann, E., and Lenart, G.: Industrial Fluorosis. Fluoride, 8:61-85, 1975.

19. Linsman, J.F.: Fluoride Poisoning. J. Am. Med. Assoc., 145:688, 1951.

20. Fry, B.W., Taves, D.R., and Merlin, R.G.: Fluorometabolites of Methoxyflurane: Serum Concentrations and Renal Clearances. Anesthesiology, 36: 38-44, 1973 (cf. Ref. 5 in Ch. 7 above, page 96).

21. Kaushik, R.: Biochemical and Metabolic Changes in Chronic Fluoride Intoxication. Thesis submitted to Punjabi University, Patiala, 1977.

22. Manocha, S.L., Warner, H., and Olkowski, Z.L.: Cytochemical Response of Kidney, Liver and Nervous System to Fluoride Ions in Drinking Water. Histochem. J., 7:343-355, 1975.

23. Bacon, J.F.: Arterial Calcification in Infancy. J. Am. Med. Assoc., 188: 933-935, 1964.

24. Waldbott, G.L.: The Arteries, in Symposium on the Non-Skeletal Phase of Chronic Fluorosis. Fluoride, 9:24-28, 1976.

25. Hodge, H.C.: Research Needs in the Toxicology of Food Additives. Food Cosmet. Toxicol., 1:25-31, 1963.

26. Weidmann, S.M., and Weatherell, J.A.: Distribution [of Fluoride] in Hard Tissues, in Fluorides and Human Health. 1970, p. 104.

CHAPTER 9

ILLNESS FROM ARTIFICIALLY
FLUORIDATED WATER

IN THE METROPOLITAN AREA of Milwaukee, an unusual illness—with a broad range of symptoms—has plagued citizens and baffled some of the city's most competent diagnosticians since 1953. On a visit to Milwaukee in April 1969, I had the opportunity to learn some of the features of this disease. Mrs. K. D., a 31-year-old woman, described her case as follows. It began in 1960 within a week after she had moved to Milwaukee from Cudahy, Wisconsin. She experienced cramp-like pains and distention in the abdomen, diarrhea alternating with constipation, and a gradually progressive deterioration of her strength. X-Ray and laboratory studies failed to provide her physician with a diagnosis. Although uncertain about the proper treatment, he placed her on tranquilizers, which added lethargy and drowsiness to her other complaints. The discomfort in the abdomen grew worse, and she developed a new set of symptoms connected with the bladder and the lower urinary tract. After a nine-month stay in Milwaukee, the patient returned to Cudahy where, to her great surprise, she recovered within two weeks without any treatment.

Shortly after her marriage in 1962, Mrs. K. D. moved back to Milwaukee. As before, her health once again began to deteriorate. This time the pains in the abdomen were more persistent regardless of diet or medication. She frequently felt nauseated, her vision became blurred, and she was plagued by persistent headaches. When standing or walking, she often felt dizzy and tended to lose her balance. Much more distressing than these symptoms, however, was her increasing loss of strength, which became so pronounced that her husband had to assist her in getting out of bed in the morning. Finally, she reached the stage where she was forced to abandon her job, which consisted of placing small screws in an appliance on a factory assembly line. By now, constant pain in the

- 110 -

lower spine radiated toward her knees and the headaches were so severe that she had to take as many as *twenty* aspirin tablets a day. An insatiable thirst caused her to drink as many as nine 4–ounce cups (more than a quart) of water at a time. Yet such excessive amounts of water rarely relieved her thirst for more than half an hour, and her mouth and throat were constantly dry and parched. By May 28, 1968, she was hospitalized at Trinity Memorial Hospital in Milwaukee because she was no longer able to stand up and had become completely bedridden. Her physicians failed to arrive at a definite diagnosis despite numerous laboratory tests. To bolster her failing strength, they injected vitamin B_{12} without noticeable benefit. However, during her four-week stay at the hospital, a new condition developed – a convulsive seizure suggestive of an epileptic attack. Such seizures continued to recur as often as two to three times weekly after she had returned home.

A Milwaukee resident, witnessing the gradual deterioration of her health, suggested to the family that she avoid Milwaukee's fluoridated water. Within a few days after she began to follow his advice by using practically fluoride–free spring water for cooking and drinking, she improved remarkably, and after one month her health had been completely restored. Mrs. K. D., however, was skeptical of this simple cure, and tried Milwaukee's water again. Within two weeks all her former symptoms, including the epilepsy-like seizures, recurred. Still not satisfied, she experimented further and switched to Milwaukee's Pryor Avenue well water (about 1 ppm) which, she had been told, would produce no ill effects because of its high calcium content. Again her illness returned. Mrs. D. was finally able to piece together the events of her dismal experience. Milwaukee's drinking water had been fluoridated since 1953 to a concentration of about 1.2 ppm, but at the time she was residing in Cudahy, fluoridation had not yet been adopted there.

There was a good reason why James F. Quirk, a lay person who had persuaded Mrs. K.D. to substitute low-fluoride spring water for Milwaukee's tap water, was able to diagnose this mysterious disease. As a real estate agent, he had an unusual opportunity to learn about many complaints of illness among newcomers to fluoridated Milwaukee. Frequently, their illness originated within days after their arrival in the city from a nonfluoridated community. Mr. Quirk's one-page advertisement in the *Milwaukee*

Journal, December 26, 1970, maintained that many Milwaukee citizens had been and were being made ill by its fluoridated water.

Mr. Quirk had also learned from several clients that they had been advised by their physicians to abstain from using city water for drinking and cooking. One eminent physician on the staff of a leading Milwaukee clinic, for instance, had mentioned to his patient (Mr. E. A.), whom he so advised, that neither he nor his daughter could tolerate the Milwaukee municipal water. This fact undoubtedly enabled him to diagnose Mr. E. A.'s disease, since none of the most widely read American medical journals provided information about this new malady. Two other physicians in the same medical group had also recommended avoidance of fluoridated water to some of their patients. Mr. Quirk stated in his advertisement that another physician, Dr. R.B. Pittelkow, the president of the Milwaukee County Medical Society during 1970, had also encountered illness due to fluoridated water and had promised an investigation by the medical society. The society requested the names of individuals whom Mr. Quirk thought had been adversely affected by the city's water, together with the names of their physicians. About three dozen such names were submitted to the society, but apparently no investigation of these cases was undertaken. One spokesman for the society indicated that they had no adequate facilities to study this disease – only a few laboratories in the country were equipped to carry out reliable tests for fluoride. Another stated that Mr. Quirk's cases were "hand-picked," a true but completely irrelevant charge. He had indeed selected some of the most dramatic cases in order to provide convincing evidence that their illness was caused by fluoridated water.

Dr. E. R. Krumbiegel, Milwaukee's former health commissioner, had made a long-standing offer to Mr. Quirk to test any patient who suspected that fluoridated water had been affecting his health adversely. Because Dr. Krumbiegel had proposed hospitalization of such cases under his exclusive care and control, Mr. Quirk would not agree to what he considered to be a one-sided investigation by a long-time advocate of fluoridation of water supplies; instead he suggested that an unbiased panel be established.

Another physician, Dr. H. T. Petraborg, a practitioner in the town of Aitkin, Minnesota, became interested in the Milwaukee illness since he too had observed in his own community similar cases that he had diagnosed as poisoning from fluoridated water. To satisfy his curiosity, he decided to ascertain whether the illness in Milwaukee was identical to that which he had encountered elsewhere in Minnesota. During a four-day period in Milwaukee, Dr. Petraborg interviewed and examined 28 individuals whom Mr. Quirk had singled out as victims of fluoridated water. The medical histories of their illness, the uniformity of their complaints, and his own personal examinations convinced Dr. Petraborg that the fluoridated water had, indeed, caused a serious progressive illness. The following are accounts of two of the cases that he studied during the period August 21 to 25, 1973.

Mr. J. B., age 40, became unusually thirsty within a few weeks after he had taken up residence in Milwaukee following his discharge from the Army Air Corps in 1957. It was not unusual for him to drink between 20 and 30 cups (approximately six quarts) of fluoridated coffee a day. This perplexing phenomenon was accompanied by muscular pains, numbness, and spasticity, especially in the right hand and in both feet, and by a gradual loss in strength. His illness persisted over several years with progressive loss of weight from 140 to 107 pounds. Increasing fatigue compelled him to resort to bedrest immediately after his eight-hour work day. Eventually, in 1964, he was hospitalized for two weeks, but laboratory tests and X-rays furnished no clues regarding the cause of his illness. Vitamins prescribed by his physician failed to restore his deteriorating strength. After his hospitalization, he moved from fluoridated Milwaukee to unfluoridated Caledonia, Wisconsin, where, to his amazement, he experienced a complete, spontaneous recovery and quickly regained the weight he had lost.

Mrs. S. T., age 42, was another of the cases studied by Dr. Petraborg. Her main complaints were extreme thirst, bloating in the stomach and continuous headaches. Numbness and muscular pains in hands and legs often compelled her to get out of bed at night and walk. While taking a bath she always experienced intense itching of her skin which subsided after several hours. Her disease began in 1959 within a week after she moved to fluoridated St. Francis, Wisconsin, from unfluoridated Cudahy, and it cleared up promptly in 1965 when she substituted spring water for fluoridated water.

According to Petraborg, every one of the 28 patients related the same story of a progressive illness characterized by a multiplicity of complaints, mainly weakness, exhaustion, excessive thirst, headaches, and gastrointestinal disturbances. Since most of these patients had not been aware that fluoride was being added to their drinking water, Petraborg felt there was no further need to carry out so-called blind and double-blind studies. He has published two clinical reports of his findings.[1,2]

MY OWN CASE STUDIES

This widespread malady in Milwaukee was not a new illness, but had appeared in other cities throughout the United States in the early 1950s.[3-7] Quite by accident, I encountered this fluoride-induced syndrome in my own patients and described it in several medical journals. The fact that only a few cities in Michigan were fluoridated at that time facilitated a correct diagnosis of the problem, for when patients visited a non-fluoridated community their health returned. In my first case, serendipity was responsible for the diagnosis.

Bay City, Michigan. In 1954, Mrs. S. S., age 40, a resident of Bay City, Michigan, was referred to me by her family physician for allergic studies because of painful spastic bowels, frequent nausea and vomiting, bloating of the abdomen, and persistent migraine-like headaches, which her physician thought were brought on by an allergy of unknown causes. All my tests, however, failed to show that food allergy was involved. During the course of examination, the patient casually mentioned that every morning upon awakening she was so thirsty that she had to drink several glasses of water. She was wondering whether or not Bay City's water could account for her stomach and bowel upsets because they usually occurred in the morning after she had consumed water. Whenever she was away from the city, her mouth and throat no longer felt dry and she was no longer thirsty, nor did the cramps in the abdomen and the headaches occur. Neither she nor I realized then that Bay City's water had been fluoridated since

1951. Soon afterward I learned that excessive thirst, polyuria (excess urination), and the other symptoms are a common feature of both acute and chronic fluoride poisoning.[7,8]

Highland Park, Michigan. A few months later, during the fall of 1954, a fortunate coincidence made it possible for me to study this unusual disease.[3] A 35-year-old woman residing in Highland Park, Michigan, had been experiencing a mysterious illness manifested by a variety of symptoms, including a very noticeable case of mottled teeth. Her condition was much more severe than that of the Bay City patient. She was constantly nauseated, vomited frequently, had periodic pains in the stomach, and suffered from diarrhea and pains in the lower back. Her general health had gradually deteriorated to the point where she was bedridden. Her dentist had identified the white and brown stains of her teeth as mottling caused by fluoride, and her physician had suggested to her that the current illness might be related to drinking water, although Highland Park's water, fluoridated since 1952, could not have been responsible for the dental condition because mottling occurs only during the tooth-forming years up to age 12.

At first, neither her dentist nor her physician appeared to be much concerned about her disease, and her condition continued to deteriorate. She reported a progressive weight loss, passed blood repeatedly from her kidneys and uterus, and had a constant and frequently unbearable pain in her head. Her eyesight had also gradually deteriorated, and she had noticed "scotomata" or "moving spots" in both eyes, which are often indicative of an organic disease of the eye. On her skin she had what she thought were bruises or hemorrhages. The muscles of her hands and arms had weakened to the extent that she was unable to grasp certain objects. For instance, when she was doing her laundry, garments often dropped from her hands, and potatoes slipped from her grip when she was peeling them. Furthermore, she often lost control of her legs and could no longer coordinate her thoughts, eventually becoming incoherent, drowsy, and forgetful. She had gradually given up her housework and was confined to bed.

These progressive symptoms suggested a brain tumor, but the uterine bleeding, the so-called hemorrhages of the skin, and the diarrhea pointed to a systemic disease rather than to involvement of a single organ such as the brain. Fortunately, her mottled teeth constituted a clue, merely a vague hint for a diagnosis. In her childhood she had lived in a natural fluoride area in China where white-spotted teeth among children were common and where the teeth of many adults had taken on a brownish yellow stain. Her illness, however, did not bear the slightest resemblance to what was then known as chronic fluoride poisoning—characterized by thickening of bone substance, calcification of ligaments and tendons, and arthritis of the spine. I wondered if mottling and a nonskeletal fluorosis might be associated.

On my advice the patient was hospitalized for diagnostic studies. Eight of Detroit's most prominent specialists were called in for consultation: a neurologist to explain the brain symptoms; an orthopedist for the backache; an ophthalmologist for the eye disease; a hematologist to assess the hemorrhages of the skin, uterus, and bladder; a cardiologist, an endocrinologist, a specialist in metabolic diseases, and a gynecologist were consulted to evaluate the individual symptoms that were covered by their specialties. All considered the illness serious but were at a loss to establish an overall diagnosis. Only one of the eight consultants suggested that this disease might be of psychosomatic (imaginary) origin. This in itself was remarkable, for physicians often resort to this explanation when they cannot diagnose a disease, perhaps in a subconscious effort to save face. Although a psychosomatic element may be superimposed upon almost every illness, only rarely does it constitute the real cause of a disease.

The case became more puzzling when the X–rays of bones, especially of pelvic bone and spine, failed to show the expected changes of chronic fluoride intoxication, and when most of the laboratory tests revealed nothing. Only the blood calcium level was slightly elevated, namely 11.6 mg per 100 cc (normally up to 11) of blood serum. One specimen of urine collected during 24 hours contained 1.38 mg of fluoride; another 1.37 mg. Experience later taught me that this examination proved very little. It showed only that the patient was eliminating some fluoride, perhaps slightly more than average in an artificially fluoridated community. It did not indicate to what extent fluoride had been stored in her system nor whether the patient was still consuming it in drinking water and from other sources. No matter how much or how little fluoride is being eliminated through the kidneys, the harm which it may have caused during its passage through the body and through vital organs can be determined by only one approach: careful clinical observation of the patient.

Until completion of the preliminary tests in the hospital, the patient was instructed to use fluoridated Highland Park water that she had brought with her to the hospital. After the tests were completed, she began drinking unfluoridated (0.1 ppm) Detroit water. Within only two days the stomach symptoms and headaches subsided, and she was soon well enough to be discharged.

Neither in the hospital nor after her discharge was she given any medication. Instead, she was instructed to avoid fluoridated water strictly, not only for drinking but also for cooking her food as well. She was also told to avoid both tea and seafood because of their high fluoride content. The headaches, eye disturbances, and muscular weakness disappeared in a most dramatic manner. After about two weeks her mind began to clear, and she underwent a complete change in personality. For the first time in two years she was able to undertake her household duties without having to stop and rest. Within a four-week period she had gained five pounds.

Subsequently, the patient was subjected to a series of tests which definitely proved that her disease was related to fluoridated water. She was given test injections of minute amounts of fluoride in drinking water and distilled water as a control. She was not aware which water contained fluoride. The fluoride solutions induced a recurrence of the symptoms, whereas the fluoride-free water showed no adverse effects. In one of the subsequent tests a classical attack of migraine headache was produced by one milligram of fluoride taken in two glasses of water. This is about one fifth to one half the average amount ingested in one day by people living in a fluoridated area.

Further laboratory and other diagnostic studies were contemplated, especially a study of the behavior of calcium, phosphorus, and magnesium, the activity of certain enzymes, and a tracing of her brain waves before and after administration of a test dose of fluoride. These plans came to an abrupt end when the patient suffered another sudden episode of excruciating pains in head, muscles and spine following an experimental dose of fluoride. The severity of her response to this so-called blind test made me stop all further testing. Fortunately, the patient recovered completely without any treatment other than the elimination of Highland Park fluoridated water for drinking and cooking.

Judging from the overall picture, this serious progressive illness might have terminated fatally within a few months, and had she died, even the most competent physician would not have been able to establish the real cause of death. Certain features, rarely found in other diseases, were remarkable. The more water the patient drank the thirstier she became. The deterioration of her brain function was progressive. The painful numbness in arms, hands and legs, and the arthritic pains in the spine were worse upon awakening in the morning. After a night's rest one would have expected the reverse. The slight, but definite, disturbance in the calcium metabolism was of paramount interest in view of reports in medical journals that fluoride interferes with the action of this vital mineral.[9]

Could something other than fluoride have caused the disease, perhaps another poison in the water? This question was definitely answered by the ease with which this disease could be reproduced at will when extremely small amounts of fluoride were administered to her. In order to ascertain the cause of her problem she was given a test dose of fluoride in water without being told the nature of the test. She had, of course, given me permission to carry out any test I saw fit.

Saginaw, Michigan. Within a few weeks after observing this unusual ailment I had another opportunity to gather more information about it. During November, 1954, at the request of a local physician in Saginaw, Michigan, I interviewed and examined some 30 people who had been ill there. They became suspicious of fluoridated water because their health improved immediately, and their illness gradually cleared up completely following termination of fluoridation in Saginaw. Nine of the 30 people described a disease which in every respect conformed to that of the Highland Park case. Some had experienced relief when they were away from Saginaw for even short periods. Most of them had not been aware that fluoride was being added to their drinking water until they were confronted with voting on fluoridation. Some of the individuals suffered exclusively from bladder and bowel symptoms which, at that time, I did not relate to fluoride.

In one of the victims, Mrs. H. M., age 49, the resemblance to the Highland Park case was particularly striking.[7] She too had mottled teeth, as did members of her family and other inhabitants of the

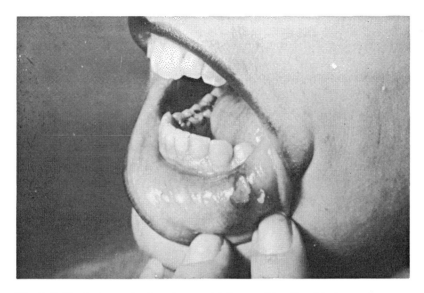

Fig. 9-1. Typical mouth ulcer (stomatitis) caused by fluoride in toothpaste.

Canadian village where she spent her childhood. In addition to constant gastric distress and muscular pains, she described the loss of control of her arms and particularly of her legs which frequently "collapsed under her." Most annoying was the persistent dryness in her mouth that led to frequent ulcers (Fig. 9-1 above) for which her physicians had no explanation. Because drinking more water aggravated the dryness, she eventually associated her illness with the Saginaw water. She learned, for the first time in October, 1953, that the water was fluoridated and shortly thereafter she began to use distilled water for drinking and cooking. Within four to six weeks, the illness had completely subsided.

Another case typical of the Saginaw group was that of a 42-year-old salesman, Mr. R.M., who was about to give up his job because of progressive pains and weakness in his hands that prevented him from grasping the steering wheel of his car. This condition became so severe that he often had to stop on the highway. He finally became suspicious of Saginaw's water because the disease invariably improved when he was on extended sales trips away from Saginaw. When fluoridation was abandoned there, he quickly recovered.

Whereas the evidence in these cases was reasonably convincing, I felt that additional studies were needed to confirm the diagnosis.

This requirement was fulfilled in the case of W. J., a 12-year-old boy who was one of the 30 persons whom I examined in Saginaw and had been under my observation for two to three years.[10] He had been suffering from convulsions that had become increasingly severe in recent months. After fluoridation had been discontinued, the seizures gradually subsided.

This case was so different from what I had learned thus far about fluoride poisoning that I would not have given it a second thought had it not been for his unusual teeth which bore some resemblance to mottling. They were underdeveloped and partially deprived of enamel, a condition termed "hypoplasia." Causes of hypoplastic teeth are fever, nutritional disturbances and also the advanced stage of chronic fluoride poisoning.[11]

According to the patient's physician, Dr. W.P.M., the boy remained fully conscious during the seizures, a feature not usually encountered in epileptic attacks. The description of the episodes and the appearance of the boy's teeth suggested to me a possible disturbance of the calcium metabolism, particularly since so-called tetaniform convulsions associated with low blood calcium are common in acute poisoning in persons who use fluoride for homicidal or suicidal purposes. Fluoride is known to combine with calcium in the system,[11] and in a few persons fluoride induces excessive calcium loss through the urine.[12] At Harper Hospital, Detroit, a pediatrician, a neurosurgeon, and a dentist were consulted to aid in establishing the diagnosis. Although these consultants had had no personal experience with fluoride poisoning, I accepted their diagnosis that the illness was epilepsy and was not related to fluoride. The neurosurgeon carried out test after test and finally did exploratory surgery on the child's brain in an effort to locate the area of disturbance and to view and remove the suspected lesion, which he thought would be a brain tumor. To his surprise, he found none.

Several weeks after the child had left the hospital, a 24-hour urine specimen contained 4.4 mg of fluoride – an extraordinary amount. Since the boy was then no longer drinking fluoridated water, fluoride had obviously been stored in his system and was now being eliminated, a well-established phenomenon.[13,14] The elimination of excess fluoride and the failure of the neurosurgeon to find a cause for the convulsions led me to reconsider the earlier diagnosis and to hospitalize the patient again for additional studies. This time a leading Detroit neurologist, Dr. G. Steiner at Wayne State University, diagnosed the boy's illness as tetany. The diagnosis hinged on the fact that the convulsions had been confined to one side of the body. The previous consultants had not been aware that this condition, resembling epilepsy, also occurs in convulsions due to a calcium (or magnesium) disturbance, a rare condition known as hemitetany. That the child remained conscious during the attacks supported the diagnosis. After elimination of fluoridated water, the child had no further attacks, and the fluoride levels of his urinary specimens gradually became negligible.*

Why was this case so different from the Highland Park case? Events in medicine are unpredictable. For instance, if a person is intolerant to iodide, he may develop one of several entirely different diseases – a toxic goiter, acne (a skin eruption), or an acute swelling of the salivary glands. Whereas all these diseases are due to the single agent iodide, rarely, if ever, do two of them occur in the same person. As indicated in Chapter 7, fluoride in large doses can induce convulsions as well as gastrointestinal symptoms.

Windsor, Ontario. In contrast to the Saginaw cases, in which the illness was recognized after cessation of fluoridation, in Windsor, Ontario, ill effects were detected after fluoride was introduced into the water supply (September 11, 1962). The local health department, fearing an adverse reaction by the citizens, did not announce when fluoridation would begin. This afforded an excellent opportunity--much better than any so-called double-blind test – to determine whether fluoridated water produces ill effects. Two weeks later, when the press announced the event to the public, eight individuals were able to diagnose their own disease.

Two of the eight, Mrs. M.H., age 57, a nurse, and Mrs. E.K., age 38, had been in the habit of drinking one or two glasses of water before breakfast. For some unknown reason, they suddenly experienced abdominal cramps and vomiting immediately after their

---

*In the hospital, urine was collected in a metal container which interferes with the correct measurement. A plastic container should have been used since metal, enamel and glass, like calcium, attract fluoride. This error, however, would have worked in favor of the diagnosis. Had some fluoride in the specimen been lost to the container the original amount in the specimen would have been even higher than that reported to me.

customary morning drink. During the course of the day, they developed headaches, pains in the lower spine, and numbness and pains in arms and legs. They had never before had any such discomfort; moreover, they were not then aware that Windsor's water was being fluoridated. The physician of Mrs. H., Dr. F.S., at first provisionally considered a stomach ailment, but his medication was of no avail. After several days of careful observation, he suspected that the water might somehow be involved in her illness and advised her to discontinue drinking it but requested her not to disclose his diagnosis to anyone lest it jeopardize his position in the eyes of some of his colleagues, especially Windsor's Medical Officer of Health. The other patient, Mrs. K., resorted to the use of distilled water on her own. Both patients recovered promptly upon eliminating fluoridated water.

One of the eight cases was subjected to a double-blind test, the technique of which was outlined by the editor of the *Journal of the American Medical Association* in a letter to me dated April 2, 1958:

> One very obvious method for testing the validity of the diagnosis would be to place the patient on a fluoride-free water supply until the symptoms have subsided. Then, unbeknown to the patient (and to the physician), add 2.2 parts per million of sodium fluoride to the water.

Two and two tenths parts of sodium fluoride per million parts of water equals 1 ppm *fluoride ion,* the concentration officially recommended for artificial fluoridation.

The patient tested was a 13-year-old schoolgirl (C.D.), who had developed increasingly severe migraine-like headaches starting in mid-September, 1962. Simultaneously, pains and numbness in arms and legs, and a distinct deterioration in her mental alertness interfered with her attendance at school. A consulting neurologist ruled out the possibility of a brain tumor. Tests to determine whether the headaches were caused by allergy, were negative. On the advice of another patient, who had been similarly afflicted, the child stopped drinking Windsor water. Her condition began to improve immediately, and her ailment subsided completely after 10 days. On Mondays and Thursdays, however, the headaches recurred when, inadvertently, after gym classes, she quenched her thirst with Windsor tap water. These recurrences ceased after she began to carry her own distilled drinking water to school.

As final proof that fluoride had caused the illness, the disease was subsequently reproduced by the above-described double-blind procedure under the guidance of the Windsor physician. This procedure clearly eliminated the possibility of personal bias on my part. The Windsor and Saginaw cases also proved beyond any doubt that no chemical other than fluoride caused the disease, in view of the fact that the illness occurred or subsided promptly following the addition or removal of fluoride from the drinking water. In most instances, the patients had no knowledge about fluoride, nor did it occur to them that it might be in their drinking water.

OBSERVATIONS BY OTHER PHYSICIANS

The two major obstacles to studies of this kind are the lack of cooperation by physicians and patients. Only an exceptionally idealistic and public-spirited patient would be willing to undergo the time-consuming and (frequently) painful tests involved in reproducing the illness for experimental purposes. Physicians, on the other hand, often hesitate to cooperate because the belief that fluoridation is harmless has seemingly been established beyond reasonable doubt. Merely to question authoritative opinions constitutes a defiance of established orthodoxy. Nevertheless, I have communications from many other physicians who have diagnosed intoxication by fluoridated water. For instance, the following is an account of a patient studied by Dr. C. D. Marsh of Memphis, Tennessee.

Mrs. W.E.A., age 62, residing in Memphis (not fluoridated at that time), invariably developed the same disease on trips to Washington, D.C., and Richmond, Virginia, during 1952 to 1956, and always improved promptly within a few days after her return home.[4] This experience drew her attention to drinking water as a possible source of her trouble. At the time, she had no knowledge whatsoever of fluoride or fluoridation. After she had learned that both Washington and Richmond were adding fluoride to the water supply, on future trips to the two cities she prevented a recurrence by taking several bottles of Memphis water with her and avoiding fluid foods.

Subsequently, Mrs. A. suddenly experienced new episodes of this illness, this time to her surprise while she was at home. Dr. Marsh, her physician, was able to trace these recurrences to a tranquilizer – trifluoperazine – prescribed by him and, on another occasion, to a new toothpaste. Neither she nor her physician had been aware that both the drug and the toothpaste contained fluoride.

After the patient had regained her health, she was given – with her consent – an intradermal injection of 1 mg fluoride, which is the equivalent of the daily amount recommended for children's teeth. She was not aware of the nature of the test. Within half an hour she developed excruciating pains in the abdomen, headaches, backache, and profuse nasal discharge, followed by diarrhea and lethargy – the same group of symptoms from which she had suffered on previous occasions from fluoridated water, from fluoride toothpaste, and from the fluoride-containing tranquilizer. Subsequently, a double-blind test carried out by Dr. Marsh confirmed that fluoride was responsible for the disease.

Among other physicians who have observed harm to their patients from fluoridated water is Dr. W. P. Murphy of Brookline, Mass., who received the Nobel Prize in 1934 for his work on pernicious anemia. He wrote me about one of his patients who had intermittent attacks of a generalized allergic edema (hives) which cleared up after he moved from a fluoridated to a nonfluoridated town. As in the above-mentioned case from Memphis, the use of a fluoride toothpaste precipitated periodic recurrences of the swellings, mainly in the face and about the mouth, which subsided completely after the toothpaste was discontinued.[15]

Extensive studies were also carried out in fluoridated Haarlem, Holland, by a group of 12 physicians under the guidance of Dr. H. C. Moolenburgh. They encountered 60 patients with the above-described symptoms in which the relationship of the disease to fluoridated water was verified by a carefully controlled double-blind test.[16] In order to rule out personal bias, these physicians devised a system by means of which only an attorney and the druggist knew which of three bottles of water contained fluoride. Thirty of the 60 individuals experienced abdominal pains, bloating of the abdomen, and diarrhea alternating with constipation. Eighteen had ulcers in the mouth, 5 suffered from persistent thirst. Joint pains, headaches, vertigo, and mental depression were other features of this ailment as shown in Table 9-1 (opposite).

Table 9-1

Summary of Ill Effects from F⁻ in 60 Selected Patients[16]

Complaints	Number	Percent
Stomach and intestinal	30[a]	50
Stomatitis	18[b]	30
Polydipsia	5	8
Joint pains	3	5
Migraine-like headaches	3	5
Visual disturbances	3	5
Tinnitus	2	3
Mental depression	2	3

[a] Including 17 patients with abdominal pain, 12 with diarrhea, 5 with flatulence, 4 with nausea, and 1 with spastic constipation.

[b] Two of these patients had symptoms after using fluoride tablets.

The evidence presented in this chapter clearly establishes that nonskeletal chronic fluoride intoxication is a serious, frequently misdiagnosed disease. Many physicians and scientists were involved in these clinical investigations, and objective diagnostic procedures were utilized. If the illness is caught in time, the symptoms are reversible and disappear when distilled or low-fluoride water is consumed. Hundreds of patients who were seriously ill have been cured by this simple procedure. To deny the proven physical basis of this disease would hardly be scientific, especially since fluoride from any source produces similar results.

REFERENCES

1. Petraborg, H.T.: Chronic Fluoride Intoxication from Drinking Water. Fluoride, 7:47-52, 1974.

2. Petraborg, H.T.: Hydrofluorosis in the Fluoridated Milwaukee Area. Fluoride, 10:165-169, 1977.

3. Waldbott, G.L.: Chronic Fluorine Intoxication from Drinking Water. Int. Arch. Allergy Appl. Immunol., 7:70-74, 1955.

4. Waldbott, G.L.: Fluoride in Clinical Medicine. Int. Arch. Allergy Appl. Immunol., 20, suppl. 1, 1962.

5. Waldbott, G.L.: Acute Fluoride Intoxication. Acta Med. Scand., 174, suppl. 400, 1963.

6. Waldbott, G.L., and Steinegger, S.: New Observations on "Chizzola" Maculae. Proceedings of the Third International Clean Air Congress. Düsseldorf, Federal Republic of Germany, Oct. 8-12, 1973, Verlag des Vereins Deutscher Ingenieure, Düsseldorf, 1973, pp. A63-A67.

7. Waldbott, G.L.: Incipient Chronic Fluorine Intoxication from Drinking Water. Acta Med. Scand., 156:157-168, 1956.

8. Whitford, G.M., and Taves, D.R.: Fluoride-Induced Diuresis: Plasma Concentrations in the Rat. Proc. Soc. Exp. Biol. Med., 137:458-460, 1971.

9. Faccini, J.M.: Fluoride-Induced Hyperplasia of the Parathyroid Glands. Proc. Roy. Soc. Med., 62:241, 1969.

10. Waldbott, G.L.: Tetaniform Convulsions Precipitated By Fluoridated Drinking Water. Confin. Neurol., 17:339-347, 1957.

11. Roholm, K.: Fluorine Intoxication: A Clinical-Hygienic Study. 1937.

12. Spencer, H., Lewin, I., Fowler, J., and Samachson, J.: Effect of Sodium Fluoride on Calcium Absorption and Balances in Man. Am. J. Clin. Nutr., 22:381-390, 1969. Cf. Elsair, J., Poey, J., Reggabi, M., Hattab, F., Benouniche, N., and Spinner, C.: Effets de l'intoxication fluorée sabaiguë du lapin sur les métabolismes fluoré et phosphocalcique et sur la radiographie du squelette. Eur. J. Toxicol., Suppl., 9:429-437, 1976.

13. Likins, R.C., McClure, F.J., and Steere, A.C.: Urinary Excretion of Fluoride Following Defluoridation of a Water Supply. Public Health Rep., 71:217-220, 1956. (Reprinted in Fluoride Drinking Waters, 1962, pp. 421-423.)

14. Siddiqui, A.H.: Fluorosis in Nalgonda District, Hyderabad-Deccan. Br. Med. J., 2:1408-1413, 1955.

15. Murphy, W.P.: Letter to George L. Waldbott, May 4, 1965.

16. Grimbergen, G.W.: A Double Blind Test for Determination of Intolerance to Fluoridated Water (Preliminary Report). Fluoride, 7:146-152, 1974.

CHAPTER 10

HEALTH EFFECTS OF AIRBORNE FLUORIDE

IN VIEW OF THE FACT that as little as 1 ppm fluoride in drinking water can produce serious debilitating illness, might not a similar effect be anticipated from various, even smaller, concentrations in the air? We have already seen that fluoride from chimneys, exhaust fans, storage bins of factories or from volcanic eruptions can damage plants and domestic animals. But can the minute amounts of fluoride that contaminate the air also affect the health and life of human beings, especially of those who work in such factories or reside nearby?

EXPOSURE TO AIRBORNE FLUORIDE

The average amounts of gaseous fluoride in the air of large U.S. cities are extremely small – usually less than $0.05 \mu g/m^3$ or 0.0625 ppb. A person living for 24 hours in such an atmosphere would inhale only 0.001 mg of fluoride a day (considering an average inhalation of 20 m^3/day). Even in grossly polluted air, such as found within 200 yards to one mile of a Scottish aluminum factory, fluoride concentrations were not higher than 0.021–0.002 mg/m^3, depending on wind direction and speed at time of sampling.[1]

Under ordinary conditions these amounts might appear to be negligible, but prolonged inhalation of similar contaminated air, day in and day out, cannot be ignored, because absorption of gaseous fluoride into the blood stream through the respiratory tract is swift, localized, and almost complete.[2] Furthermore, as already shown in Chapter 3, fluoride particulates settle on edible vegetation, thus accounting for a considerable increase of the fluoride burden of the body.

Under unfavorable conditions such as inversions, high barometric pressure, sudden episodes of excessive pollution brought on

by increased production in a factory, air stagnation in valleys —
where many factories are located — substantial amounts of airborne
fluorides may reach the bloodstream. Even more severe contamination of air may be encountered inside an industrial facility as
illustrated in Table 10-1 (opposite). Levels as high as 137 ppm
or 112 mg/m^3 have been reported, varying with the type of building, the effectiveness of ventilation equipment, cleanliness of the
premises of the factory, work practices, and many other factors.

Fruit and vegetables grown near factories contain many times
the anticipated average levels of fluoride as seen in Table 10-2
(page 130), compiled from my own studies in a polluted area near
an Ontario fertilizer factory.[3] Indeed, near a pollutant source
practically everything is likely to be contaminated by fluoride, as I
discovered when visiting farms adjacent to aluminum factories in
Bolzano, Italy (Fig. 10-1 below), and Clarington, Ohio (Table 10-
3 below, page 131).[4] Under these conditions it is not surprising
that the medical literature reveals many instances of fluorosis in
exposed workers and reports of poisoning among persons residing
nearby.

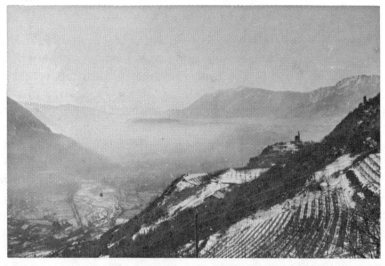

Fig. 10-1. Accumulation of fluoride-containing clouds
in a "kettle" surrounded by high mountains
(Bolzano, Italy).

Table 10-1

Atmospheric Fluoride Inside Factories

Industry	Concentration	
	ppm	mg/m³
Aluminum plant		
Potroom[a]	4.0	3.3
General[b]	1.3	1.1
Magnesium foundry[c]		
Mixing mill	7.8	6.4
General	0.2-0.9	0.1-0.7
Steel smelter[d]		
Ladle crane area	1.2-62	1-52.
General	0-17.	0-14.
Phosphate fertilizer manufacturer[e]	0.6-10.2	0.5-8.3
Pottery manufacturing[f]	4.3	3.5
Fluorspar mine [g]	0-1.1	0-0.9
Chemical plant[h]		
Room samples	0.08-10.0	0.06-8.2
General	1.8-1.9	1.5-1.6
Welding		
Welder's stand (gaseous)[i]	3.8	3.1
Welder's stand (particulate)[i]	0.6	0.5
Confined area (unvented)[j]	1.2-137	1.0-112
Confined area (vented)[j]	7.7-50	6.3-41

[a] Ref. 21 below. [b] N. Hiszek et al., *Banyasz. Kohasz. Lapok,* Kohasz, (Hungary), 103:514-517, 1970. [c] R. E. Bowler et al., *Br. J. Ind. Med.,* 4:216-222, 1947. [d] USPHS Bull. 229, 1948. [e] Ref. 20 below. [f] S. G. Luxon, *Ann. Occup. Hyg.,* 6:127-130, 1963. [g] W. D. Parsons et al., *Br. J. Ind. Med.,* 21:110-116, 1964. [h] N. A. Leidel et al., HEW Publ. No. (NIOSH) 76-103, p. 149. [i] L. K. Smith, *Ann. Occup. Hyg.,* 10:113-121, 1967. [j] J. Krechniak, *Fluoride,* 2: 13-24, 1969.

Table 10-2

Food Polluted by Fluoride in the Port Maitland, Ontario, Area[3]

	"Polluted" (ppm)	"Unpolluted" (ppm)
Wheat (grain)	2.6	0.7 to 2.0
Apples	6.6	0.8
Carrots	7.0	2.0
Beets	7.0	0.7 to 2.8
Squash	10.4	
Corn	1.3	0.7
Sauerkraut	10.7	
Currants	8.0	0.7
Cabbage Leaves	9.6	
"Chicken vegetable soup"	4.6	
"Hamburger with onions"	2.4	
Potatoes (boiled)	7.7	0.4
Beans (cooked)	17.3	1.7
Strawberries (frozen)	4.6	
Oatmeal (cooked)	5.1	0.2
Lettuce	44.0	0.1 to 0.3

INDUSTRIAL FLUOROSIS

Clinical Data. The first reliable description of industrial fluorosis was recorded in 1932 by P.F. Møller and S.V. Gudjonsson, who detected on X-ray examination increased, but varying, bone density in 30 of 78 workers engaged in the crushing and refining of cryolite.[5] Fourteen of these workers had been employed less than ten years; in one individual severe bone changes had already occurred after only five years. The two persons with the most advanced bone lesions—their spines were entirely immobile—had been employed in the factory for 25 and 11 years, respectively. It is especially noteworthy that this first description of the disease emphasized rheumatic pains, nausea, loss of appetite, and frequent vomiting in 42 of the 78 workers, the very same preskeletal symptoms that are now being encountered in patients made ill by artificially fluoridated water.

Table 10-3

Fluoride in Items Other than Food in Two Polluted Communities[4]

BOLZANO, ITALY	ppm
Rabbit (tibia, fibula ashed)	3650-3730
Soil (0 to 20 cm in depth)	1690-1530
Flydust	
Aluminum smelter	5420-6200
Magnesium factory	≤3300
Water	
Wells	0.8-25.0
Effluent from factory (ditch)	14.0-35.0
CLARINGTON, OHIO	
Pear leaves	>148
Wild cherry leaves	>77
Grass	>120
Bones of cow	3300-4560
Bones of rabbit	980-1500
Water	
Deep wells	0.098-0.164

Four years after this report appeared, P. A. Bishop, a Philadelphia roentgenologist, described a case of skeletal changes from industrial fluorosis in a 48-year-old laborer employed in a fertilizer factory for 18 years.[6] The bones contained from 2900 to 6900 ppm fluoride, but there was no history of gastric disturbances. Bishop reported that the patient died of a syphilitic heart disease.

Then, in 1937, the clinical, experimental, and toxicological aspects of the new disease were thoroughly investigated by Kaj Roholm, whose classical study covered data on 68 workers, 47 males and 21 females, aged 20 to 67.[7] He distinguished three different phases of skeletal fluorosis according to the degree of density and enlargement of the bones. He also recorded nonskeletal manifestations of the disease: mainly headaches, dizziness, stiffness, rheumatic pains, insomnia, fatigue, diarrhea, constipation, nausea, vomiting, and shortness of breath (Table 8-3, page 105).

Several striking descriptions of individual cases of industrial fluorosis have appeared in Switzerland and France,[8-10] where the disease has been recognized since 1936. E. Spéder, a French radiologist, recorded the typical bone changes in seven workers at the phosphate mines in French Morocco.[11] The occurrence of respiratory symptoms, mainly hoarseness, frequent sore throats, nasal congestion, cough, dyspnea, and asthmatic wheezing, were emphasized by subsequent investigators.[12-14]

In a 1970 Swiss survey of 17 male aluminum workers (aged 52 to 66) afflicted with skeletal fluorosis, the major complaints were arthritis, joint stiffness, and muscular pains. Fluoride levels in biopsied bones averaged 3320 ppm.[15] That arthritis is the most consistent manifestion of skeletal fluorosis was also recognized by another Swiss physician, H. H. Schlegel, who diagnosed the disease in 16 of 61 aluminum workers exposed to air with a fluoride content of 3 to 4 mg/m³.[16]

In recent years our knowledge of the disease has been greatly expanded by experimental, clinical, and histochemical studies of J. Franke, an orthopedic surgeon at the University of Halle, D.D.R. In 1967, he had encountered a patient whose illness was diagnosed as Bechterev Disease, a bone disease causing complete stiffening of the spine. The X–rays also revealed a marble-like condensation of pelvic bones that did not fit the diagnosis. He was considering reporting the unusual simultaneous occurrence of the two conditions, Bechterev Disease and Marblebone (or Albers-Schönberg) Disease, when he recalled that the patient was being exposed to fluoride in an aluminum smelter where he was employed. When he reviewed the literature, a single sentence in a textbook alerted him to fluoride as one of the sources of sclerotic bones. In his attempt to confirm his suspicion and to arrive at a correct diagnosis, he biopsied the iliac crest for a fluoride assay; the bone was so hard that the biopsy needle broke and the piece of bone had to be chiselled out. It contained over 4000 ppm fluoride. Once the diagnosis of skeletal fluorosis was thus verified, he embarked on extensive studies of the disease, which yielded a remarkable body of data on industrial fluorosis.

Subsequently, his examination of 300 workers revealed 35 with similar changes. The first signs of the disease appeared after an average of 10.7 years of employment and the most advanced changes after 19.5 years.[17] Franke emphasized the highly individual response to fluoride intake: in one of two workers employed for 15 years in the same area of the plant, the skeletal disease was far advanced; in the other it was hardly noticeable. In three autopsies he verified that the bone changes (Fig. 10-2, next page) are identical with those found in endemic areas from fluoride in drinking water (see Figs. 8-1 to 8-4 above, pages 99-101).[18]

E. Czerwinski and W. Lankosz have also observed typical skeletal fluorosis in 60 retired disabled aluminum workers, mainly exostoses, and ossification of the interosseous membranes and of muscle attachments. All but one case exhibited respiratory and circulatory manifestations, and about one half of the workers had gastrointestinal disorders, including a high (12%) incidence of gastric ulcers. Kidney stones and gallstones were found in 8 patients (see Table 10-4 below).[19]

Statistical Studies. Industrial exposure to fluoride has also been investigated in several large-scale statistical studies relating the magnitude of exposure to fluoride to the health of the worker. In 1963, physicians at the Tennessee Valley Authority fertilizer plant at Wilson Dam estimated the degree of exposure of 74 workers by comparing their urinary fluoride values with those of 67 other employees who had been exposed less.[20] In 23% of the "exposed" group, X-rays showed minimal or questionable degrees of increased bone density characteristic of fluorosis. The "exposed" group also had a higher incidence of respiratory disease (25.7% vs. 11.9%), of albuminuria (12.2% vs. 4.5%), and of musculoskeletal conditions than the presumably "unexposed" group.

Table 10-4

Nonskeletal Changes in 60 Retired Aluminum Workers[19]

Manifestations	Frequency of Occurrence	
Respiratory and circulatory system	58	(97%)
Digestive system	31	(52%)
Gastric ulcer	7	(12%)
Stasis after stomach resection	5	(8%)
Urolithiasis and cholelithiasis	8	(13%)
Dental changes	44	(73%)
Psychiatric disturbances	14	(23%)

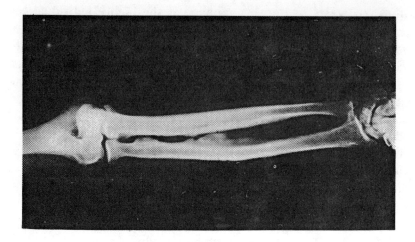

Fig. 10-2. X-Ray of forearm in advanced industrial fluorosis showing thickened bones and calcification of interosseous ligament. (Courtesy Dr. J. Franke, Halle, D.D.R.)

On the other hand, several studies suggest little or no damage to workers' health inside fluoride-emitting factories. For instance, a 1944 survey on 698 pot workers of a Canadian aluminum smelter disclosed no excessive incidence of respiratory illness, rheumatism, digestive, kidney, and cardiovascular disorders, compared with the respective condition in unexposed workers.[21] Another five-year survey published in 1976 by the medical staff of the Aluminum Company of America (ALCOA) did not "reveal any evidence of fluoride-associated bony change" in 56 aluminum smelter workers with 10- to 43-year occupational exposure.[22] The fluoride content of 56,000 urine specimens from 6500 workers averaged 2.24 ppm before they started their eight-hour shift compared with 7.7 ppm at the end of the shift. Despite such high temporary exposure to airborne fluoride, the ALCOA physicians found no abnormally high incidence of albumin, sugar, ketones, or occult blood in the urine.

Consequently, it is difficult to obtain a clear picture of the extent of harm created inside factories polluted with fluoride. In reviewing these reports we must consider that in such manufacturing processes the presence of other airborne pollutants modifies the symptomatology of the disease either synergistically or by attenuating the effect of fluoride. Little information is currently available on these matters, which may account for the divergence of the observations reported. Furthermore, the slow, insidious onset and individual variability of the patients' complaints and the absence of reliable diagnostic laboratory criteria, especially during the incipient stage of the disease, tend to confuse the picture further.

These features are illustrated in the case of K.M., a 57-year-old man, who was exposed to hydrogen fluoride fumes practically every day for 10 years (1961-1971). He consulted me on August 10, 1976, about a multiplicity of complaints which started in the early sixties and which had been thoroughly studied by numerous physicians at several hospitals and diagnosed as chronic emphysema, osteoarthritis, gastroduodenitis, pyelonephritis, and diabetes. The hospital records indicated that he had undergone surgery twice: in 1969 for a diseased lumbar disc, and in 1972 for an osteotomy of the left knee joint. Not one of the numerous medications either brought substantial relief or impeded the steady progression of the disease, particularly the ever-increasing general debility. In 1974 he sustained a minor injury when he tripped on an oil pipe and fractured the fifth metacarpal bone in his left foot. Prior to his employment he had been in perfect health.

On his job at the alkylation unit of an oil company, he was exposed to hydrogen fluoride fumes of varying intensity from a "neutralizer pit," from leaky pipes and valves, and from defective seals on pumps. On several occasions, sudden bursts of fumes precipitated nausea, vomiting, and excruciating headaches. Some of the manifestations pointing to nonskeletal fluorosis involved the urinary tract (polydipsia—up to 3 gallons of water a day—polyuria, hematuria), the neuromuscular system (pains and paresthesias in arms and legs—his legs frequently collapsed under him—urinary and fecal incontinence, visual and hearing defects, tinnitus aureum), the gastrointestinal tract (diarrhea—6 to 10 bowel movements daily), lapse of memory, and inability to concentrate.

The principal feature of the examination was evidence of osteoarthritis, especially in the spine and both knees. Blood and urinary fluoride in 1974—four years after he had stopped working—were within normal limits; the iliac crest, however, still contained 1125 ppm fluoride (normal up to 300 ppm). Three of the attending physicians concurred independently of each other in the diagnosis nonskeletal fluorosis, whereas the medical consultants for the oil company failed to attribute the multiple manifestations to a single cause. Litigation, however, led to an out-of-court settlement in which the company conceded that the illness was probably related to fluoride exposure.[23]

NEIGHBORHOOD FLUOROSIS

If it is difficult for physicians to diagnose the early stage of fluorosis in industrial workers, how much more diagnostic skill is required to recognize the disease among residents in the neighborhood of factories? That populations might be at risk due to fluoride emission from an individual plant was emphasized in 1939 by M. Klotz, a German clinician, who reported the case of an infant residing near a fertilizer factory.[24] The baby had gastric disturbances indicative of pyloric stenosis (vomiting, abdominal cramps) and muscular spasm especially in the upper parts of the legs. X-Rays showed thickening of the periosteum of leg bones of the kind described in skeletal fluorosis. At the age of six months, the rigidity of muscles extended over the whole body and the child expired during a convulsion. Klotz observed a similar condition in three children of a family in the same area who also had mottled, stained, and fragile teeth, which he diagnosed as dental fluorosis.

In 1946, M. M. Murray and D. C. Wilson coined the term "neighborhood fluorosis" for a disease they encountered among nine members of a farmer's household near a fluoride-emitting iron-stone works in South Lincolnshire, England.[25] The symptoms associated with 1 to 14 years of fluoride air pollution were persistent aches and pains, headaches, blurred vision, stiffness in muscles and joints, gastric upsets, cough, and a tendency to frequent upper respiratory infections. The fluoride content of the urine ranged from 1.6 to 4.2 ppm. On the side facing the factory, the windows were etched, a characteristic sign of air pollution by hydrofluoric acid. Seven horses and eleven cows had died of fluoride poisoning. Grass samples within a few hundred yards of the burning ironstone mounds contained over 2000 ppm fluoride in dry matter, and the exterior of a straw stack about 0.5 miles away showed 490 ppm.

Unfortunately, there was no follow-up on the subsequent fate of these nine cases.

The same disease was experienced in 1955 by a farm family of three residing near an aluminum smelter in Troutdale, Oregon.[26] Litigation of this case revealed muscular pains, general fatigue, arthritis in conjunction with liver and kidney damage, and evidence of hypothyroidism. The court action established a definite relationship between the disease and fluoride ingested from food grown in the contaminated area. Neither the British nor the Oregon patients displayed signs of the skeletal changes with which fluorosis is usually identified.

The hematological findings of neighborhood fluorosis were described in 1969 in children 6 to 14 years old residing close to an aluminum factory in Czechoslovakia. Significantly lower hemoglobin but higher than normal red blood cell values were recorded, a condition often encountered in certain lung diseases caused by inhalation of toxic agents.[27]

The medical literature reveals a limited number of other reports on damage to the health of residents in the vicinity of fluoride-emitting factories. In 1967, J. Herbert et al.[28] reported the case of a 46-year-old worker residing 10 km from an aluminum plant who showed advanced skeletal fluorosis on X-ray examination. In the city of Dohna, D.D.R., C. W. Schmidt[29] studied the X-rays of 20 residents living close to an aluminum smelter and found minor periosteal changes in 11, as well as definite skeletal fluorosis in 5. None of these persons were occupationally exposed to fluoride. Near the smelter, the following fluoride levels were found: air – 0.75 mg/m³ fluoride (maximum allowable concentration, 0.03 mg/m³); leaves of fruit trees – 119 to 580 mg/kg (dry); and hay – 8.8 to 9.1 mg/100 gm.

Currently, it is difficult to estimate the incidence of neighborhood fluorosis because few physicians are aware of its existence and because its symptoms mimic a number of other diseases. Furthermore, those who do diagnose it may not be unduly concerned because of the subtlety of the manifestations and because of the absence of clear, objective, diagnostic criteria. It is pertinent, therefore, to record my own data which are remarkably in accord with those encountered from artificially fluoridated water.

PERSONAL OBSERVATIONS

My own observations on neighborhood fluorosis pertain to the nonskeletal phase of the disease in residents near fluoride-emitting factories and workers employed in such facilities. Altogether I have encountered 133 cases in five different areas.

Near an Ontario phosphate fertilizer factory in 1968, I interviewed 28 persons, 15 of whom were examined and 3 hospitalized. During November 1971, I examined another 24 individuals in the city of Bolzano in northern Italy where the air was contaminated by an aluminum and magnesium factory. Bolzano is located in a deep valley surrounded by high mountains, conditions favorable to persistent stagnation of polluted air (Fig. 10-1 above, page 128; see also Table 10-3 above, page 131). In 1972 in a southern Ohio village situated in a valley exposed to smoke from an aluminum smelter, I observed another 36 persons, four of whom were subsequently studied thoroughly in my clinic. During April 1971, I encountered the same disease in 22 adults (18 males and 4 females), including 2 children ages 5 and 7 respectively, whom I interviewed in Kitimat, British Columbia. Their illness originated from fumes and smoke emitted from a nearby aluminum smelter. In the 18 male adults, however, the disease could not be designated neighborhood fluorosis, since all were employed at the smelter; 13 of them had been working in the potrooms where the contamination was at its worst.

In 1977 a Chicago medical team conducted a major survey of 1242 workers at the Kitimat aluminum plant and found that there were "large numbers with abnormalities of function and disease, particularly of the lungs and skeletal system."[30] Over 25% of the workers had significant pulmonary impairment or "back trouble," including numerous cases of slipped disc, spinal fusion, and history of cervical and lumbar surgery. On December 27-28, 1977, I interviewed 27 persons (I examined 10) living near a fluoride-emitting enamel factory in Urbana, Ohio. Twenty-three of them had typical symptoms of nonskeletal fluorosis. In all but one of these the respiratory tract was involved; 17 had paresthesias in the arms and legs; the same number had gastrointestinal symptoms; 9 had muscular fibrillation; and 3 had Chizzola maculae (see page 141).

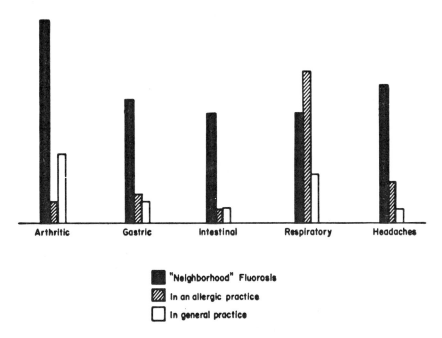

"Neighborhood" Fluorosis

▨ In an allergic practice

☐ In general practice

Fig. 10-3. Relative incidence of symptomatology in 32 cases of "neighborhood" fluorosis. (From G. L. Waldbott and V.A. Cecilioni: "Neighborhood" Fluorosis. *Clin. Toxicol.,* 2:387-396, 1969.)

The following are examples I encountered in the Ontario area. Mrs. V. F., the 54-year-old wife of an Ontario farmer, experienced progressive malaise and debility, constant pain in the lower spine, and frequent migraine-like headaches. She frequently dropped dishes and glasses because numbness and pain in her fingers and hands prevented her from gripping objects firmly. She had continuous painful distention of the abdomen and diarrhea, alternating with periods of constipation. Her strength had gradually declined, and eventually she was bedridden most of the time (Fig. 10-3).

The illness of her 13-year-old son, M. F., was similar to hers. He had always enjoyed good health until the phosphate fertilizer factory began operations one-quarter mile northeast of their home. Pains in the shoulders and below the ribs, in the knee joints, and in the lower spine severely limited his activities. His legs frequently stiffened, his big toes cramped and, on several occasions, his knees collapsed under him. He experienced involuntary, uncontrollable twitching of muscles in various parts of the body—a phenomenon known as muscular fibrillation, suggestive of a temporary deficiency of calcium and/or magnesium in the blood stream. His nose was constantly running, his eyes were bloodshot, especially on windy days, and he was constantly troubled with what he called small "bruises" all over his body.

On their 50-acre farm, the family had witnessed gradual deterioration and eventual destruction of their strawberry and rhubarb plants, currant bushes, and apple and pear trees. Eighty-three of their 86 colonies of bees had been wiped out. Burns had appeared on the tips and margins of begonia and geranium leaves growing on a one-acre garden plot. Lilac bushes wilted early in spring even before they had borne flowers. The window glass of their house showed the characteristic fluoride etching, and the finish of their new automobile had become pitted and cracked. The cistern water that the family used for drinking contained as much as 37.8 ppm of fluoride.[31] Both patients improved remarkably after avoiding fluoride-contaminated water and produce.

In 10 afflicted individuals who derived much of their principal staple food from produce grown in their own polluted area, I have encountered another most disturbing sign of the disease, namely episodes of acute gastrointestinal upsets with pains and vomiting so severe that their physicians have mistakenly diagnosed their illness as intestinal obstruction, appendicitis, or acute gall bladder attacks—ailments which usually require surgical intervention. Yet the disease, which lasted only one to three days, cleared up spontaneously; laboratory tests as a rule were non-diagnostic. Careful inquiry proved that these persons seemed to have been acutely poisoned by the high-fluoride content of vegetables or fruit produced on their farms. The following case suggests this conclusion.

Mrs. M. McK., one of the Ohio patients, age 54, was examined in my clinic on February 12, 1972. She lived on a farm in a valley less than a mile by air from an aluminum factory. Fumes and smoke from the factory had burned off the leaves of grape vines, trees, and flowers, and had etched the glass of her windows. Dustfall was so heavy that it penetrated into her home even when doors and windows were closed, and her front porch was constantly covered with a layer of dust. The bark of a maple tree close to her house contained 47 ppm fluoride; dust collected inside the house had 74 ppm. Two of her dogs had died in convulsions for no known reason, and dead birds were frequently found lying on her lawn.

During the summer of 1971 Mrs. M. McK. herself experienced frequent attacks of excruciating abdominal pains with nausea and vomiting accompanied by abdominal distention for which her physician had no explanation. These episodes were also accompanied by chest pains, arthritis in her knees and fingers, pains and numbness in the legs, and were often followed by bladder disturbances. She was so thirsty that she had to drink "gallons of water." When she was mowing her lawn she experienced burning in the throat and burning and itching on the exposed parts of the skin. This condition progressed rapidly, and gradually led to severe weakness accompanied by impairment of vision, mental confusion, and loss of memory. Eventually she was completely incapacitated. On one occasion, like her two dogs, she too had a convulsion. Laboratory tests were unrevealing, and sedatives and vitamins given her by her physician were of no avail.

On November 27, 1972, she moved to Owosso, Michigan (municipal water fluoridated January 1972), where she was instructed to drink nonfluoridated water. Her condition improved considerably, and the abdominal episodes disappeared. On December 29th of that year she returned to her Ohio home for only a few hours. Within this short time she again experienced the above-described symptoms. Five 24-hour urine tests during the interval between May 3, 1972, and February 16, 1973, showed fluoride values in the range of 1.03 to 2.86 mg, which suggested that her body was excreting excess amounts of stored fluoride as long as 14 months after her departure from the polluted area.

The striking feature in this and similar cases that I have observed is the alarming acute abdominal episodes. Therefore, whenever such acute abdominal emergencies arise in a polluted area, the possibility of excessive ingestion of fluoride should be strongly considered.

CHIZZOLA MACULAE

During the above-mentioned studies I observed another feature of the disease — peculiar skin lesions, which deserve special mention because they have become an important clue to the early diagnosis of fluorosis, whether from fluoride in air, food, or water. They were first recognized and reported by an Italian general practioner, Dr. M. Cristofolini, in the neighborhood of an aluminum factory near the village of Chizzola in northern Italy.[32] Health authorities have subsequently established that exposure to fluoride was related to the lesions, which they described as follows:

They [the lesions] resemble bruises except that they gradually become paler and disappear without changing color. The appearance of the lesion is sometimes preceded by pronounced headache, sudden episodes of sharp pain and aching of the bones and joints at or near the point where the lesions appear. Each mark lasts for about five to six days and then disappears. If the patient remains in the contaminated zone the symptoms recur in other areas of the skin. On palpation the larger marks appear like a sponge.

When the lesions were first observed they cleared up within five to six days after the patient was removed from the contaminated zone. Lately, however, (Spring 1967), it has taken up to 20 days for the symptoms to disappear. As in 1933 to 1937, the condition mainly affects women and children. During the acute phase, the histological examination of the biopsied skin revealed an edematous-fibrinous leucocytic exudate in the interstice of the adipose lobules. It is most pronounced at the dividing line between dermis and hypodermis. It is associated with degeneration of the adipose cells, partial reabsorption of the fat and formation of frothy, basophilic cells. The regressive phase of the lesions is characterized by mild perivascular infiltration. These histological changes resemble those of erythema nodosum but cannot be identified as such.[33]

On my visit to Chizzola in 1971, Largaiolli, the collaborator of Cristofolini, was able to demonstrate these lesions to me in several residents in whom they had recurred following increased emissions from the smelter after 30 years of low levels. The skin lesions are always round or oval in shape and rarely larger than a 25-cent piece (1 inch or 2.5 cm in diameter)[34] (Fig. 10-4 opposite). Because of their similarity to bruises (Table 10-5 opposite) and because they clear up spontaneously after about seven to ten days, physicians and patients have paid little attention to them.

As of January 1978, I have observed 55 cases of "Chizzola" maculae among persons in my own medical practice. It could not

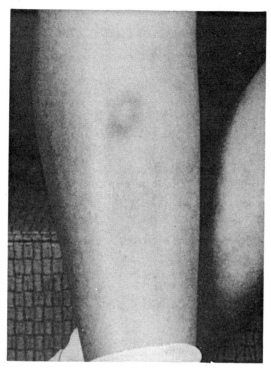

Fig. 10-4. Chizzola macula in an 8-year-old girl residing near a West Virginia aluminum smelter. Other symptoms: muscle pain, arthralgia, bilateral headaches, stomatitis, persistent nasal and sinus congestion, diarrhea alternating with constipation, and convulsions.

Table 10-5

Differentiation of Chizzola Maculae from Bruises[4]

Feature	Chizzola Maculae	Bruises
History	Exposure to fluoride	Trauma
Shape	Round or oval	Any shape
Size	1 to 2.5 cm in diameter	Any size
Color		
At first	Pinkish or bluish red	Blue
When fading	Pale pinkish or bluish red	Brown, then yellow
Histology	Pericapillary inflammation	Extravasation of blood through broken veins

always be established in each case whether the cause was fluoridated water or fluoride-contaminated food or air.

How these seemingly harmless skin lesions can serve clinicians in the diagnosis of fluorosis regardless of whether it is caused by airborne fluoride or by drinking water is illustrated by the following case.[4]

Miss C. C., age 24, had been under my care since February 27, 1971, because of allergic nasal disease caused by certain pollen, fungi, and food. She had undergone extensive investigation by several specialists because of a diversity of complaints—arthritis in the lower and cervical spine, dizziness, and nystagmus (a spasmodic, involuntary movement of the eyes). Pain and numbness in arms, fingers, and legs made her frequently drop things; her legs tended to collapse while she was walking. Often, she had ulcers in the mouth, diarrhea alternating with constipation, bladder trouble, and irregular vaginal bleeding. She was subject to constant headaches, progressive lethargy, loss of memory, and inability to concentrate. Habitually she had been consuming 10 to 15 glasses of fluoridated water per day (a total of 2.5 mg to 4 mg of fluoride) and about 6 cups of tea containing about another 3 mg of fluoride.

On October 22, 1971, one of the above-described lesions was noted on the right arm and three on the shins. Because she had observed these so-called "bruises" on many occasions before, her former hospital records and consultations were reviewed. It was determined in retrospect that the illness began in fall 1967, shortly after fluoridation was started in Detroit (August 1967). On October 23, 1971, an X-ray disclosed degenerative changes in the lower spine and narrowing of the joint space. An electroencephalogram revealed evidence of a right-sided inner ear disorder indicative of a disturbance in the area of the brain that maintains the body's equilibrium. Other tests, including those for liver and kidney disease, and an analysis of a 24-hour urine specimen for fluoride, were within normal range. On October 23, 1972, the patient began using distilled water for drinking and cooking exclusively, and she avoided tea. The skin lesions disappeared promptly, and within 2 to 3 weeks all but the spinal symptoms were relieved. By late November 1972, the patient was symptom-free.

On March 15, 1973, the maculae reappeared on the left forearm and on the left thigh simultaneously with pains in the lower spine, dizziness, blurred vision, ulcers, and persistent dryness in the mouth. The patient had become lax in the use of distilled water for nearly a month and had been using fluoridated city water. This episode, however, was aggravated by the inadvertent use of a fluoridated toothpaste, which had precipitated vomiting and cramps in the upper abdomen after brushing her teeth in the morning. Return to the low-fluoride regime promptly cleared up the skin lesions and the accompanying symptoms. On August 12, 1977, the patient reported that she had only minor short-lived recurrences of the lesions, always accompanied by systemic symptoms following inadvertent consumption of fluoridated water.

A few isolated cases of this kind would perhaps not be significant, but they become highly important when numerous patients from different fluoridated cities have essentially the same complaints and when their disease — as will be further shown in subsequent chapters — correlates with the findings of acute fluoride intoxication. We are dealing, therefore, with what is undoubtedly a widespread and seriously debilitating ailment.

The question obviously arises: why are so few physicians apparently aware of these preskeletal toxic effects of waterborne and airborne fluoride? One of the major reasons that makes the diagnosis difficult is the nature of the disease itself, a topic I shall discuss in the following chapter.

REFERENCES

1. Agate, J.N., Belo, G.H., Boddie, G.F., Douglas, T.H.J., and de V. Weir, J.B.: Industrial Fluorosis—A Study of the Hazard to Man and Animals near Fort William, Scotland. Med. Res. Council Memorandum No. 22. His Majesty's Stationery Office, London, 1949.

2. Collings, G.H., Jr., Fleming, R.B.L., and May, R.: Absorption and Excretion of Inhaled Fluorides: Further Observations. Arch. Ind. Hyg. Occup. Med., 6:368-373, 1952.

3. Waldbott, G.L., and Cecilioni, V.A.: "Neighborhood" Fluorosis. Clin. Toxicol., 2:387-396, 1969.

4. Waldbott, G.L., and Steinegger, S.: New Observations on "Chizzola" Maculae, in Proceedings of the Third International Clean Air Congress, Düsseldorf, Federal Republic of Germany, Oct. 8-12, 1973, Verlag des Vereins Deutscher Ingenieure, Düsseldorf, 1973, pp. A63-A67.

5. Møller, P.F., and Gudjonsson, S.V.: Massive Fluorosis of Bones and Ligaments. Acta Radiol., 13:269-294, 1932.

6. Bishop, P.A.: Bone Changes in Chronic Fluorine Intoxication. A Roentgenographic Study. Am. J. Roentgenol. Radium Ther., 35:577-585, 1936.

7. Roholm, K.: Fluorine Intoxication: A Clinical-Hygienic Study. 1937.

8. DeSepibus, C., and DeChastonay, J.L.: Un cas de Fluorose en Valais. Radiol. Clin. Biol., 32:340-348, 1963.

9. Champeix, M.J.: Observations récentes d'ostéopétrose fluorée professionnelle. Arch. Mal. Prof. Med. Trav. Secur. Soc., 21:357-361, 1960.

10. Ravault, P.P., Vignon, G., Roche, L., Lejeune, E., Maitrepierre, J., and Lambert, R.: Deux nouvelles Observations d'ostéopétrose fluorée. Rev. Rhum. Mal. Osteo-Artic., 27:158-161, 1960.

11. Spéder, E.: L'ostéopétrose généralisée ou "marmorskelett" n'est pas une maladie rare: sa fréquence dans l'intoxication fluorée. J. Radiol. Electrol., 20:1-11, 1936.

12. Bruusgaard, A.: Astmalignende Sykdom Blant Norske Aluminiumsarbeidere. Tidsskr. Nor. Laegeforen., 80:796-797, 1960.

13. Midttun, O.: Bronchial Asthma in the Aluminium Industry. Acta Allergol., 15:208-221, 1960.

14. de Vries, K., Lowenberg, A., Coster van Hoorhout, H.E.V., and Ebels, J.H.: Long-Term Observations in Exposure to Fluorides. Pneumonologie, 150:149-154, 1974.

15. Vischer, T.L., Bernheim, C., Guerdjikoff, C., Wettstein, P., and Lagier, R.: Industrial Fluorosis, in T.L. Vischer, Ed.: Fluoride in Medicine. Hans Huber, Bern, 1969, pp. 96-105.

16. Schlegel, H.H.: Industrielle Skelettfluorose. Vorlaufiger Bericht über 61 Falle aus Aluminiumhütten. Soz. Praeventivmed., 19:269-274, 1974.

17. Franke, J.: Histological Changes of Human Fluorosis, Experimental Fluorosis in Animals and Osteoporosis Following Sodium Fluoride Therapy. Fluoride, 5:182-199, 1972.

18. Franke, J.: Scanning Electron Microscopic Studies in Human Industrial Fluorosis. Fluoride, 9:127-138, 1976.

19. Czerwinski, E., and Lankosz, W.: Fluoride-Induced Changes in 60 Retired Aluminum Workers. Fluoride, 10:125-136, 1977.

20. Derryberry, O.M., Bartholomew, M.D., and Fleming, R.B.L.: Fluoride Exposure and Worker Health: The Health Status of Workers in a Fertilizer Manufacturing Plant in Relation to Fluoride Exposure. Arch. Environ. Health, 6:503-514, 1963.

21. Tourangeau, F.-J.: La santé du travailleur dans l'industrie de l'extraction de l'aluminium. Laval Med., 9:548-561, 1944.

22. Dinman, B.D., Bovard, W.J., Bonney, T.B., et al.: Prevention of Bony Fluorosis in Aluminum Smelter Workers. Absorption and Excretion of

Fluoride Immediately After Exposure–Part 1. J. Occup. Med., 18:7-13, 1976; cf. Parts 2-4, ibid., 18:14-23, 1976.

23. Waldbott, G.L., and Lee, J.R.: Toxicity Due to Repeated Low-Grade Exposure to Hydrogen Fluoride (Case Report). Clin. Toxicol., in press, 1978.

24. Klotz, M.: Über einen eigentümlichen Fall von Periostitis hyperplastica ungeklärter Ursache (Fluor-Schädigung?) bei einem Säugling. Arch. Kinderheilkd., 117:267-272, 1939.

25. Murray, M.M., and Wilson, D.C.: Fluorine Hazards with Special Reference to Some Social Consequences of Industrial Processes. Lancet, 2:821-824, 1946.

26. Reynolds Metals Corp. vs. Paul Martin et al.: Transcript of Record. U.S. Court of Appeals, Ninth District, Nos. 14990-14992, June, 1958.

27. Balazova, G., Macuch, P., and Rippel, A.: Effects of Fluorine Emissions on the Living Organism. Fluoride, 2:33-36, 1969.

28. Herbert, J., Françon, F., and Grellat, P.: L'ostéopétrose fluorée en Savoie. Rev. Rhum. Mal. Osteo-Artic., 34:319-331, 1967.

29. Schmidt, C.W.: Auftreten von Nachbarschaftsfluorose unter der Bevölkerung einer sächsischen Kleinstadt. Dtsch. Gesundheitswes., 31:1271-1274, 1976.

30. Carnow, B.W., and Conibear, S.A.: Report: CASAW Study of the Effects of Aluminum Smelting on the Health of ALCAN Workers in Kitimat, British Columbia, Canada. Univ. Illinois School of Public Health, Chicago, Nov. 1977.

31. Mills, W.C.B., Medical Officer of Health: Ontario Water Resources Commission, Chemical Laboratories, Sherbrooke Township, Analyses Nov. 30 through Dec. 6, 1965.

32. Cristofolini, M., and Largaiolli, D.: Su di una probabile tossidermia da fluoro. Rivista Med. Trentina, 4:1-5, 1966.

33. Colombini, M., Mauri, C., Olivo, R., and Vivoli, G.: Observations on Fluorine Pollution Due to Emissions from an Aluminum Plant in Trentino. Fluoride, 2:40-48, 1969.

34. Waldbott, G.L., and Cecilioni, V.A.: "Chizzola" Maculae. Cutis, 6:331-334, 1970.

CHAPTER 11

FLUORIDE IN SOFT TISSUES

THE BROAD SPECTRUM of symptoms in chronic fluoride poisoning, whether from water, air, food, or drugs, has been confusing and perplexing to most investigators. Indeed, some critics of reported ill effects from fluoridation have suggested that we are not dealing with a clear-cut disease entity at all, but rather with imaginary illness.[1] Episodic pains in many parts of the body, headaches, persistent fatigue, and upset stomach are of course among the principal complaints of persons who become ill because of psychological trauma. How can fluoride affect so many organs of the body and produce such a wide variety of symptoms?

We have already seen in Chapter 1 that multiple, wide-ranging complaints and ailments are characteristic of the initial stage of many kinds of chronic intoxication that precede the characteristic features of the particular kind of poisoning. For instance, the "lead line" of the gums and the palsy of the radial nerve of the arm, which are the two hallmarks of chronic lead poisoning, the softening of bones in chronic cadmium poisoning, and the changes in the thyroid gland in cobalt poisoning are always preceded, or accompanied by, various symptoms of the kind encountered in incipient chronic fluoride poisoning. These multiple hidden effects of slow poisoning contradict widespread, excessively optimistic beliefs in "safe limits" of toxic substances in our environment. Actually, subclinical poisoning can harm vast numbers of people before obvious clinical symptoms appear.

Although two conspicuous and readily diagnosable signs of chronic fluorosis are the changes in bones and teeth, neither is a prerequisite or an infallible criterion of the disease. The small size of the fluoride ion and its high charge density enable it to penetrate into every cell of the body and to combine with other ions, especially polyvalent positive ions. Its interference with the metabolism of calcium and phosphorus and with the function of the parathyroid glands is a reflection of its marked affinity for calcium ions. Moreover, because of its tendency to bind with magnesium and manganese ions, fluoride interferes with the activity of many enzyme systems that require these two cations, especially those enzymes involved in carbohydrate metabolism, in bone formation, and in nerve-muscle physiology.

ENZYMES

The sensitivity of different enzymes to the action of fluoride varies considerably. Some are inhibited; others are activated. Some systems such as nucleoside diphosphokinases are only slightly affected, whereas, under appropriate conditions, others such as the lipases and phosphatases are extremely sensitive to fluoride. Although most studies have been carried out under *in vitro* conditions on isolated enzyme preparations, there is now a substantial body of data on the *in vivo* effects of fluoride on enzymes in living organisms.

Enzyme Inhibition. Since the classical experiments by O. Warburg and W. Christian in 1942,[2] it has been recognized that fluorides are strong inhibitors of glycolysis, due to interference with the glycolytic enzyme enolase.[3,4] Another enzyme involved in glycolysis, phosphoglucomutase, which catalyzes the reaction between glucose-1-phosphate and glucose-6-phosphate, is also inhibited by fluoride ions, presumably through formation of a magnesium fluoride complex with glucose-1-phosphate.[5]

Two important *in vivo* studies related to glucose metabolism may have considerable bearing on water fluoridation. In 1962, W. D. Sullivan and A. J. von Knobelsdorff reported that 1-ppm sodium fluoride in the drinking water caused a 6.4% decrease in the activity of succinate dehydrogenase in liver tissue, and a 47.8% decrease in the kidneys of golden hamsters after nine months.[6,7] Recently, Kaul has observed – both in experimental animals and in patients with skeletal fluorosis – a marked inhibition of succinate dehydrogenase activity.[8] This effect can account for impairment of oxidative metabolism in skeletal muscles and is undoubtedly responsible for the muscular weakness and muscle wasting encountered in chronic fluoride poisoning, even in the preskeletal phase.

Table 11-1

In Vitro Inhibition of Mammalian Enzymes by Fluoride[11]

Enzyme	Fluoride Concentration Molarity	Ppm	Percent Inhibition
Human salivary acid phosphatase	2×10^{-4}	3.8	55
Erythrocyte inorganic pyro- phosphatase	2×10^{-5}	0.38	52
Sheep brain glutamine synthetase	5×10^{-5}	0.95	50
Liver esterase (lipase) pH 8.0	5×10^{-3}	95.0	50
″ ″ ″ pH 3.0	6×10^{-7}	0.011	50
Human plasma cholinesterase	5×10^{-5}	0.95	61
″ ″ ″	5×10^{-6}	0.095	12
″ ″ ″	2×10^{-6}	0.038	7
″ ″ ″	5×10^{-7}	0.0095	1

Fluoride has also been shown to cause a decrease in the active ion transport at the cell membrane and an increase in the membrane permeability of cells because of its inhibition of pyrophosphatase activity.[3,9] This inhibition also interferes with fatty acid oxidation.[10] Examples of *in vitro* inhibition of selected mammalian enzymes at extremely low concentrations are presented above in Table 11-1.[11]

Enzyme Activation. Clinicians have given much attention to alkaline phosphatase, an enzyme involved in the growth of bones and the function of the liver, which may be drastically affected by low-level fluoride intake. In advanced chronic fluoride poisoning and following large doses of sodium fluoride (100 mg daily up to three years) in the treatment of osteoporosis, alkaline phosphatase activity usually remains elevated in the blood serum.[12,13] In my own case studies of incipient chronic fluoride poisoning, serum alkaline phosphatase was often elevated, but this finding was not a consistent diagnostic criterion of the disease.[14] On the other hand, in 33 students at Newcastle, England, who consumed 1-ppm fluoridated water, the alkaline phosphatase of the serum decreased to 86% of the initial control values after four weeks of fluoridation, but after eight weeks it returned to pre-test levels.[15] Such initial disturbance of alkaline phosphatase activity, and then its return to normal, suggests a certain degree of adaptation to fluoride by the body, but the long-term effect is still unknown.

Among other seemingly contradictory findings, similar enzymes from different parts of the same organism may show varying degrees of sensitivity to fluoride. For instance, at very low concentrations fluoride inhibits the esterase in human liver but apparently not in the pancreas and the bowels.[16] Similarly, the administration of sodium fluoride to rabbits in doses of 50, 30, and 10 mg per kg of body weight for a period of 3 months inhibited the phosphorylase activity of the liver and the myocardium but not of skeletal muscle.[17] Likewise, although isocitric dehydrogenase levels are lowered in rats,[18] they are slightly elevated in squirrel monkeys[19] after long-term exposure to low levels of fluoride, but other enzymes are only mildly affected. Clearly, many factors control the action of fluoride on enzyme systems: the concentration and dose, the duration of exposure, the ease of penetration (pH-dependent), the type of organism, the nature and susceptibility of the enzyme, etc. Since virtually every vital function of the body is dependent on enzymes, and since fluoride readily reaches every organ in the body, it is not surprising that this halogen produces a wide range of toxic symptoms.

SOFT TISSUES: RANGE OF F⁻ LEVELS

For years, many scientists have assumed that bones and teeth are the only major targets for fluoride. For instance, Hodge and Smith categorically state: "No soft tissue stores fluoride."[20] This view is still widely accepted, but contrary evidence has been growing steadily, mainly from investigations carried out for other purposes. For example, in patients with kidney stones in New York City with little or no fluoride in the drinking water prior to fluoridation in September 1965, analyses of organ tissue for fluoride revealed 181 ppm in kidneys and 290 ppm in skin.[21] The aorta of an infant with extensive generalized calcification of arteries who died shortly after birth in fluoridated Ames, Iowa, contained 59.3 ppm of fluoride at autopsy.[22] Clinicians have recorded 61 ppm in the liver of a Texan who died with skeletal fluorosis at age 64.[23] In a cataract lens, removed surgically, I found 77.3 ppm[24] (see Fig. 11-1 below, page 152).

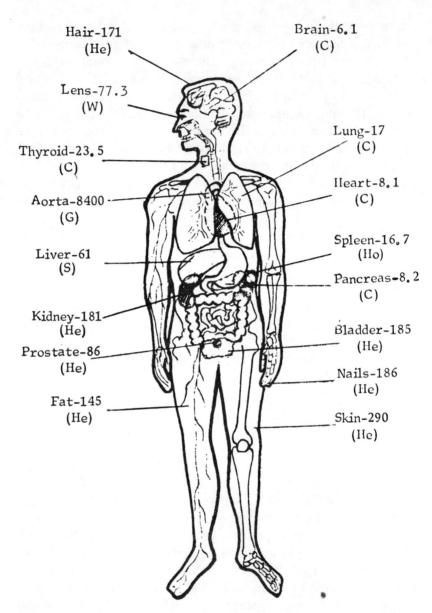

Hair-171
(He)

Brain-6.1
(C)

Lens-77.3
(W)

Lung-17
(C)

Thyroid-23.5
(C)

Heart-8.1
(C)

Aorta-8400
(G)

Spleen-16.7
(Ho)

Liver-61
(S)

Pancreas-8.2
(C)

Kidney-181
(He)

Bladder-185
(He)

Prostate-86
(He)

Nails-186
(He)

Fat-145
(He)

Skin-290
(He)

Fig. 11-1. Highest reported fluoride concentrations (ppm) in soft tissues. (C = Call, R.A., et al., *Public Health Rep.,* 80:529-538, 1965; G = Geever et al.[25] ; He = Herman et al.[21,46]; Ho = Hodge and Smith[20]; S = Sauerbrunn et al.[23] ; W = Waldbott.[14,60]

The highest fluoride value in soft tissue organs recorded to date is 8,400 ppm in the aortas of persons who had lived in fluoridated Grand Rapids and 2,340 ppm in the aorta of a person who had lived in an unfluoridated city in New York State.[25] Such high levels exceed those generally found in the bones, even in advanced skeletal fluorosis.

Observations of this nature demonstrate that fluoride is stored in soft tissue and that fluoride levels vary unpredictably from person to person and even within the organs themselves. The question then arises: how does the storage of fluoride in such organs or its passage through them affect their function? Most research on this subject in the past has dealt with doses larger than those involved through drinking artificially fluoridated water. Nevertheless, the data in the following sections warrant careful consideration since they provide a biological basis for the symptoms I have described in Chapters 9 and 10 on chronic fluoride poisoning.

KIDNEYS

One of the most striking features in the early stage of fluorosis is the craving for fluids, accompanied by excess production of urine. Indeed, the more water the patient drinks the thirstier he or she becomes.[26] Polyuric nephropathy (a kidney disease characterized by excess urination) has been established as a major manifestation of fluoride toxicity in its early stage.[27] This fact and the important role of the kidneys in the elimination of fluoride from the body have led to extensive studies of the action of fluoride on kidneys.

Experimental Data. For instance, the presence of 500 ppm of sodium fluoride in the diet of rats for 21 to 28 days produced damage to the kidney tubules which regulate homeostasis (the equilibrium of ions) in the blood.[28] Similar levels of fluoride intake resulted in impaired kidney function and accounted for retention of non-protein nitrogen and of creatinine in the blood.[29] Such high intakes of fluoride also affect the glomeruli, the filtering units of the kidneys.[30] Fluoride in amounts of 2 to 7.5 mg given daily to rats for 18 to 48 weeks induced excessive thirst, frequent urination, and increased elimination of nitrogen through the urine. It also lowered the kidney threshold for sugar. Histologic

examination showed vascular, glomerular, and tubular degeneration leading finally to interstitial fibrosis.[31]

In contrast to these short-term, relatively large-dose experiments, three Cornell University scientists more closely approached
conditions of fluoridation by giving 0, 1, 5, and 10 ppm of fluoride
in drinking water to 86 albino rats throughout 520 days or their
approximate lifetime.[32] In these prolonged experiments with
small amounts of fluoride corresponding to the daily human
intake from fluoridated water, they found changes in the tubules
which were similar to those from larger doses in short-term experiments; the kidneys of the control rats drinking nonfluoridated
water remained normal. In a follow-up study, the same abnormalities were observed, but this time the authors concluded that the
changes were due to "old age."[33,34] Such a difference in interpretation of the same results could have been easily resolved had the
affected kidneys been analyzed for their fluoride content and compared with those of the control animals. Since no analyses were
made, these studies did not rule out the possibility that consuming fluoridated water at the 1 ppm concentration throughout a
person's lifetime can damage the kidneys. In fact, electron microscopic examination of the kidneys of monkeys drinking fluoridated
water at a concentration of 1 and 5 ppm for 18 months reveals
definite cytochemical abnormalities compared to controls on fluoride-free water.[19]

Observations on Humans. Related observations are also available
on humans with skeletal fluorosis, where kidney disease is not uncommon. In persons drinking water containing 5 to 16.2 ppm fluoride (about 7 to 25 mg per day), kidney function was impaired,
as indicated by depressed clearance of urea, lowered rate of filtra-
tion, and enhanced elimination of amino acids—products of protein metabolism.[35-37]

Unfortunately, it can rarely be determined whether a coexisting
kidney dysfunction is actually the result of long-term fluoride intake or whether, on the other hand, the skeletal changes are precipitated by excessive fluoride storage in the body, because of a
pre-existing kidney disorder. For instance, the autopsy of a 22-
year-old Texas soldier with extensive skeletal fluorosis, who had
been drinking natural fluoride water at concentrations from 1.2 to
5.7 ppm during most of his life, revealed complete destruction of

both kidneys, as discussed in Chapter 8 (above).[38] In two other kidney patients, ages 17 and 18, bone changes typical of fluorosis as well as increased water consumption – up to 7.6 liters a day – were reported by two Mayo Clinic physicians.[39] Throughout his life the younger patient had consumed water containing 1.7 ppm fluoride; the older one drank water from two different sources containing 2.6 ppm and 0.4 ppm. These concentrations are very close to those recommended for artificial fluoridation. It is of course difficult to establish the cause and effect relationship, but the occurrence of skeletal fluorosis so early in life in teenagers who were consuming relatively low-fluoride water is certainly noteworthy.

In my medical practice I have encountered two cases in which fluoridated water interfered with kidney function. One of these,[40] Miss G. L., 27 years old, had been under my care from July 1966 to September 1969 for allergic nasal and sinus disease. She had a congenital cystic kidney necessitating consultation with a urologist. As shown by its inability to excrete indigo carmine, a dye employed as an indicator of kidney function, the left kidney was not working and was slated for removal. This patient also reported having pains and numbness in arms and legs, spasticity of the bowels, ulcers in the mouth, headaches, and a progressive general disability – symptoms of possible intolerance to fluoride – for about 15 years. Her water supply (Highland Park, Michigan) had been fluoridated since September 1952. On February 1, 1967, I instructed her to avoid fluoridated water for drinking and cooking. Within a few weeks *all* the above-mentioned symptoms disappeared, and another kidney dye test on June 12, 1967, astonishingly revealed that the left kidney had begun to function again! A follow-up 5 years later revealed that the patient had remained in good health as long as she refrained from drinking fluoridated water.

The other patient, Mrs. E. P., 39 years old, who visited me on August 25, 1969, had advanced pyelitis of the left kidney, beginning osteosclerotic changes in the pubic bones, and exostosis at the sternum, accompanied by the same clinical picture as in the patient just discussed. The function of the diseased kidney and the other symptoms improved markedly within six weeks after she stopped drinking the municipal water in Midland, Michigan (fluoridated since January 1946). Twenty-four-hour urinary fluoride excretions before and after the tests were 2.39 and 4.20 mg, respectively. For most of her life she had resided in Lubbock, Texas (water supply fluoride then 4.4 ppm). The development of osteosclerosis in this case was not surprising, since – as recorded in fluoridated Evanston, Illinois,[41] and also in a fluoridated Finnish community[42] –kidney patients retain as much as 60% more fluoride than do persons in normal health. In the Finnish work blood fluoride levels were 3 to 4 times higher than normal in the patients with renal disorders.

In marked contrast to these clinical observations of individuals with kidney disease, a USPHS survey reported no loss of kidney function among 116 persons in "natural fluoride" (8 ppm) Bartlett, Texas, compared with a control group of 121 residents of nearby "low-fluoride" Cameron (0.4 ppm).[43] Likewise, no significant difference in the albumin content, number of red blood cells, and casts were found in the *pooled* urine specimens of 12-year-old boys in Newburgh, N.Y., compared with those who had used nonfluoridated water in Kingston.[44] The urine volumes of the boys in fluoridated Newburgh, however, were slightly larger than those of the controls in nonfluoridated Kingston, thus suggesting greater water intake in the fluoridated city. Another statistical study of 728 necropsies in Colorado Springs with 2.5 ppm fluoride naturally in water reported that "comparative statistical analyses of the pathologic findings" of the kidneys and other organs "revealed no significant differences which could be related to prolonged residence" in that area.[45] Unfortunately, however, electron microscopic findings were not presented in these surveys, and kidney pathology cannot be ruled out; indeed, it should be anticipated. In this connection it should be mentioned that certain kinds of kidney stones have been found to contain fluoride ranging up to 1795 ppm.[46,47] The physiological significance of these findings has not yet been determined.

Although USPHS statistical data seem to rule out any gross pathological effect of waterborne fluoride on kidneys, my clinical findings clearly indicate that artificially fluoridated water can impair kidney function. Moreover, there is much irrefutable evidence that a person with renal insufficiency not only retains and stores more fluoride in the skeleton but also has significantly higher levels of fluoride in the soft tissues and blood. Obviously, such a person is more susceptible to systemic poisoning from fluoridated water than a person with normal kidney function.

HEART

Besides the kidneys, the heart and blood vessels are also potential targets for damage from fluoridated water. This conclusion is suggested by the findings of fragmentation or breakage (Fig. 11–2 below) of elongated cells of the heart muscle in acute fluoride poisoning from massive doses[48] and also of cardiac irregularities and low blood pressure observed in experimental poisoning with large

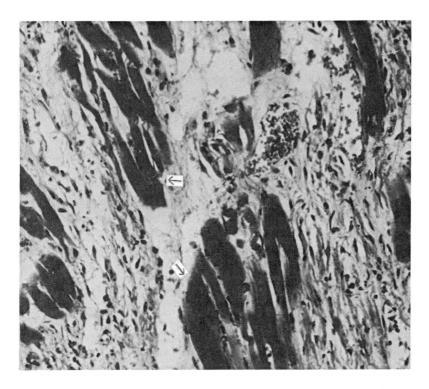

Fig. 11–2. Microphotograph of heart muscle of a 37-year-old man poisoned by magnesium fluorosilicate.[48] Note breakage of muscle fibers (arrows), interstitial edema, and cellular infiltration.
(Courtesy O. Pribilla, Kiel, West Germany.)

doses.[49] In a naturally "high-fluoride" area in Japan (6 to 13 ppm in drinking water), changes in the electrocardiogram and enlargement of the heart in children have been linked to fluoride in the water.[50] Because of a sparsity of data on the effect of fluoridated water on the heart, however, we must again refer to statistical studies.

When the mortality rates for cancer, kidney, liver, and heart diseases in 32 "natural-fluoride" cities were compared in 1954 with those of 32 "non-fluoride" cities, no significant differences were reported.[51] On the other hand, by 1950, five years after the introduction of fluoridation in the experimental city of Grand Rapids, Michigan (January 1945), the number of deaths from heart disease had nearly doubled: from 585 in 1944 to 1059 in 1950.[52] Mortality rates for heart and other chronic diseases (Table 11–2 opposite) were 25% to 50% above those of Michigan as a whole.[53] Although other large (but nonfluoridated) cities in Michigan such as Flint did not show such excess mortality, one perhaps cannot place too much reliance on these data because of differences in the age structure of the population and other factors in Grand Rapids at the time. (For further discussion, see Chapter 19, pp. 359-360.)

ARTERIES

More dependable are the available data on the action of fluoride on blood vessels. In at least six widely separated "natural-fluoride" areas, clinicians have observed calcification of arteries in association with skeletal fluorosis[54 – 58] (Fig. 11–3 opposite). When such damage occurs in persons consuming natural fluoride water at 3 or more parts per million, it is logical to anticipate that less conspicuous changes in the arteries will occur at slightly lower concentrations.

In support of this view I have already mentioned in Chapter 8 the striking case of a newborn infant in Ames, Iowa, whose arteries had accumulated extraordinary amounts of fluoride (59.3 ppm).[22] A careful inquiry revealed no appreciable sources of fluoride intake other than the fluoridated drinking water. Because of the absence of any other causes for this unusual finding, there is strong reason to suspect that the death of this child was related to artificially fluoridated water the parents had been drinking for 4 years.

Table 11-2

1950 Mortality in Grand Rapids and the State of Michigan[53]

Cause of Death	DEATHS PER 100,000 POPULATION	
	Grand Rapids	Entire State
Heart disease	403.9	322.1
Cancer	189.2	136.3
Intracranial lesions	149.6	100.1
Diabetes	32.3	22.6
Arteriosclerosis	26.1	20.3

Another indication of the vulnerability of arteries to fluoride is the microscopic appearance of the bruise-like skin lesions, Chizzola maculae, described in Chapter 10, which display inflammatory areas around capillary blood vessels suggestive of a toxic reaction. These early signs of fluorosis probably should be interpreted as the beginning of a life-long process that may eventually result in the above-described calcifications.

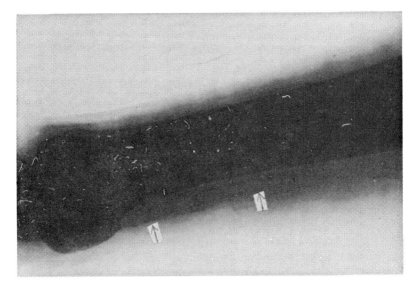

Fig. 11-3. X-Ray showing calcified artery associated with sclerosis of tibia and fibula in a 55-year-old male residing in a high natural fluoride (3-5 ppm) area of Sicily.
(Courtesy Drs. G. Nalbone and F. Parlato, Palermo, Italy.)

The extraordinary storage of fluoride in the aorta, the largest artery of the body, has been documented repeatedly. J.L. Steinfeld, former Surgeon General of the USPHS, has explained that high concentrations of fluoride in arteries might simply be the result of natural calcification accompanying the aging process: "it has been shown that fluoride accumulates as an adventitious constituent in the mineral phase during calcification of both soft and hard tissues."[59] However, in 16 cases which I selected at random in 1966 from autopsy material at Hutzel Hospital, Detroit, no correlation between fluoride and calcium in the aortas was found.[60] In other words, the degree of fluoride accumulation in the aorta was *not* dependent upon the amount of calcium. This observation was further corroborated by a review of the fluoride and calcium values on 59 cases in industrial Utah communities in which the fluoride levels of the aorta varied erratically.[60] Therefore, fluoride in arteries appears to attract calcium and thus can contribute directly to their hardening.

CENTRAL NERVOUS SYSTEM

The manifestations of the initial phase of fluorosis also indicate injury to the central nervous system – the brain and the spinal cord. Indeed, in many of my patients afflicted with fluorosis, the neurological manifestation – especially episodes of excruciating headaches, vertigo, spasticity in the extremities, visual disturbances, and impaired mental acuity – had suggested to the attending physicians a brain tumor, multiple sclerosis, or a similar ailment.

Partial and complete paralysis of arms and legs in advanced fluorosis is usually related to pressure upon the spinal cord of newly-formed bone protruding into the spinal canal, and upon nerves at the point of their exit from the spine, which can be demonstrated by X-ray. J. Franke, a clinician in Halle, D.D.R., has presented important evidence in a fatal case of industrial fluorosis, that the fluoride ion can damage nerve tissue without physical pressure upon the spinal cord. For the first time, he and his colleagues observed tissue damage to a certain portion of the spinal cord – the cells of the anterior horns – without the presence of newly formed bone in the respective vertebral area.[61]

Soviet physicians have detected neurological symptoms in 79% of patients with occupational fluorosis, thus also suggesting direct nerve involvement by fluoride. This work indicated that fluoride caused a "higher nervous activity and dysfunction of subcortical axial nonspecific structures of the brain."[62] Moreover, Polish investigators have reported intensified activity of the enzymatic complexes in the Purkinje cells of the cerebellar cortex of guinea pigs following daily intramuscular administration of sodium fluoride in large doses (4 mg/kg in a 1% aqueous solution) for three months.[63] If such a direct action of fluoride upon nerve tissue should be confirmed by further studies, it would explain some of the diverse neurological complaints in arms and legs, such as numbness, muscle spasms and pains, and the frequent headaches as well as damage to the optic nerve and the retina that I and others have encountered in the early stage of fluoride poisoning before bone changes occur. There is also evidence that fluoride-induced reduction in circulating magnesium and/or calcium may play a role in these effects.

That fluoride affects muscle tissue as well as nerves, and thus accounts for muscular atrophy and weakness, has been unequivocally demonstrated by the administration of large doses (50 mg/kg body weight) of sodium fluoride to rabbits daily for a maximum of 45 days.[64] In another investigation a reduction of muscle fibers and deterioration of nuclei in muscles in humans with skeletal fluorosis as well as in experimental animals was observed.[65] Upon electron microscopic examination, every component of muscle tissue – the muscle fiber filaments, the mitochondria. and the nuclei – showed damage. No unusual changes were noted, however, in nerve tissue. These experiments furnish a plausible explanation for the marked muscular weakness and fibrillation of the extremities and muscles throughout the body that I have reported in preskeletal fluorosis.[26]

GASTROINTESTINAL TRACT

Stomach and bowel disorders are cardinal features of intolerance to fluoride, undoubtedly because the stomach and the upper portions of the bowels are the major pathway through which the halogen enters the blood stream. Free hydrochloric acid, which is normally present in the stomach at a concentration of ca. 0.1 molar (0.2% to 0.4%) and is considerably increased in persons with gastric ulcers, reacts with fluoride compounds to form highly corrosive hydrofluoric acid.[66] This fact undoubtedly accounts for the common occurrence of hemorrhages and other corrosive changes in the upper gastrointestinal tract in acute fluoride poisoning from large doses (Fig. 7-2 above, page 92). Even with small amounts of fluoride sufficient hydrofluoric acid can form in the stomach and produce gastric pains, nausea, and vomiting common in preskeletal fluorosis. This has also been established by R. Feltman and G. Kosel, who observed stomach and bowel upsets in about 1% of 1,100 pregnant women and young children receiving fluoride tablets for prevention of tooth decay in doses corresponding to those supposedly obtained from the average daily consumption of fluoridated water.[67] It is not surprising, therefore, that 12 out of 60 retired aluminum workers afflicted with skeletal fluorosis were found to have gastric ulcers.[68]

Apparently the delicate lining of the gastrointestinal tract in young children and infants is particularly susceptible to injury from fluoride. For instance, five infants who received 0.5 mg of fluoride per day in drops—an amount equal to the intake from 500 ml of fluoridated water—developed hemorrhages in the stomach and bowels (as evidenced by bloody stools) that promptly disappeared when this medication was discontinued.[69] Gastric hemorrhages were also discovered in five newborn infants whose mothers had been exposed during pregnancy to fluoride fumes in a Czechoslovakian aluminum factory.[70]

I have had occasion to review the record and the microscopic findings of a dramatic instance of fluoride-induced stomach damage. On August 24, 1962, the chief surgeon of one of the large southern hospitals consulted me about a nine-year-old boy, W.B.B., Jr. Gastric hemorrhages had necessitated the removal of a large portion of the stomach. After the boy's return home from the hospital, he promptly suffered another hemorrhage so severe that a part of the upper bowel had to be removed. This time, careful questioning revealed that several hours before the second incident, the boy had taken a 1 mg fluoride tablet for prevention of tooth decay. The attending physicians concluded that the fluoride tablet had caused the hemorrhages and thus was responsible for the child losing much of his digestive tract.[71]

The microscopic sections of the boy's stomach revealed another remarkable and rare phenomenon – the presence of so-called teleangiectasis, areas of widened capillary blood vessels below the surface of the stomach. This unusual finding supports the causal relationship to fluoride, since teleangiectasis also occurs on the skin of patients treated with fluorine-containing cortisone medications, but not if the cortisone molecule lacks fluorine.[72]

THYROID GLAND

One of the most outstanding features of preskeletal fluorosis is the extraordinary general fatigue experienced by most sufferers. Such marked weakness is usually linked by physicians to a low activity of the thyroid gland. The role of this gland in fluorosis has been subject to controversy since 1854 when the French physiologist E. Maumené, who was studying the toxicity of fluoride, observed a tumor, presumably a goiter, on the neck of a dog to which he had administered 20 to 120 mg of sodium fluoride daily for four months. In the early part of this century several clinicians, convinced that fluoride intake reduces the activity of the gland, administered sodium fluoride on a large scale, particularly in Germany, Switzerland, and Argentina, for the control of hyperthyroidism (overactive thyroid).[73] On the advice of a Vienna clinician, patients with toxic goiter have reportedly benefited by bathing in a highly diluted solution of hydrofluoric acid, which is known to reach the blood stream after penetrating normal skin.[74]

A high incidence of goiter has been observed by some, and denied by others, in countries where skeletal fluorosis is endemic.[75] In India, for example, small visible goiters have been connected directly to high concentrations of fluoride in drinking water in persons 14 to 17 years of age.[76] In the vicinity of Rome, Italy, A. Benagiano and colleagues compared the thyroid function (circulating thyroid hormone) of 20 residents of Campagnano (2.1 ppm fluoride in water) and 21 of Anguillara (1.7 ppm) to the thyroid function of residents in an "optimal" (1 ppm) fluoride community. In the high fluoride areas, they found both significant increases and decreases in thyroid function.[77]

The most plausible explanation of such paradoxical findings is that fluoride does not impede the normal capacity of the thyroid gland to synthesize the thyroid hormone if there is abundant iodine in the blood.[78] When the total iodine pool of the body is low, however, fluoride interferes with the function of the gland and thereby produces a fluoride-iodine antagonism. This interpretation is further supported by a survey on 648 people in 13 mountainous villages of Nepal where the iodine content of water is low (0.001 ppm or less) and where goiter is prevalent. There was a close correlation between fluoride intake and the incidence of goiter.[79]

In most cases of poisoning from fluoridated water in which I had occasion to study the action of the thyroid gland, its function was low. For instance, a 33-year-old male, A.B., who had been drinking fluoridated water for 8 years, exhibited typical manifestations of preskeletal fluorosis and a basal metabolism rate of -22, indicative of hypothyroidism (depressed thyroid activity). Within 3 months after he ceased consuming fluoridated water, the thyroid function had returned to normal (BMR = 0). Simultaneously, other symptoms associated with low-grade fluoride poisoning — including excessive thirst, headaches, blurred vision, arthritis in shoulders, elbows and knees, and gastrointestinal disturbances — also disappeared.

PARATHYROID GLANDS

The endocrine glands that regulate the distribution of calcium and phosphorus in the body are the parathyroids. These four cherry-sized glands located in the neck on both sides of the thyroid gland are extremely sensitive to excessive intakes of fluoride, which upset the delicate balance of calcium and phosphorus in the blood and produce epilepsy-like convulsions. In lambs with about 200 ppm fluoride in their drinking water for one week, the parathyroid glands became enlarged, and an excess of parathyroid hormone appeared in the blood.[80] Moreover, clinicians studying endemic fluorosis in India have found a close relationship of skeletal fluoride poisoning with hyperparathyroidism (over-activity of the parathyroid glands).[81]

Scientists in an endemic area of Algeria offer a reasonable explanation for the involvement of the parathyroid glands. In rabbits that received 21.4 mg fluoride per day for 10 months they observed a lowered intestinal absorption of Ca and P which, combined with excess urinary excretion of these two elements due to a decrease in their reabsorption in the renal tubules, led to secondary hypocalcemia and to stimulation of the parathyroid glands (hyperparathyroidism).[82]

PITUITARY GLAND

Situated at the base of the brain, the pituitary gland, which controls water and sugar metabolism and the rate of growth, has also been connected with fluoride poisoning.[83] Excessive thirst and an increased output of urine in patients intolerant to fluoridated water[14] might be related to a reduced release of vasopressin from this gland. Pituitary diabetes insipidus, it should be noted, is associated with diminished vasopressin.[84] Sauerbrunn's patient with advanced skeletal fluorosis consumed 4 to 10 liters of water per day[23] (normal is about 2 liters). In guinea pigs fed large amounts of fluoride, the pituitary gland is enlarged.[85] Furthermore, less than normal amounts of thyroid hormone are deposited in the pituitary gland when rabbits are given fluoride in water at levels corresponding to that of artificially fluoridated water.[85] The role of the pituitary as well as that of the adrenal glands in fluorosis, however, has not been sufficiently explored.

EYES

The eyes may serve as a valuable guidepost in diagnosis, since they often reflect what occurs inside the body. Blurred vision, inability to focus, and the presence of moving spots (scotomata) in the eyes have occurred frequently in my fluorosis patients. Examination by ophthalmologists has revealed distinct widening of retinal vessels, an early sign of retinitis. I recall especially the case of W.P.D., 45 years old, in whom the severity of these symptoms almost forced him to abandon his avocation of flying until his condition was completely remedied simply by his avoidance of fluoridated water.[14] Objective vascular changes in the retinal arteries were associated with his condition.

A more advanced case of retinitis has been reported following administration of 60 mg daily in three doses (20 mg each) of sodium fluoride for six weeks to a patient in the treatment of osteoporosis.[86] Furthermore, animal experimentation has confirmed the production of retinitis by fluoride in large doses.[87,88] Since the retina is genetically a part of the central nervous system, it is likely to be involved by a toxic process affecting nerve substance.

Fluoride involvement in diseases of the lens of the eye is less certain in light of current knowledge. The presence of up to 77.3 ppm fluoride in cataracts,[24] however, as discussed earlier in this chapter, strongly suggests that the halogen could take part in their production, and other observations support this view. In the often quoted Bartlett-Cameron study, the incidence of cataracts in subjects of 15 or more years' residence was high—10.1% in Bartlett and 14.1% in Cameron[43] —compared to an estimated U.S. average of less than 5% for adults over age 35.[89] In a survey of the high-fluoride Province of Punjab, India, the prevalence of cataracts was significantly higher than in low-fluoride regions of the upper and lower Himalayas, namely 7.2% vs. 3.8% and 5%, respectively.[90] Furthermore, an above average rate of blindness caused by senile cataracts in naturally high-fluoride Green Bay, Wisconsin, together with the strikingly high incidence of cataracts among adult mongoloids (67 out of 95 cases in one of the Wisconsin institutions), were observed in work leading to studies on the relationship of fluoride in drinking water to the appearance of mongolism (see Chapter 13, below).[91,92]

EARS

Minute amounts (0.1 mg) of sodium fluoride given twice daily for 10 days to guinea pigs have been reported to cause no apparent damage to the structure of the ear on microscopic investigation. In the organ of Corti, however, a deficiency in several enzymes, especially acid phosphatase, was observed.[93] Impairment of enzyme activity in the ear could be the reason for such symptoms as vertigo and tinnitus that I have often found in my cases. On the other hand, comparatively large doses of sodium fluoride have been administered for limited periods for the control of otosclerosis, and in some individuals this treatment seems to have been beneficial.[94]

SKIN

The pinkish to bluish-brown skin lesions called "Chizzola" maculae—inflammation around capillary blood vessels—described in the previous chapter, are often the earliest signs of chronic fluoride poisoning in children and women. Other skin lesions such as acne eruptions and allergic reactions are generally known to be caused by iodides and bromides. It is not surprising, therefore, that the much more reactive fluoride ion also causes these disorders, especially since some fluoride is eliminated from the body through the skin. However, only limited data on this point are recorded in the literature. In 1956, a German clinician described "fluoride acne" in a worker at a glass factory following exposure to hydrogen fluoride.[95] On the other hand, a California dermatologist gave lozenges containing 2.0 mg of calcium fluoride (ca. 0.97 mg of fluoride ion) to 20 acne patients every day for an average of six weeks, and concluded that fluoride neither aggravated nor alleviated the eruptions.[96] Since he administered other remedies concurrently with the calcium fluoride, his results cannot be considered conclusive.

In fact, the opposite results are more often observed. For example, dermatitis and hives are not uncommon following intake of, or bathing in, fluoridated water.[97] The occurence of contact dermatitis from the use of fluoridated toothpaste containing approximately 0.1% (1000 ppm) fluoride which I have described has been confirmed by several other investigators; moreover, controlled patch tests for sodium and stannous fluoride were positive.[98,99] I have encountered—as have other allergists—patients who developed severe urticaria following the use of fluoride toothpaste and after topical application of fluoride to teeth. The following is a typical case:

On May 19, 1975, K. W., a 9-year-old girl allergic to pollen and fungi, experienced severe itching in the mouth while her dentist was applying a 2% sodium fluoride solution to her teeth for prevention of tooth decay. The child had previously shown Chizzola maculae on arms and legs and had "mild" mottling of teeth. Within 10 minutes after the fluoride treatment, her lips and face swelled up, followed by the appearance of ulcers in the lining of the mouth—some as large as a pea—and by swelling of lymph glands with fever up to 102°F. It took three weeks for the condition to subside. Interestingly, the maculae on her arms and legs recurred on the second day following the fluoride treatment; they have since been controlled by strict avoidance of Detroit's fluoridated water.

The intake of fluoride, even in amounts as small as those consumed in fluoridated communities, produces a kaleidoscope of adverse effects. Yet most studies on fluoride today generally emphasize its action on teeth and bones and largely disregard the clear fact that, with such broad systemic toxic properties, fluoride *must* involve other organs as well. The evidence in this chapter leaves no doubt on this matter. As the spectre of danger looms ever greater year by year, doctors and dentists must recognize the contradictions of making patients ill, rather than alleviating their sickness, by allowing the fluoride burden of the body to increase beyond prudence and reason. These dedicated health bringers face a great dilemma.

REFERENCES

1. Hornung, H.: Fluoridation: Observations of a German Professor and Public Health Officer. J. Am. Dent. Assoc., 53:325-326, 1956.

2. Warburg, O., and Christian, W.: Isolierung und Kristallisation des Gärungsferments Enolase. Biochem. Z., 310:384-421, 1942.

3. Klahr, S., Kantrow, C., and Bricker, N.S.: Effect of Metabolic Inhibitors and Strophanthin on Sodium Transport and Metabolism of the Isolated Turtle Bladder. Comp. Biochem. Physiol., 33:773-782, 1970.

4. Hamilton, I.R.: Studies with Fluoride-Sensitive and Fluoride-Resistant Strains of *Streptococcus Salivarius*. II. Fluoride Inhibition of Glucose Metabolism. Can. J. Microbiol., 15:1021-1027, 1969.

5. Slater, E.C., and Bonner, W.D., Jr.: The Effect of Fluoride on the Succinic Oxidase System. Biochem. J., 52:185-196, 1952.

6. Sullivan, W.D., and Von Knobelsdorff, A.J.: The *In Vitro* and *In Vivo* Effects of Fluoride on Succinic Dehydrogenase Activity. Broteria Ser. Trimest. Cienc. Nat., 31:3-13, 1962.

7. Sullivan, W.D.: The *In Vitro* and *In Vivo* Effects of Fluoride on Succinic Dehydrogenase Activity. Fluoride, 2:168-175, 1969.

8. Kaul, R.D.: Fluoride Toxicity and Muscular Manifestations: Histoenzymic and Ultrastructural Effects in Man and Animal. Ph.D. Dissertation submitted to the All-India Institute of Medical Sciences, 1976.

9. Daniel, E.E.: Potassium Movements in Rat Uterus Studied *In Vitro*. II. Effects of Metabolic Inhibitors, Ouabain, and Altered Potassium Concentration. Can. J. Biochem. Physiol., 41:2085-2105, 1963.

10. Batenburg, J.J., and van den Bergh, S.G.: The Mechanism of Inhibition by Fluoride of Mitochondrial Fatty Acid Oxidation. Biochim. Biophys. Acta, 280:495-505, 1972.

11. Wiseman, A.: Effect of Inorganic Fluoride on Enzymes, in F.A. Smith,

Ed.: Pharmacology of Fluorides, Part 2, Vol. XX/2 of Handbook of Experimental Pharmacology. Springer-Verlag, Berlin, Heidelberg, and New York, 1970, pp. 48-97.

12. Merz, W.A., Schenk, R.K., and Reutter, F.W.: Paradoxical Effects of Vitamin D in Fluoride-Treated Senile Osteoporosis. Calc. Tissue Res., 4 (Suppl.): 49-50, 1970.

13. Srikantia, S.G., and Siddiqui, A.H.: Metabolic Studies in Endemic Fluorosis. Clin. Sci. (Oxf.), 28:477-485, 1965.

14. Waldbott, G.L.: Fluoride in Clinical Medicine. Int. Arch. Allergy Appl. Immunol., 20, Suppl. 1, 1962.

15. Ferguson, D.B.: Effects of Low Doses of Fluoride on Serum Proteins and a Serum Enzyme in Man. Nat. New Biol., 231: 159-160, 1971.

16. Gomori, G.: Histochemistry of Human Esterases. J. Histochem. Cytochem., 3:479-484, 1955.

17. Iwase, T.: Studies on the Glycogen and Phosphorylase Variations in Myocardium, Skeletal Muscle, and Liver in Experimental Fluorosis. II. Influence of Fluorine on Phosphorylase. Shikogu Ikagu Zasshi, 12:624-629, 1958.

18. Doberenz, A.R., Kurnick, A.A., Kurtz, E.B., Kemmerer, A.R., and Reid, B.L.: Effect of Minimal Fluoride Diet on Rats. Proc. Soc. Exp. Biol. Med., 117:689-693, 1964.

19. Manocha, S.L., Warner, H., and Olkowski, Z.: Cytochemical Response of Kidney, Liver and Nervous System to Fluoride Ions in Drinking Water. Histochem. J., 7:343-355, 1975.

20. Hodge, H.C., and Smith, F.A.: Metabolism of Inorganic Fluoride, in J.H. Simons, Ed.: Fluorine Chemistry, Vol. IV. Academic Press, New York and London, 1965, p. 143.

21. Herman, J.R., Mason, B., and Light, F.: Fluorine in Urinary Tract Calculi. J. Urol., 80:263-267, 1958.

22. Bacon, J.F.: Arterial Calcification in Infancy. J. Am. Med. Assoc., 188:933-935, 1964. For fluoride levels in tissues, see Waldbott (in Ref. 40, below).

23. Sauerbrunn, B.J.L., Ryan, C.M., and Shaw, J.F.: Chronic Fluoride Intoxication with Fluorotic Radiculomyelopathy. Ann. Intern. Med., 63:1074-1078, 1965.

24. Waldbott, G.L.: Comments on the Symposium: "The Physiologic and Hygienic Aspects of the Absorption of Inorganic Fluorides." Arch. Environ. Health, 2:155-167, 1961.

25. Geever, E.F., McCann, H.G., McClure, F.J., Lee, W.A., and Schiffmann, E.: Fluoridated Water, Skeletal Structure, and Chemistry. Health Serv. Mental Health Admin., Health Rep., 86:820-828, 1971.

26. Waldbott, G.L.: Incipient Chronic Fluorine Intoxication from Drinking Water. Acta Med. Scand., 156:157-168, 1956.

27. Whitford, G.M., and Taves, D.R.: Fluoride-Induced Diuresis: Plasma Concentrations in the Rat. Proc. Soc. Exp. Biol. Med., 137:458-460, 1971; Fluoride-Induced Diuresis: Renal Tissue Solute Concentrations, Functional, Hemodynamic, and Histologic Correlates in the Rat. Anesthesiology, 39:416-427, 1973.

28. Pindborg, J.J.: The Effect of 0.05 Per Cent Dietary Sodium Fluoride on the Rat Kidney. Acta Pharmacol. Toxicol., 13:36-45, 1957.

29. Kawahara, H.: Influence of Sodium Fluoride on the Urine Changes and Non-Protein Nitrogen, Creatinine and Sodium Chloride in Serum of Rabbits. Shikoku Acta Med., 8:266-272, 1956. (Abstracted in Fluoride, 5:46-48, 1972.)

30. Kawahara, H.: Experimental Studies on the Changes of the Kidney Due to Fluorosis. Part 3. Morphological Studies on the Changes of the Kidney of Rabbits and Growing Albino Rats Due to Sodium Fluoride. Shikoku Acta Med., 8:283-288, 1956. (Abstracted in Fluoride, 5:50-53, 1972.)

31. Bond, A.M., and Murray, M.M.: Kidney Function and Structure in Chronic Fluorosis. Br. J. Exp. Pathol., 33:168-176, 1952.

32. Ramseyer, W.F., Smith, C.A.H., and McCay, C.M.: Effect of Sodium Fluoride Administration on Body Changes in Old Rats. J. Gerontol., 12:14-19, 1957.

33. Bosworth, E.B., and McCay, C.M.: Pathologic Studies of Rat Kidneys: Absence of Effects Ascribed to Fluoride Following Long-Term Ingestion of Drinking Water Containing Fluoride. J. Dent. Res., 41:949-960, 1962.

34. Lovelace, F., Black, R.E., Kunz, Y., Smith, C.A.H., Bosworth, E.B., Wang, C.N., Austria, L., Park, R.L., and McCay, C.M.: Metabolism of Fluoride in Old Rats and Hamsters. J. Appl. Nutr., 12:142-151, 1959.

35. Shortt, H.E., McRobert, G.R., Barnard, T.W., and Mannadi Nayar, A.S.: Endemic Fluorosis in the Madras Presidency. Indian J. Med. Res., 25:553-568, 1937.

36. Siddiqui, A.H.: Fluorosis in Nalgonda District, Hyderabad-Deccan. Br. Med. J., 2:1408-1413, 1955.

37. Singh, A., Jolly, S.S., Bansal, B.C., and Mathur, C.C.: Endemic Fluorosis. Epidemiological, Clinical and Biochemical Study of Chronic Fluorine Intoxication in Punjab (India). Medicine, 42:229-246, 1963; 44:97, 1965.

38. Linsman, J.F., and McMurray, C.A.: Fluoride Osteosclerosis from Drinking Water. Radiology, 40:474-484, 1943; correction of misprint, 41:497, 1943.

39. Juncos, L.I., and Donadio, J.V., Jr.: Renal Failure and Fluorosis. J. Am. Med. Assoc., 222:783-785, 1972.

40. Waldbott, G.L.: Hydrofluorosis in the U.S.A. Fluoride, 1:94-102, 1968.

41. Yudkin, E.P., Czerniejewski, J., and Blayney, J.R., and Zoller, W.G.:

Evanston Dental Caries Study. XIII. Preliminary Report on Comparative Fluoride Retention in Human Tissue. J. Dent. Res., 33:691-692, 1954 (Abstract).

42. Hanhijärvi, H.: Comparison of Free Ionized Fluoride Concentrations of Plasma and Renal Clearance in Patients of Artificially Fluoridated and Non-Fluoridated Drinking Water Areas. Proc. Finn. Dent. Soc., 70, Suppl. 3, 1974; Inorganic Plasma Fluoride Concentrations and Its Renal Excretion in Certain Physiological and Pathological Conditions in Man. Fluoride, 8:198-207, 1975. For further data and comment, see Marier, J.R.: Some Current Aspects of Environmental Fluoride. Sci. Total Environ., 8:253-265, 1977.

43. Leone, N.C., Shimkin, M.B., Arnold, F.A., Jr., Stevenson, C.A., Zimmerman, E.R., Geiser, P.B., and Lieberman, J.E.: Medical Aspects of Excessive Fluoride in a Water Supply. Public Health Rep., 59:925-936, 1954. (Reprinted in Fluoride Drinking Waters, 1962, pp. 402-411.)

44. Schlesinger, E.R., Overton, D.E., and Chase, H.C.: Study of Children Drinking Fluoridated and Nonfluoridated Water. Quantitative Urinary Excretion of Albumin and Formed Elements. J. Am. Med. Assoc., 160:21-24, 1956.

45. Geever, E.F., Leone, N.C., Geiser, P., and Lieberman, J.: Pathologic Studies in Man After Prolonged Ingestion of Fluoride in Drinking Water. I. Necropsy Findings in a Community with a Water Level of 2.5 p.p.m. J. Am. Dent. Assoc., 56:499-507, 1958. (Reprinted in Fluoride Drinking Waters, 1962, pp. 437-441.)

46. Herman, J.R.: Fluorine in Urinary Tract Calculi. Proc. Soc. Exp. Biol. Med., 91:189-191, 1956.

47. Spira, L.: Urinary Calculi and Fluorine. Exp. Med. Surg., 14:72-88, 1956.

48. Pribilla, O.: Four Cases of Acute Silicofluoride Intoxication. Clinical and Pathological Findings. Fluoride, 1:102-109, 1968.

49. Leone, N.C., Geever, E.F., and Moran, N.C.: Acute and Subacute Toxicity Studies of Sodium Fluoride in Animals. Public Health Rep., 71:459-467, 1956. (Reprinted in Fluoride Drinking Waters, 1962, pp. 539-544.)

50. Okushi, I.: Changes of the Heart Muscle Due to Chronic Fluorosis. Part I. Electrocardiogram and Cardiac X-Rays in Inhabitants of a High Fluoride Zone. Shikoku Acta Med., 5:159-165, 1954. (Abstracted in Fluoride, 4:194-198, 1971.)

51. Hagan, T.L., Pasternack, M., and Scholz, G.C.: Waterborne Fluorides and Mortality. Public Health Rep., 69:450-454, 1954.

52. Miller, A.L.: Fluoridation of Water—Extension of Remarks. Congressional Record, March 24, 1952, pp. A 1899-A 1901.

53. Prothro Plans Year-Long Probe of City's High Chronic Disease Toll. The Grand Rapids Press, July 27, 1955; also, Why is GR's Death Rate

Above Rest of State's? The Grand Rapids Herald, July 28, 1955.

54. Pinet, F., Pinet, A., Barrière, J., Bouché, B., and Bouché, M.M.; Les ostéopathies fluorées endemique d'origine hydrique – 49 observations d'ostéoses condensantes du Souf (Sud-Algérien). Ann. Radiol. 4:589-612, 1961.

55. Kumar, S.P., and Harper, R.A.K.: Fluorosis in Aden. Br. J. Radiol., 36:497-502, 1963.

56. Soriano, M.: Periostitis Deformans Due to Wine Fluorosis. Fluoride, 1:56-64, 1968.

57. Chawla, S., Kanwar, K., Bagga, O.P., and Anand, D.: Radiological Changes in Endemic Fluorosis. (Brief Review of the Literature and Analysis of Seventeen Cases.) J. Assoc. Physicians India, 12:221-228, 1964.

58. Khan, Y.M., and Wig, K.L.: Chronic Endemic Fluorosis (With Bone Affections) in the Punjab. Indian Med. Gaz., 80:429-433, 1945.

59. Steinfeld, J.L.: Letter to the Editor. Fluoride, 6:69-70, 1973.

60. Waldbott, G.L.: Fluoride and Calcium Levels in the Aorta. Experientia (Basel), 22:835-837, 1966.

61. Franke, J., Rath, F., Runge, H., Fengler, F., Auermann, E., and Lenart, G.: Industrial Fluorosis. Fluoride, 8:61-85, 1975.

62. Popov, L.I., Filatova, R.I., and Shershever, A.S.: Aspects of Nervous System Affections in Occupational Fluorosis. Gig. Tr. Prof. Zabol., 5:25-27, 1974.

63. Czechowicz, K., Osada, A., and Slesak, B.: Histochemical Studies on the Effect of Sodium Fluoride on Metabolism in Purkinje's Cells. Folia Histochem. Cytochem., 12:37-44, 1974.

64. Kaul, R.D., and Susheela, A.K.: Evidence of Muscle Fiber Degeneration in Rabbits Treated with Sodium Fluoride. Fluoride, 7:177-181, 1974.

65. Kaul, R.D., and Susheela, A.K.: The Muscle, in Symposium on the Non-Skeletal Phase of Chronic Fluorosis. Fluoride, 9:9-18, 1976.

66. Roholm, K.: Fluor und Fluorverbindungen, in W. Heubner and J. Schüller, Eds.: Handbuch der experimentellen Pharmakologie, Ergängzungswerk, Vol. 7. Julius Springer, Berlin, 1938, p. 20.

67. Feltman, R., and Kosel, G.: Prenatal and Postnatal Ingestion of Fluorides – Fourteen Years of Investigation – Final Report. J. Dent. Med., 16:190-199, 1961.

68. Czerwinski, E., and Lankosz, W.: Fluoride-Induced Changes in 60 Retired Aluminum Workers. Fluoride, 10:125-136, 1977.

69. Shea, J.J., Gillespie, S.M., and Waldbott, G.L.: Allergy to Fluoride. Ann. Allergy, 25:388-391, 1967.

70. Kauzal, G.: Fluoróza ako etiopatogenetický factor pri vzniku gastroduodenálnych lézlii u novorodencov [Fluorosis as an Etiopathogenic Factor in the Development of Duodenal Ulcers in the Newborn]. Rozhl. Chir., 42: 379-382, 1963.

71. Waldbott, G.L.: Editorial. Gastric Ulcer and Fluoride. Fluoride, 10: 149-151, 1977.

72. Snyder, D.S., and Greenberg, R.A.: Evaluation of Atrophy Production and Vasoconstrictor Potency in Humans Following Intradermally Injected Corticosteroids. J. Invest. Dermatol., 63:461-463, 1974.

73. Roholm (in Ref. 66, above), pp. 38-39.

74. Gorlitzer von Mundy, V.: Einfluss von Fluor und Jod auf den Stoffwechsel, insbesondere auf die Schilddrüse, in T. Gordonoff, Ed.: The Toxicology of Fluorine. Schwabe & Co., Basel/Stuttgart. 1962, pp. 111-117.

75. McLaren, J.R.: Editorial. Fluoride and the Thyroid Gland. Fluoride, 2:192-194, 1969.

76. Siddiqui. A.H.: Incidence of Simple Goiter in Areas of Endemic Fluorosis in Nalgonda District. Andhra Pradesh, India. Fluoride, 2:200-205, 1969.

77. Benagiano, A., Colasanti, A., and De Simone, G.: Studio della funzionalità tiroidea in soggetti residenti in zone fluorotiche. Ann. Stomatol., 1:5-13, 1959.

78. Galletti, P.M., and Joyet, G.: Effect of Fluorine on Thyroidal Iodine Metabolism in Hyperparathyroidism. J. Clin. Endocrinol. Metab., 18:1102-1110, 1958.

79. Day, T.K., and Powell-Jackson, P.R.: Fluoride, Water Hardness, and Endemic Goitre. Lancet, 1:1135-1138, 1972.

80. Faccini, J.M.: Fluoride-Induced Hyperplasia of the Parathyroid Glands. Proc. R. Soc. Med., 62:241, 1969.

81. Teotia, S.P.S., and Teotia, M.: Hyperactivity of the Parathyroid Glands in Endemic Osteofluorosis. Fluoride, 5:115-125, 1972. Cf. Spira, L.: Fluorosis and the Parathyroid Glands. J. Hyg., 42:500-504, 1942.

82. Elsair, J., Poey, J., Reggabi, M., Hattab, F., Benouniche, N. and Spinner, C.: Effets de l'intoxication fluorée sabaiguë du lapin sur les métabolismes fluoré et phosphocalcique et sur la radiographie du squelette. Eur. J. Toxicol., Suppl., 9:429-437, 1976.

83. Cristiani, H.: Modifications histologiques de la glande hypophysaire dans la cachexie fluorique. C. R. Séances Soc. Biol. Fil., 103:981-982, 1930.

84. Klein, H.: Dental Fluorosis Associated with Hereditary Diabetes Insipidus. Oral Surg., 40:736-741, 1975.

85. Jentzer, A.: Action du fluor sur le relais thyroïdenhypophysaire démontrée par l'iode 131. Bull. Schweiz. Akad. Med. Wiss., 10:211-220, 1954.

86. Geall, M.G., and Beilin, L.J.: Sodium Fluoride and Optic Neuritis. Br. Med. J., 2:355-356, 1964.

87. Babel, J., and Avanza, C.: Degenerescence retinienne expérimentale provoquée par le fluorure de sodium. Experientia (Basel), 17:180-181, 1961.

88. Sorsby, A., and Harding, R.: Experimental Degeneration of the Retina. V. Fasting and Metabolic Accelerators in Degeneration Produced by Sodium Fluoride. Br. J. Ophthalmol. 44:213-224, 1960.

89. Based on age distribution in 1970 U.S. Census and figures in Table 2, Chapter 4, in Summary and Critique of Available Data on the Prevalence and Economic and Social Costs of Visual Disorders and Disabilities. Prepared for

the Dept. of Health, Education, and Welfare, USPHS National Eye Institute, by Westat, Inc., Rockville, Md., Feb. 16, 1976 (Contract No. NOl EY 52108).

90. Chatterjee, A.: Cataract in Punjab, in The Human Lens — in Relation to Cataract. Ciba Found. Symp., 19:265-279, 1973.

91. Rapaport, I.: Contribution à l'étude etiologique du mongolisme. Rôle des inhibiteurs enzymatiques. Encephale, 46:468-481, 1957.

92. Rapaport, I.: Les opacifications du crystallin mongolisme et cataracte sénile. Rev. Anthropol. (Paris), Ser. 2, 3:133-135, 1957.

93. Schätzle, W., and von Westernhagen, B.: Enzymhistochemisches Verhalten des Cortiorgans unter der experimentellen Einwirkung von Natriumfluorid. Arch. Klin. Exp. Ohren- Nasen-Kehlkopfheilkd., 200:292-299, 1971.

94. Shambaugh, G.E., Jr.: The Diagnosis and Treatment of Active Cochlear Otosclerosis. J. Laryngol. Otol., 85:301-314, 1971.

95. Andermann, I.: Zur Kenntnis der Fluorakne. Dermatol. Wochschr., 133:245-247, 1956.

96. Epstein, E.: Effect of Fluorides in Acne Vulgaris. Stanford Med. Bull., 9:243-244, 1951.

97. Waldbott, G.L.: Allergic Reactions to Fluoride. J. Asthma Res., 2:51-64, 1964.

98. Saunders, M.A., Jr.: Fluoride Toothpaste: A Cause of Acne-Like Eruptions. Arch. Dermatol., 111:793, 1975.

99. Mellette, J.R., Aeling, J.L., Nuss, D.D.: Fluoride Toothpaste—A Cause of Perioral Dermatitis. Arch. Dermatol., 112: 730-731, 1976.

CHAPTER 12

THE GREAT DILEMMA

AFTER FLUORIDATION BEGAN in the mid-1940s, many people believed that a new and glorious age had dawned for preventive dentistry. At last, with a minimum effort and no essential change in diet, tooth decay would be reduced by an average of 65%! The prospect of extending such an enormous dental benefit to the population at large was breathtaking, and vigorous efforts were begun to promote fluoridation everywhere. At the same time, because of the well-known cumulative toxicity of fluoride, serious doubts naturally arose about the safety of fluoridation. With the ever-increasing spread of fluorides into the environment from constantly expanding industrial and commercial sources, might not fluoridation create a threat to health of unknown magnitude that could outweigh even the most optimistic hopes for dental improvement? From these circumstances The Great Dilemma unfolded.

THE TEETH

Dental Fluorosis. From the very beginning of the fluoridation program, scientists attempted to balance two factors: (1) maximum protection against tooth decay and (2) minimum harm to both the body and the teeth.[1] Indeed, F. F. Heyroth, Cincinnati's Commissioner of Health and Assistant Director of the Kettering Laboratory at the University of Cincinnati, described fluoridation as a "calculated risk."[2] Dental authorities, in fact, had long known that fluoride in drinking water was responsible for the objectionable and irreversible dental defect called "mottled teeth."

In 1916 G. V. Black and F. S. McKay had presented their classic description of mottled teeth in Colorado Springs, where the water contained 2.5 ppm fluoride:

When not stained with brown or yellow, they [mottled teeth] are a ghast-
ly, opaque white that comes prominently into notice whenever the lips
are opened, which materially injures the expression of the countenance of
the individual. When this opaque white color is mingled with spots of
brown, or a very large proportion of brown, the injury is still greater. In
very many cases the teeth appear absolutely black as one sees them in ordinary social intercourse.[3]

In a later publication G. A. Kempf and McKay quoted Black's
technical description:

Mottled enamel is distinguished especially by the absence of cementing
substance between the enamel rods in the outer fourth, more or less, of
the enamel, and presenting great variety of color, rendering it totally different from anything else I have known.[4]

Black and McKay had a strikingly pessimistic outlook about the
prognosis of teeth exhibiting this abnormality:

But when the teeth do decay, the frail condition of the enamel makes it
extremely difficult to make good and effective fillings.
    For this reason many individuals will lose their teeth because of caries,
though the number of carious cavities is fewer than elsewhere. . . . This is
much more than a deformity of childhood. If it were only that, it would
be of less consequence, but *it is a deformity for life*. The only escape from
the deformity is by the placing of crowns, and possibly of bridges or
artificial dentures later in life.[3] [Emphasis added.]

In 1940 M. C. and H. V. Smith, two other early workers in dental fluoride research, concurred with these observations when they
stated:

There is ample evidence that mottled teeth, though they be somewhat
more resistant to the onset of decay, are structurally weak, and that unfortunately when decay does set in, the result is often disastrous.[5]

In St. David, Arizona, with 1.6 to 4.0 ppm fluoride in the drinking water and a high incidence of mottling, the Smiths observed
that although only 33% of the childern 12 to 14 years of age had
any caries,

Beyond the age of 21, there were relatively few individuals in which caries had not developed. That the result of the onset of caries was especially severe is reflected in the high percentage of all age groups with extracted teeth. . . . Steps taken to repair the cavities in many cases were unsuccessful, the tooth breaking away when attempts were made to anchor the fillings, so that extraction was the only course. That decay was widespread and repair was highly unsuccessful among the young adults is shown by an incidence of more than 50 per cent of false teeth in the age group 24 to 26 years. *Very rarely, adults were found whose teeth, though mottled, were free from caries.*[5] [Emphasis added.]

The Smiths remarked further that Cox's recommendation to fluoridate water, food, or medicine "seems, to put it mildly, unsafe." Roholm's ominous warning in 1938 had emphasized the same point: "Because of the harmful effect of fluoride upon tooth formation, it is contraindicated to administer fluoride compounds to children and pregnant and nursing women."[6]

Years later, however, when he visited the experimentally fluoridated city of Newburgh, N.Y., in 1954, and examined "representative members in the grade school," H. V. Smith reported that he found no "mottled teeth."[7] By "mottled" he was probably referring to what advocates of fluoridation euphemistically term "cosmetically objectionable mottling," which they claim does not occur from artificially fluoridated water. In view of the secondary discoloration that often occurs later in life, however, even the "mild" degrees of mottling must be considered "objectionable" from the esthetic point of view (see Figs. 5-6 and 5-7 above, pages 67 and 68).

Index of Dental Fluorosis. In the light of such seemingly contradictory views, a crucial problem had to be solved: what was the optimal amount of fluoride in a water supply that would produce the soundest teeth without the disfigurement of mottling? In 1934 Dean had classified dental fluorosis into six (later five) categories as a basis for estimating a "community index of dental fluorosis."[8] This index was calculated by multiplying the number of afflicted individuals in each category by a weighting factor corresponding to the severity of the mottling and dividing the sum of the result by the total number of persons examined. Dean's categories and weighting factors for classifying dental fluorosis are presented in Table 12-1 on the following page.

Table 12-1

Classification of Degrees of Dental Fluorosis[8,9]

Category	Nature of Affliction[a]	Weighting Factor
Questionable	Slight aberrations from translucency with a few white flecks or occasional white spots	0.5
Very mild	Small, opaque, paper-white areas involving less than 25% of the surfaces of the two most affected teeth; may acquire brownish tint in adulthood	1.0
Mild	More extensive dull white opacities involving less than 50% of the surfaces of the two most affected teeth; brown staining often present	2.0
Moderate	All enamel surfaces affected; distinct brown staining frequent	3.0
Severe	Teeth show marked hypoplasia, attrition, and pitting; brown or black staining widespread	4.0

[a]Normal enamel has a smooth, glossy, natural, pale creamy white translucency and is assigned a weighting factor of 0 in calculating the community index of dental fluorosis.

According to Dean, it is preferable that the community index of dental fluorosis not exceed 0.4; at 0.6 "it begins to constitute a public health problem." From his surveys in Illinois (temperate climate), he found that water supplies containing 1.3 to 1.9 ppm fluoride resulted in an index of 0.5 to 0.7, while those with 0.9 to 1.2 ppm had an index of about 0.3.[9] Astonishing though it may seem, Dean recognized early in the 1940s that the 0.7-1.2 ppm fluoride concentration recommended for fluoridation was *at the borderline that produces disfiguring degrees of dental mottling in a community.*

Although in theory such calculations are attractive, in reality they are misleading. The community index of dental fluorosis does not accurately represent the true state of mottling in a community. It gives the same weight to eight questionable (0.5) cases as to one severe case (4.0); it counts three mild (2.0) or six very mild (1.0) cases as equal to two moderate (3.0) ones (see Figs. 5-5 through 5-8 above, pages 66 through 69). For the individual with an unsightly degree of mottling, it is of no comfort to know that the community index of dental fluorosis is below 0.6 or even below 0.4! This dilemma was clearly perceived by Cox, who first explicitly advocated fluoridation, when he wrote: "With the threat of the Scylla and Charybdis of dental caries and mottled enamel, great caution must be observed in the means of administration of fluorides and in the control of such procedures as may be adopted."[10]

In fact, objectionable degrees of dental fluorosis had been encountered by Dean himself where fluoride concentrations were below 1.0 ppm. He found not only "very mild" but also "mild" dental fluorosis (see Figs. 5-5 and 5-6 above, pages 66 and 67) in midwestern cities with as little as 0.4-0.5 ppm fluoride in the water supply. In Marion, Ohio (0.4 ppm), for example, he observed these degrees of mottling in 6.1% of the 12- to 14-year-old children, and in Kewanee, Illinois (0.9 ppm), he detected them in 12.2% of the children in this age group.[9]

My own survey of 2,000 patients admitted to my allergy clinic between 1955 and 1960 also agrees with these findings. Although Detroit's water supply at that time contained only 0.1 ppm fluoride, I found objectionably fluorosed teeth in 21 allergic patients born and raised in low-fluoride metropolitan Detroit. Their defective enamel may have resulted from fluoride in food or vitamins ingested during early childhood, but extreme sensitivity to very low fluoride water cannot be ruled out. Photographs of some of these teeth (Figs. 12-1 and 12-2, pages 180 and 181) were identified by Dean himself as typical fluoride mottling.[11] Often such dental opacities in "low-fluoride" communities are designated as "idiopathic," i.e., mottling of unknown cause. But in view of the many sources of fluoride intake apart from drinking water, it is quite possible that the halogen is responsible for such mottling in

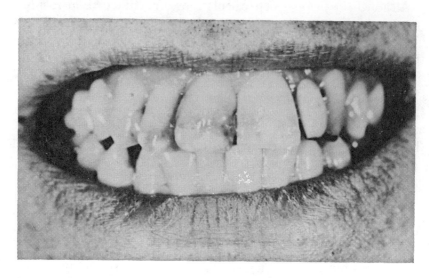

Fig. 12-1. Mottled teeth of a 32-year-old asthmatic male who had lived all his life in low-fluoride (0.1 ppm) Detroit. (Identified as dental fluorosis by H. Trendley Dean at the AMA Council hearing in Chicago, August 7, 1957.)

most cases. As McKay astutely remarked: "Fluorine is the *only* agent ordinarily included in the diet that is capable of exerting a modifying influence on the structure of the enamel."[12] [Emphasis added.]

Surprisingly high incidences of what appears to be dental fluorosis have been encountered elsewhere, in contrast to Dean's findings, even with relatively low concentrations of fluoride in the drinking water. On Tristan da Cunha, for example, 30% of persons six to nine years of age had mottling in 60% of their upper incisors, although the drinking water on this South Atlantic volcanic island contained a maximum of only 0.2 ppm fluoride.[13] In rural areas of Lucknow in north-central India, with 0.4-0.8 ppm fluoride in the drinking water, the incidence of definite fluorosis among 499 children was 24%, including a total of 6% in the "very mild" category or worse.[14] Moreover, in some North African communities with 0.5 ppm fluoride in the water supplies, 25% of the children were afflicted with dental fluorosis, and where the fluoride content was 1.0 ppm the frequency rose to 100%.[15] Although such a high incidence is usually related to the increased water consump-

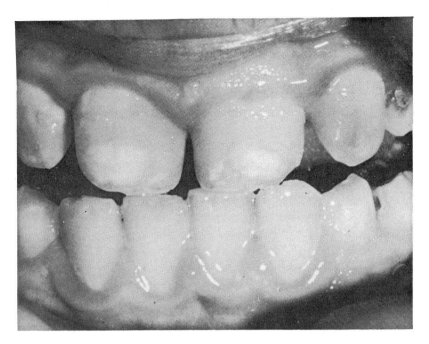

Fig. 12-2. Mottled teeth of an adult female allergy patient who had lived all her life in low-fluoride (0.1 ppm) Detroit. (Identified as dental fluorosis by H. Trendley Dean at the AMA Council Hearing in Chicago, August 7, 1957.)

tion caused by warmer climates, equally high frequencies have been reported from cooler areas. In two low-fluoride (0.05 to 0.41 ppm) districts in Finland, 41% and 74% of the children, respectively, had enamel mottling (including the "questionable" category), and in a fluoridated (1.08 ppm) community the incidence was 98%.[16]

Likewise, in Massachusetts, "enamel fluorosis" was found in 63% of 7- to 12-year-old children living from birth in a fluoridated community near Boston.[17] In this group, 30% had questionable, 22% had very mild, 9% had mild, and 2% had moderate mottling. The authors of this study also reported that fluoride tablets in doses comparable to those obtained from drinking fluoridated water produced even more fluorosis in 7- to 12-year-old children: 17% questionable, 34% very mild, 19% mild, and 14% moderate — a total incidence of 84% mottling! Admitting that the appearance of some of the teeth "was considered undesirable," the authors suggested that "less fluorosis and equivalent caries protection of the permanent teeth might be achieved by decreasing the dose before age 3 yr and increasing the dose after the age of 5-6 yr when most of the tooth crowns are formed."

Other investigations have also revealed a conspicuous lack of consistency in the amount and degree of dental fluorosis in relation to the fluoride content of drinking water. In the Province of Punjab in India, 81% of 5- to 15-year-old children in the village of Mandi Baretta (0.73 ppm fluoride) had definite mottling; in Khara, with 9.4 ppm fluoride in the water, or over ten times as much, the percentage was essentially the same – 80%.[18] A comparison of the incisors of 15-year-old children in fluoridated (1.0 ppm) Anglesey, Wales, with low-fluoride (<0.1 ppm) Bangor and Caernarvon revealed about equal incidences of mottling in both areas, namely 35% (88 persons) in Anglesey and 37% (97 persons) in the other two cities. The authors therefore concluded that there was "no association between mottling in Anglesey with either the fluoride content or the hardness of the drinking water."[19] But the habitual consumption by British children of substantial quantities of tea that is high in fluoride[20] undoubtedly accounts for much of the mottling in the "low-fluoride" cities. A comparable percentage of "fluoride opacities" was reported by A. L. Russell in 1962 for Grand Rapids, Michigan, after 16 years of fluoridation, namely 19.3% in the white and 40.2% in the Negro children.[21] The community index of fluorosis, however, was only 0.15 for the white and 0.31 for the Negro groups – well below the 0.40 level regarded by Dean as "borderline."

In 1949 V. O. Hurme had anticipated Russell's findings by also observing significantly more enamel opacities in the upper incisors of Negro children in low-fluoride (<0.25 ppm) New Haven, Connecticut.[22] Russell considered such mottling "unimportant from the esthetic point of view,"[21] but in my experience most children with fluoride opacities become self-conscious about the defective appearance of their teeth, especially as they grow older, when the white lesions often take on a brownish tint. Nevertheless, some dental proponents of fluoridation go so far as to claim that the "very mild" and "mild" classifications of Dean (Figs. 5-5 and 5-6 above, pages 66 and 67; cf. Figs. 12-1 and 12-2 above, pages 180 and 181) are actually "desirable degrees ... of fluorosis for all children."[23] How such levels of disfiguring dental fluorosis can be considered *unobjectionable,* let alone "desirable," is impossible to comprehend. Even so, these same authors clearly recognize the dilemma of mottling in fluoridation when they admit: "It is not possible, however, to adjust the fluoride level in a water supply to insure that all children in a region will exhibit only the desirable [!] degrees of enamel fluorosis."[23] Furthermore, their own data show that the levels of fluoride they recommend for different mean maximum temperatures *produce community indexes of dental fluorosis in the excessively high range of 0.5 to 0.6!*

Concentration Not Optimally Beneficial. The above evidence amply demonstrates that fluoridation at the "optimal" concentration does *not* provide a sufficient margin of safety with respect to dental health; moreover, it is doubtful whether this concentration even provides maximum benefit to teeth. In Qiryat Haiyim, a suburb of Haifa, Israel, with a mean maximum temperature of 78°F. and an "optimal" concentration of 0.76 ppm fluoride in water naturally, the number of DMF teeth in all age groups was not any lower than in the major low-fluoride cities of Israel, but the incidence of dental fluorosis was "higher than expected."[24] In 18 West German communities and in 27 places around Jena in East Germany, the incidence of dental caries failed to show any decrease with increasing concentrations of fluoride (up to 0.8 ppm) in the drinking water.[25,26]

In Lucknow, India, a large-scale survey disclosed more tooth decay – as well as mottling – with 0.8–1.2 ppm fluoride in the water supply than with 0.3–0.4 ppm.[14] Likewise, a study of over 20,000 Japanese school children revealed less tooth decay where the fluoride level in the water was only 0.2-0.4 ppm than where it exceeded 0.4 ppm.[27] These investigations sharply underscore the impossibility of having, simultaneously, both an innocuous and an optimally effective concentration of fluoride in drinking water -- a dilemma indeed!

Calcifications in and about Teeth. The prospect of another disturbing problem further compounded the dilemma, namely the irregular distribution of calcifications in and about the teeth. The behavior of fluoride as a bone and tooth seeker is highly erratic, and enhanced calcification is not limited to the enamel and dentin: in natural fluoride areas the halogen produces new deposits of

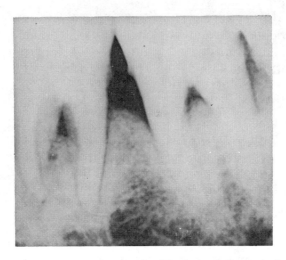

Fig. 12-3. Dental changes associated with skeletal fluorosis involving hyper-
cementosis around the roots of the teeth with loss of lamina dura and resorption of alveolar bone due to secondary hyperparathyroidism.
(Courtesy Dr. S.P.S. Teotia, Meerut, India.)

bone or bone-like material both inside the pulp chamber and ex-
ternally on the roots of teeth (Fig. 12-3 above) in a manner similar
to the fluoride-induced calcifications that appear on the inner and
outer surfaces of bones.[28] When such newly formed calcified material is localized inside the dental pulp, it narrows the pulp chamber, interferes with the tooth's nutrition, and rarifies the dentin
adjoining the plug.[29,30]

Periodontal Problems. Around the roots new, irregular, bone deposits loosen the tooth in its socket and attract bacteria, a process
that predisposes persons to periodontal (gum) disease. Promotion
of this condition by fluoride has been demonstrated experimentally in rats having a 520-day exposure to drinking water containing
only 1.0 ppm fluoride.[31] In humans, periodontal disease has been
linked to "high-fluoride" water by Dean[32] and by others,[33,34] although opposite findings have also been claimed.[35]

In October 1955, at a medical conference in Lubbock, Texas
(formerly 4.4 ppm fluoride in the water supply), local dentists and
physicians informed me that *most* lifetime residents of the town
had lost all their teeth because of gum disease by the time they

had reached age 35! At lower fluoride levels, such as in artificial fluoridation, the limited data are inconclusive. In 1957 a USPHS study showed no significant association of periodontal disease with either "fluoride" or "non-fluoride" cities,[36] but other reports have claimed slight improvement in periodontal health among children with fluoridation.[35] In 1974 a comparison of 12- to 14-year-old boys in a phosphate mining area of Morocco showed no significant difference in gum disease between a community with 0.25-0.54 ppm fluoride in the water and one with 0.93 ppm.[37] Conceivably, the beneficial effect of increased dietary phosphate in the area contributed to the prevention of periodontal disorders; the differences in fluoride intake, as in many other studies, were probably too small to create much dissimilarity in the periodontal status of the two groups.

Delayed Dentition. Another effect associated with increased fluoride intake and with mottling is a delay in the eruption of teeth. This was recognized by a number of early investigators[38] and was later attributed to fluoride-induced suppression of thyroid function,[39] which laboratory studies have shown to be a direct cause of retarded tooth eruption.[40] In Colorado Springs (2.5 ppm fluoride) the permanent teeth of the children exhibited "an appreciably lower eruption rate" than in low-fluoride cities.[41] This finding was confirmed in a long-term investigation of the administration of fluoride tablets to pregnant mothers and to children up to age 9, resulting in a marked "delay in the eruption of the teeth, in some cases by as much as a year from the accepted eruption dates."[39]

In fluoridated cities a delay in the eruption of the permanent teeth – attributed by certain authors to decreased caries in the deciduous teeth rather than to thyroid inhibition – has been observed in some studies but not in others.[42] After ten years of fluoridation, the average number of erupted permanent teeth per 9- to 12-year-old child in Newburgh, N.Y., was 9.35, compared with 9.82 in the nonfluoridated control city of Kingston.[43] In Brazil, "a delay in tooth eruption" was found with fluoridation,[44] but in a study at Evanston, Ill., the authors concluded that fluoridation "does not retard the normal shedding of deciduous teeth or the eruption of the permanent dentition."[45]

Caries Statistics. Although delayed dentition might not be a matter of much concern *per se*, retardation in the eruption of

teeth by as much as one to three years, as found in many areas of
endemic fluorosis,[38] does create serious problems in the interpretation of caries-reduction data in fluoridated communities. Figures
for DMF (decayed, missing, filled) permanent teeth in such cities
suggest that there is a one- to three-year delay in the *onset* or *recognition of caries* and that the *rate of decay* (i.e., the number of
new cavities per year) does not differ appreciably from that in
low-fluoride communities. This fact was first pointed out by R.
Weaver in comparing decay rates in naturally fluoridated (1.4 ppm)
South Shields, England, with those in low-fluoride (0.25 ppm)
North Shields.[46] The 12-year-old children in South Shields in 1943
had 56% fewer DMF teeth than those in North Shields—"a remarkable result," but then he added:

> I suggest, however, that such a comparison can be most misleading. The
> question which really needs to be answered is: How many years does it
> take for the figure 2.4 DMF permanent teeth in South Shields to reach 4.3
> in North Shields? The answer is approximately three years. . . . the fact re-
> mains that children 15 years of age in South Shields have the same average
> amount of caries as is found in North Shields at 12 years of age.[46]

Weaver's investigation also indicated a longer postponement
period of about five years for the DMF rates of adults in South
Shields to equal those of persons in North Shields. In the United
States, K. K. Paluev, a professional statistician and research
engineer, carried out a similar analysis of the 10-year DMF figures
from fluoridated Grand Rapids and Newburgh and showed that
the same interpretation applied.[47] In Austria, R. Ziegelbecker has
extended this approach to other fluoridation studies and has
shown that the annual increments in tooth decay among older
children in the nonfluoridated control communities decline faster
than in the fluoridated ones, thus gradually nullifying the apparent
initial benefit of fluoridation.[48]

The effect of delayed onset of caries in combination with a similar annual decay increment is well illustrated by the official
results after 11 years of fluoridation in the United Kingdom.[49] As
seen in Table 12-2 (opposite), the amount of caries *increases* in
the permanent teeth from age 8 through 14 are practically the
same in both the fluoridated study areas and the nonfluoridated

Table 12-2

Results After Eleven Years of Fluoridation
in the United Kingdom[49]

Age (years)	DMF Teeth (latest year)	
	Fluoridated Areas	Nonfluoridated Areas
8	1.2	2.0
9	1.8	2.7
10	2.4	3.3
11	3.0	4.0
12	4.0	5.6
13	5.4	6.9
14	6.3	7.2
Increase from age 8 through age 14	5.1	5.2

control areas — 5.1 and 5.2 DMF teeth per child (for the latest year of data)! In other words, fluoridation evidently delayed the initiation of the decay process by a year or two but did not appreciably change the *rate* of decay.

Inconsistency in the data is also a major problem in fluoridation statistics. Examiner variability and differences in time, diet, environment, and other factors all combine to make comparisons uncertain and unreliable. For example, when Weaver examined the teeth of 12-year-old children in low-fluoride North Shields in 1949, he found that his 1943 DMF count of 4.3 had decreased to 2.3 – the same figure he had determined in naturally fluoridated South Shields in 1943. During the same period the DMF count in South Shields decreased to 1.3, and he concluded that these reductions were primarily the effect of the less cariogenic nature of the British war and postwar diet.[50]

Data from Grand Rapids, Michigan, furnish another example. When M. Klerer, a computer scientist at New York University, compared the DMF rate (0.234) of 6-year-old children in that city in 1946 with that (0.380) in 1949, after four years of fluoridation, he noted that there had "been an *increase* in decay of 62 per cent."[51] In 1951 the rate was lower but still 10% higher than in

1946. "Clearly," he commented, "the decay rate, as a function of time elapsed during fluoridation, is anything but 'mathematically precise'. These variations are found consistently in the data for the other age groups as well. . . . the *apparent* over-all pattern must be subject to doubt if its individual elements are in contradiction to each other and inconsistent with that pattern."

Klerer also pointed out additional inconsistencies:

> The figures presented for Muskegon, the "control city" (no fluorine), generate an even more horrible statistical nightmare. . . . we find a reported *increase* of decay of over 200 per cent in the five-year-old group between 1946 and 1949; a reported *decrease* in decay of 40 per cent between the base year [1944-1945] and 1946 for the six-year-olds, and an *increase* in decay of 66 per cent between 1946 and 1951. . . . The ten-year-olds shown an *increase* of 35 per cent between 1947 and 1948 although the base year to 1951 comparison shows a *decrease*. The variations are similarly evident for the eleven through fifteen-year-old groups. The sixteen-year-old group shows a magnificent decay *decrease* of nearly one-third from 1946 to 1947. . . ."[51]

Further inconsistency is evident in the National Research Council report of 1952, which pointed out that at the time Muskegon began to fluoridate its water supply in July 1951 the 6- and 7-year-old children were showing a decrease in dental caries of 22% and 28%, respectively, even without fluoridation.[52]

Preliminary results from Ottawa, Kansas, also illustrate these contradictions. There C. A. Scrivener found that the percentage of children five and six years of age who had caries-free teeth *decreased* from 82% in 1946 to only 45% in 1949 after three years of fluoridation (and the introduction of municipal water softening).[53] On the other hand, the official State survey claimed an overall *increase* in decay-free teeth for the six- and seven-year-old children for the period 1946-1951, together with a 15% and 11% decline, respectively, in the DMF rates for these two age groups.[54] In his article Klerer also discussed similar inconsistencies in the data from the Kingston-Newburgh, Evanston, and Charlotte, N.C., pilot fluoridation studies.[51]

When DMF data from different regions and different countries are compared, even more glaring inconsistencies come to light. For example, in 1965 an official Kansas study indicated that the DMF count for 10-year-old children in three nonfluoridated control

cities was 2.22, and in three fluoridated cities it was 1.19.[55]   But
in the 1974 Massachusetts study[17] referred to above (page 181),
the DMF count for children of this average age in a fluoridated
community near Boston was 3.16 — a figure that is 42% higher
than that of the *non*fluoridated group in Kansas! In Yamashima,
Japan, after eleven years of fluoridation (0.6 ppm), the average
DMF rate of the 12- and 13-year-old children *rose* from 1.67 to
2.55, *an increase of 53% with fluoridation!* On the other hand,
since the decay rate for this age group in the control town of
Shugakuin increased by 187% (DMF from 1.43 to 4.10) over this
same period, it was concluded that fluoridation had exerted some
protective benefit.[56]

In still another example, DMF rates of children and of adults up
to age fifty were actually lower in areas of Hungary with less than
0.35 ppm fluoride in the water than those reported for "optimally" fluoridated (natural or artificial) communities in the United
States, Canada, and England.[57]   Although the Hungarian data also
indicated 61% less tooth decay among young adults (age 20-25)
living in a 1.1 ppm fluoride area as compared with persons living in
low-fluoride control areas, by age 50-55 this difference had decreased to only 11%. Therefore, the decay-preventive effect of fluoride is neither uniform nor permanent.

Another crucial factor to be considered in evaluating caries
statistics is the variability and possible bias of the examiner. One
investigation demonstrated, for example, that repeated examinations of the same tooth by the same examiner yielded widely varying caries scores from one examination to another.[58] In a different
study, when each of the 33 patients was examined by three of
eight different dentists, a deviation of 89% in the number of cavities was recorded.[59] In one case two of the dentists found 12 cavities, while the third found only five. In another case one dentist
found 13 cavities, the second found six, and the third found only
five. Overall, the average difference in assessment for the 33
patients was 4.2 carious teeth and 5.8 carious surfaces. With such
large and glaring discrepancies, it is obvious that any conclusion
based on differences of only two or three DMF teeth, as is often
the case in fluoridation studies, has only marginal value at best.
Realistically speaking, such conclusions are highly questionable,
perhaps even worthless.

Still another shortcoming of DMF scores as a reliable measure of dental caries is the fact that missing teeth, especially in older subjects, are often lost or extracted for reasons other than decay.[60] Likewise, a tooth that has one small filling counts the same as one with several large fillings; the amount of decay is clearly quite different, yet both teeth count as only *one* DMF tooth. Moreover, in modern dental practice fillings in molars are often "prophylactic" in nature and are made to seal fissures rather than to repair actual cavities; nevertheless, they count the same as "decayed" teeth. Such fillings, like orthodontic work, often reflect socio-economic conditions more than any absolute measure of dental conditions. It is also reasonable to assume that dental examiners in most official fluoridation studies have usually already been convinced of the dental benefits of fluoride, and this conviction can hardly fail to affect their assessments.

That bias may well have played a part in the favorable results reported from the original pilot studies is evident from the trenchant criticisms dental researchers such as P. R. N. Sutton of the University of Melbourne have leveled against them. Sutton drew attention to "omission of relevant data, arithmetical errors, misleading comments, doubtful or inadequate controls," and even the counting of unerupted teeth as "decay-free" teeth.[61] Interim reports on the Evanston study, he noted, gave different figures for the base-year sample size, reported as 4,375 children in 1946. (In the final report of 1967 it was given as 3,682.[45]) His conclusion: "The sound basis on which the efficacy of a public health measure must be assessed is not provided by these five crucial trials." Sutton's criticisms naturally sparked some lively responses, to which he replied in the second edition of his book.[61]

Other Minerals. A further complication in the fluoride-caries relationship was the possible role of minerals other than fluorides in the water or diet. Dean and co-workers showed their awareness of this fact when, in connection with their first report on the Galesburg-Quincy (Illinois) study, they wrote:

> While on the basis of our present knowledge it appears reasonable to associate the low caries rates observed at Galesburg and Monmouth with the presence of small amounts of fluorides in the domestic water, the possibility that the composition of the water in other respects may also be a factor that should not be overlooked.[62]

The importance of compositional differences in water and food can be observed in a New Zealand study in which children (six, seven, and eight years old), after 4.5 years of fluoridation in the city of Hastings, actually had *more* tooth decay than in the non-fluoridated control city of Napier with only 0.15 ppm fluoride in the water.[63] The lower caries rates in Napier were attributed primarily to higher levels of molybdenum (a similar effect had been observed in Hungary[64]) and other minerals in the Napier water and food compared with those in Hastings. By ages nine and ten, however, the protective factors in Napier seem to have been balanced by fluoridation in Hastings, for by then the differences in decay rates between the two cities virtually disappeared.

Vanadium and strontium are two other trace elements that evidently have significant decay-reducing properties. Lower cavity scores have been related to vanadium in drinking water "even in concentrations as low as 0.007-0.09 ppm."[65] Low-caries experience has also been correlated with strontium in regions (about one ppm in water,[66]) where it appears to accumulate optimally to about 200 ppm in the inner enamel, along with a similar amount of fluoride. High-caries individuals, on the other hand, were found to have enamel-strontium levels that are appreciably higher or lower than 200 ppm.[67]

In contrast to the favorable effects of these minerals, a marked caries-promoting action has been demonstrated from excess intake of selenium (mainly from foods in certain areas).[65,68] Likewise, too much copper in the water or diet seems to "negate" the anti-caries benefit of molybdenum.[67,69] Indications of trace-element effects appear in the data for six Illinois cities originally studied by Dean (Table 12-3, next page).[70] Although the DMF rates decreased roughly in proportion to the increasing fluoride content of the water, they also showed an even better inverse correlation with increasing strontium levels (and, to a lesser extent, the amount of boron). On the other hand, as the copper content rose, the caries rates also increased. Obviously, not all the caries reduction can be safely ascribed to fluoride in the water.

The beneficial effect of other minerals in the water and diet received special emphasis at Hereford, Texas, which in 1942 was heralded as "The Town Without a Toothache."[71] Although the drinking water contained 2.3-3.2 ppm fluoride, it also had

Table 12-3

Relation of Trace Elements in Drinking Water to
Tooth Decay in Children Aged 12 to 14 in
Six Illinois Cities[70]

City	Sr (ppb)	B (ppb)	Cu (ppb)	F (ppm)	DMF Teeth
Waukegan	20	20	10	0.0	8.10
Quincy	30	10	10	0.1	7.06
Oak Park	100	20	20	0.0	7.22
Joliet	500	500	5	1.3	3.23
Aurora	1000	300	5	1.2	2.81
Galesburg	2000	500	5	1.9	2.36

generous amounts of calcium, magnesium, and other minerals. Wheat grown in the area contained 600% more phosphorus than the national average and was also exceptionally high in calcium, magnesium, and other nutrients.[72] In the opinion of Dr. G. W. Heard, Hereford's dentist, the role of fluoride had been much over-emphasized. After 35 years of practice in the community he was certainly well acquainted with the condition of teeth in Hereford, and in 1956 he wrote:

> I believe that fluoride in water naturally does, in a mild way, retard caries, but I also believe Dean's survey of 21 natural fluoride cities mini-mized the importance of this [other minerals] factor. There is no doubt that other minerals in water, especially calcium and magnesium, enhance the action of fluoride and that *the damage it [fluoride] does is far greater than the good it may appear to accomplish.* It even makes the teeth so brittle and crumbly that they can be treated only with difficulty, if at all.[72] [Emphasis added.]

The exceptionally nutritious character of food produced in the Hereford region of western Texas has been confirmed by labora-tory studies at the Massachusetts Institute of Technology.[73] Ham-sters fed corn and milk produced in that area were healthier and had only half as much tooth decay as those fed corn and milk pro-duced in New England. The authors concluded, however, that the fluoride content of the Texas food was too low to have had much effect on the teeth.

The importance of these nonfluoride factors is further underscored by Russell's comment: "Colorado Springs has a high level of fluorine [2.5 ppm] in its water, yet its citizens have caries incidence far higher than do people in [areas such as] southeast Asia."[74] The same observation also applies to Hereford, Texas. In Colorado Springs the water is exceptionally soft (low in calcium and magnesium) and does not contain anywhere near the amount of buffering minerals found in the Hereford water. C. F. Deatherage observed a similar situation in Illinois in connection with waters that produced the most dental fluorosis: "This shale contained glauconite, a natural greensand, which softens the water percolating through it and also furnishes fluorides. It is these soft waters which cause the most severe mottling."[75]

The dental problems associated with fluoridation are numerous, serious, and vexing. Dentists everywhere have investigated possible solutions that will conquer, not merely delay or slightly diminish, tooth decay. Fluoridation has been offered as a miraculous cure-all. A vast quantity of negative evidence, however, emphasizes that it is not a panacea. Quite the contrary, fluoridation actually endangers human health, both dental and general, without offering more than a superficial, limited reduction of caries in return—a mirage at best. Over 30 years ago the American Dental Association itself best epitomized this great dental dilemma:

> Because of our anxiety to find some therapeutic procedure that will promote mass prevention of caries, the seeming potentialities of fluorine appear speculatively attractive, but, in the light of our present knowledge or lack of knowledge of the chemistry of the subject, the potentialities for harm far outweigh those for good.[76]

Time has not changed the truth of this statement. Scientific advances have merely underscored its wisdom.

*

THE BODY

Physicians, too, have had serious misgivings about fluoridation. On September 18, 1943, the *Journal of the American Medical Association* stated editorially:

> Fluorides are general protoplasmic poisons, probably because of their capacity to modify the metabolism of cells by changing the permeability of the cell membrane and by inhibiting certain enzyme systems. The exact mechanism of such actions is obscure. The sources of fluorine intoxication are drinking water containing 1 part per million or more of fluorine, fluorine compounds used as insecticidal sprays for fruits and vegetables (cryolite and barium fluosilicate), and the mining and conversion of phosphate rock to superphosphate, which is used as fertilizer.[77]

Early in the 1940s the ADA and AMA united in expressing strong reservations about fluoridation. Yet by 1951 both organizations had endorsed the procedure. Why? Had new scientific evidence been discovered to allay fears or cancel known physical laws indicating the serious hazards of fluorides? Since *no new favorable scientific evidence* had appeared between 1943 and 1951, we must look elsewhere for the reasons why spokesmen for the two foremost health professions did an about-face and endorsed a program formerly regarded as dangerous.

As for the strictly medical side of the argument, at least five major questions should have been resolved before fluoridation was approved and implemented:

(1) Could fluoridated water bring about an attenuated form of the serious bone disease now being recognized as a widespread health hazard in "high-fluoride" areas, especially in India?
(2) How do other minerals in water supplies modify the action of fluoride on the human body?
(3) Does its toxicity differ when fluoride is given at a certain *concentration* in water instead of in an exact *dosage*?
(4) How much does fluoride from sources other than drinking water contribute to the body's total fluoride burden?
(5) Can these other sources by themselves produce fluoride intoxication?

1. Bone and Joint Involvement. Although the skeletal changes of fluorosis are often considered relatively harmless and may indeed produce little or no discomfort to the patient,[78,79] extensive research from India has revealed severe arthritic changes and crippling neurological complications even where the fluoride concentration in water naturally is as low as 1.5 ppm.[80] Relying primarily on the Bartlett (8 ppm) study, American health authorities have repeatedly stated that no harm to the body has ever been observed from water containing up to 8 ppm fluoride. On April 23, 1954, Dr. G. F. Lull, an administrative officer of the AMA, wrote to me: "It is a well known fact, however, that no untoward effects are shown in individuals taking as high as ten parts per million in the water supply, except some mottling of the enamel of the teeth, while one part per million will not cause this mottling."[81] As recently as 1975 D. C. Fletcher of the AMA Council on Foods and Nutrition echoed this same view.[82]

Such views stand in sharp contrast to newer data on skeletal fluorosis presented in Chapter 8 (above). Even though extensive bone deformities may not be found on a large scale from fluoride in water at the 1-ppm concentration, some of the early signs of the disease, such as calcifications of ligaments, joint capsules, and muscle attachments, are likely to occur. Indeed these conditions are characteristic of osteoarthritis, in which the formation of microcrystals of apatite (known to be promoted by fluoride) has now been clearly demonstrated.[83] Among the elderly, arthritis of the spine is an especially common ailment that is customarily attributed to "aging." Since fluoride retention in bones increases as a person grows older, how can we disregard the possibility that this "old age" disease might be linked with fluoride intake? For example, Pinet and Pinet described in detail X-ray changes encountered in skeletal fluorosis in North Africa that are in every respect identical with those present in the arthritic spine of the elderly elsewhere.[15]

While bones and joints are likely to be damaged by the long-term use of artificially fluoridated water, there is considerable literature on the apparent benefit of fluoride in the treatment of osteoporosis in doses far exceeding those consumed by drinking fluoridated water.[84,85] Some "studies suggest a beneficial effect of fluoride on skeletal tissue when its use is accompanied by adequate calcium and vitamin D."[86] By itself, however, fluoride is of doubtful value and may even give rise to further bone softening (osteomalacia). Even with what was considered a proper calcium intake, prophylactic administration of fluoride (25 mg/day for five months) led to twice as many spontaneous fractures in elderly patients compared with controls.[87] Furthermore, undesirable deposition of fluoride in ligaments, joints, and arteries can cause arthritis and calcification of arteries.

2. Effects of Other Minerals. Another important factor determining the action of fluoride on general health is the presence of other minerals in water. In 1940, a survey of 75 cities with "natural fluoride" water having high levels of total hardness, i.e. an abundance of calcium and magnesium, pointed to the protective action of these two minerals in fluoride toxicity.[88] In the Eastern part of the Sahara desert, where endemic fluorosis occurs at 1.5 to 4.0. ppm fluoride in water, other minerals greatly influence the course of skeletal fluorosis:

> The waters in these districts have a high calcium content and are relatively low in magnesium, thus yielding a high Ca/Mg ratio; they are also high in sulfate and low in alkaline components. In contrast, the waters with inverse characteristics typify regions in which osteosclerosis is extremely rare. ... In the Sahara, the high level of calcium and sulfate in the "osteosclerosis" regions strikes us as being of prime importance.[15]

3. Concentration vs. Dose. Fluoridation is the addition of fluorides to water to achieve a fluoride concentration of about 1 ppm. There is absolutely no control over the amount of the dose that anyone consumes. The assumption when fluoridation began was that healthy adults living in a temperate climate would ingest about 1.0-1.5 mg of fluoride per day from the water (and children about half this amount).[89] *No one, however, can predict the precise amount of liquid anyone will imbibe under all circumstances, nor will the amount always remain the same for the same person.*

For example, a healthy person working in overheated areas such as a foundry or a steel mill—particularly in very warm climates— usually drinks at least five times the normal amounts of water. A study of soldiers under exertion recorded daily water intakes as high as 12 liters, an amount that would contribute up to 12 mg of fluoride per day if the water is fluoridated.[90] Furthermore, we have already seen that persons who are intolerant to fluoride have an unusual demand for water (polydipsia) for which *no* allowance was or has been made. That large intakes of fluoride can lead to adverse health effects was acknowledged even by McClure: "The data suggest that these [4.0 to 5.0 mg daily] may be the limits of fluorine which may be ingested daily [by healthy adults] without an appreciable hazard of body storage of fluorine."[91]

In young children and infants the situation is particularly critical because they are generally less tolerant to toxic agents than are adults. An infant weighing 5 kg, who is fed dried milk, will consume 800 ml of 1-ppm fluoridated water daily (four feedings of 200 ml each) containing 0.8 mg fluoride.[92] This amount corresponds to a daily intake of 11.2 mg for an adult weighing 70 kg; such a dose is very likely to induce adverse effects. On the other hand, when children are older, and fluoride might benefit their permanent teeth, they usually drink mainly milk, fruit juices, and other beverages, and often imbibe less than 500 ml (0.5 mg fluoride) of water per day.

Persons with nephrogenic diabetes insipidus, whose illness is characterized by an intractable thirst, are likewise especially vulnerable. Two such children, 10 and 11 years old, residing in two different artificially fluoridated communities, developed skeletal fluorosis and mottled teeth.[93] In one of the children the lateral deciduous incisor contained 285 ppm fluoride and in the other, a molar tooth showed 591 ppm fluoride, almost six times that in normal controls. Besides diabetes insipidus, which had caused the excess water consumption in the two cases, the authors named the following diseases that also give rise to polydipsia and polyuria: renal medullary disease including hypercalcemic and hypokalemic nephropathy; psychogenic water ingestion; anatomic and vascular disturbances; and diseases causing solute diuresis. They stated:

Consumption of water in any of these disorders is excessive and could lead to fluoride toxicity in a community with acceptable fluoride concentration. Therefore, a portion of the ingested water that these children consume should be supplied from a nonfluoridated source.[93]

Dispensing fluoride in uncontrolled concentrations and doses cannot help but have serious implications and further aggravate the dilemma created by fluoridation.

4. Contribution of Fluoride in Food. Another fundamental assumption on which the addition of fluoride to water supplies was based must now be revised in the light of new research – the belief that only a little fluoride reaches our system from sources other than water. As early as 1925, the famous nutritionist E. V. McCollum recognized the importance of fluoride in food when he stated after concluding an experimental study of the effect of fluoride on teeth and jawbones in rats:

> We have, in the present study, a clear demonstration that over-ingestion of an element [fluorine] which is regularly found in both food and tissues in small amounts may exert a detrimental effect when the amount ingested is increased to but little more than certain samples of foods are known to contain.[94]

In 1949 McClure estimated that the average daily fluoride intake through food exclusive of drinking water is only 0.3 to 0.5 mg.[95] He arrived at these values from analysis of a limited number of foods, using methods now recognized as outdated.[96] To make matters worse, even then McClure's data were obsolete. As shown in Chapter 3 (above), many subsequent studies have revealed considerably more fluoride in food – at least a two- to three-fold increase – than previously estimated, especially since many food items are being processed and prepared with fluoridated water and because of increased fluoride uptake by vegetation through contaminated air and soil. H. Spencer and co-workers determined the daily intake of fluoride from food alone at 0.07 mg/kg in infants up to four weeks of age and at 0.16 mg/kg in six-month-old infants.[97] *By itself, therefore, food already supplies more than the recommended 0.5 mg. of fluoride per day to infants for prevention of tooth decay.* Moreover, in 1977 these same authors extended their earlier analyses and reported an average fluoride intake of 1.8 mg/day by adult males (in a fluoridated community), *in addition to* 2.1 mg from the drinking water.[98]

5. Fluoride Intoxication from Non-Waterborne Fluoride. Under ordinary conditions can substances we eat or drink — in addition

to water – produce chronic fluoride intoxication? When fluoridation was first proposed, this question was of little concern. In
1968 in Barcelona, Spain, however, advanced skeletal fluorosis
associated with extraordinary bone fragility and destruction of
joints was reported in 29 alcoholics who had been consuming daily
8 to 10 mg of fluorine illegally added to wine to retard fermentation (See Figure 12-4, below, and 12-5, on the next page).[99]

In England, a well-substantiated case of arthritis was markedly
alleviated when the patient stopped drinking tea.[100] I encountered
a similar condition in Mrs. F. O., age 55, of Pontiac, Michigan (0.4
ppm) with features indicative of chronic fluorosis such as arthritic
changes in the lower spine, gastritis, ileitis, lower urinary tract disease, headache, paresthesias in arms and legs, and ulcers in the
mouth. She habitually drank 15 to 20 cups of tea (ca. 8 to 10 mg
fluoride) daily for 25 years. The 24-hour urinary fluoride excretions ranged from 1.7 to 6.3 mg (six determinations).[101] More advanced fluorosis with typical skeletal changes has been reported in
a "heavy" tea-drinking man in Hampshire England, who throughout his life had consumed water with little or no fluoride.[102]

Polluted air is now emerging as another potent hidden source of
fluoride intake because of the great expansion of its use in many
industries. As shown in Chapter 10, workers as well as persons
residing near fluoride-emitting factories are liable to become
afflicted with fluorosis due mainly to inhalation and to food
contaminated by atmospheric fluorides.

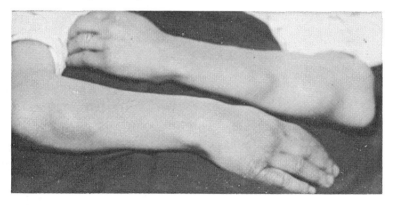

Fig. 12-4. Conspicuous exostoses (bony protrusions) caused by fluoride in
wine. (Courtesy Prof. M. Soriano, Barcelona, Spain.)

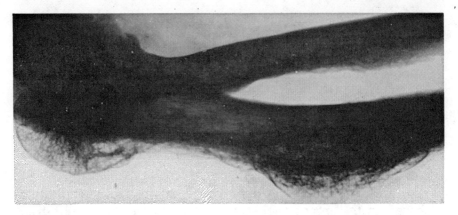

Fig. 12-5. X-Ray of forearm showing nature of periosteal growths (exostoses) caused by fluoride in wine. (Courtesy Prof. M. Soriano, Barcelona, Spain.)

The widespread use of drugs containing fluorine has dramatically increased today's fluoride burden, especially among chronically ill persons. I have records of several individuals whose habitual use of such tranquilizers and steroids produced toxic symptoms attributable to the fluoride metabolized from the drug. One of these patients had been taking a tranquilizer containing 16% of the halogen three times daily for three months, which provided a total daily fluoride intake of 2.4 mg. The free fluoride ion in his daily urine specimen ranged from 1.86 to 2.76 mg., representing 76% and 90%, respectively, of the total fluoride present in the urine.[103] It must be concluded that fluoride ion had split from the drug and thus caused damage, an assumption which is supported by recent research on other organo-fluorine pharmaceuticals, especially the anesthetic methoxyflurane. In patients with post-anesthesia kidney failure, Taves has demonstrated that free ionized fluoride appears in the blood in excess.[104] Polyuria—a characteristic feature of fluoride poisoning—occurs promptly, sometimes even while the patient is still in the recovery room following surgery; blood urea nitrogen rises, and creatinine and sodium excretion through the urine is reduced.[105] Laboratory studies have confirmed that "inorganic fluoride is responsible for the acute polyuric renal lesion which occurs after methoxyflurane administration."[106]

*

CONCLUSION

The Great Dilemma arose from the sincere desire by dentists and physicians to combat a serious disease of growing proportions — tooth decay. They long recognized many dangers from consumption of fluoride in food, water, and air, but for reasons that will be discussed later in this book, these health bringers cast aside evidence of acute and chronic fluoride toxicity in their optimistic belief that dental benefits outweighed potential harm. Somehow, they thought, the precise, beneficial general concentration and individual dose of fluoride — with no accompanying harm — could be discovered. But adverse scientific evidence had not changed; indeed, it continued to grow with greater and greater momentum just as the fluoride burden of the body has increased since fluoridation began. Difficult though it is to believe, the deleterious effects on health have been even worse than anticipated at first, and today many scientists suspect that fluoridated water causes or increases chromosome damage, birth defects, and even cancer.

REFERENCES

1. Hodge, H.C.: The Concentration of Fluorides in Drinking Water to Give the Point of Minimum Caries with Maximum Safety. J. Am. Dent. Assoc., 40: 436-439, 1950.

2. Heyroth, F.F.: Hearings Before Select Committee to Investigate the Use of Chemicals in Foods and Cosmetics Pursuant to H.R. 74 and 447, Part III, January 10 through March 10, 1952, p. 1803.

3. Black, G.V., and McKay, F.S.: An Endemic Developmental Imperfection of the Enamel of the Teeth, Heretofore Unknown in the Literature of Dentistry. Dent. Cosmos, 58:129-156, 1916.

4. Kempf, G.A., and McKay, F.S.: Mottled Enamel in a Segregated Population. Public Health Rep., 45:2933-2940, 1930. (Reprinted in Fluoride Drinking Waters, 1962, pp. 2-10.)

5. Smith, M.C., and Smith, H.V.: Observations on the Durability of Mottled Teeth. Am. J. Public Health, 30:1050-1052, 1940.

6. Roholm, K.: Fluor und Fluorverbindungen, in W. Heubner and J. Schüller, Eds.: Handbuch der experimentellen Pharmakologie, Ergänzungswerk, Vol. 7. J. Springer, Berlin, 1938, p. 62.

7. Smith, H.V.: Letter, September 17, 1954, to R. J. Munch, Greenwich, Conn., written at the request of Univ. of Arizona President Harvill. Copy in my possession.

8. Dean, H.T.: Classification of Mottled Enamel Diagnosis. J. Am. Dent. Assoc., 21:1421-1426, 1934. (Reprinted in Fluoride Drinking Waters, 1962, pp. 23-26.)

9. Dean, H.T.: Investigation of Physiological Effects by the Epidemiological Method, in F.R. Moulton, Ed.: Fluorine and Dental Health. 1942, pp. 23-31.

10. Cox, G.J.: New Knowledge of Fluorine in Relation to Dental Caries. J. Am. Water Works Assoc., 31:1926-1930, 1939.

11. Dean, H.T.: Personal communication to the author, at Hearings before Am. Med. Assoc. Councils on Pharmacy and Chemistry and on Foods and Nutrition, Chicago, Ill., August 7, 1957.

12. McKay, F.S.: Mottled Enamel: Early History and Its Unique Features, in F.R. Moulton, Ed.: Fluorine and Dental Health. 1942, pp. 1-5.

13. Sognnaes, R.F.: A Condition Suggestive of Threshold Dental Fluorosis Observed in Tristan da Cunha. I. Clinical Condition of the Teeth. J. Dent. Res., 20:303-313, 1941.

14. Nanda, R.S., Zipkin, I., Doyle, J., and Horowitz, H.S.: Factors Affecting the Prevalence of Dental Fluorosis in Lucknow, India. Arch. Oral Biol., 19:781-792, 1974.

15. Pinet, A., and Pinet, F.: Endemic Fluorosis in the Sahara. Fluoride, 1: 86-93, 1968.

16. Haaviko, K., and Helle, A.: The Prevalence and Distribution of Enamel Defects in Four Districts with Different Fluoride Contents in Drinking Water. Proc. Finn. Dent. Soc., 70:178-185, 1974.

17. Aasenden, R., and Peebles, T.C.: Effects of Fluoride Supplementation from Birth on Human Deciduous and Permanent Teeth. Arch. Oral Biol., 19: 321-326, 1974.

18. Jolly, S.S., Prasad, S., Sharma, R., and Chander, R.: Endemic Fluorosis in Punjab. II. Dental Aspect. Fluoride, 6:106-112, 1973.

19. Jackson, D., James, P.M.C., and Wolfe, W.B.: Fluoridation in Anglesey. Br. Dent. J., 138:165-171, 1975.

20. Cook, H.A.: Fluoride Intake Through Tea in British Children. Fluoride, 3:12-18, 1970.

21. Russell, A.L.: Dental Fluorosis in Grand Rapids During the Seventeenth Year of Fluoridation. J. Am. Dent. Assoc., 65:608-612, 1962.

22. Hurme, V.O.: Developmental Opacities of Teeth in a New England Community: Their Relation to Fluorine Toxicosis. Am. J. Dis. Child., 77:61-75, 1949.

23. Richards, L.F., Westmoreland, W.W., Tashiro, M., McKay, C.H., and Morrison, J.T.: Determining Optimum Fluoride Levels for Community Water Supplies in Relation to Temperature. J. Am. Dent. Assoc., 74:389-397, 1967.

24. Rosenzweig, K.A., and Abkewitz. I.: Prevalence of Endemic Fluorosis in Israel at Medium Fluoride Concentration. Public Health Rep., 78:77-80, 1963.

25. Kantorowicz, A.: Kariesbefall von Gemeinden in Nordrhein-Westfalen und der Fluorgehalt ihrer Trinkwässer. Dtsch. Zahnaetztl. Z., 7:1017-1020, 1952.

26. Rost, A.: Was erwarten wir von einer Trinkwasserfluorierung? Zahnaerztl. Rundschau, 64:83-87, 1955.

27. Imai, Y.: Relationship Between Fluoride Concentration in Drinking Water and Dental Caries in Japan. Koku Eisei Gakkai Zasshi, 22:144-196, 1972. (Abstracted in Fluoride, 6:248-251, 1973.)

28. Teotia, S.P.S., Teotia, M., and Teotia, N.P.S.: Skeletal Fluorosis: Roentgenological and Histopathological Study. Fluoride, 9:91-98, 1976.

29. Singh, A., Jolly, S.S., Bansal, B.C., and Mathur, C.C.: Endemic Fluorosis. Epidemiological, Clinical and Biochemical Study of Chronic Fluorine Intoxication in Punjab (India). Medicine, 42:229-246, 1963; 44:97, 1965.

30. Dillon, C.: Fluorosis and Dental Caries. 1969, pp. 103-114.

31. Ramseyer, H.F., Smith, C.A.H., and McCay, C.M.: Effect of Sodium Fluoride Administration on Body Changes in Old Rats. J. Gerontol., 12;14-19, 1957.

32. Dean, H.T., and Arnold, F.A., Jr.: Endemic Dental Fluorosis or Mottled Enamel. J. Am. Dent. Assoc., 30:1278-1283, 1943.

33. Day, C.D.M.: Chronic Endemic Fluorosis in Northern India. Br. Dent. J., 68:409-424, 1940.

34. Latham, M.C.: Nutritional Studies in Tanzania (Tanganyika). World Rev. Nutr. Diet., 7:31-71, 1967.

35. Russell, A.L., and White, C.L.: Fluorides and Periodontal Health, in J.C. Muhler and M.K. Hine, Eds.: Fluorine and Dental Health: The Pharmacology and Toxicology of Fluorine. Indiana Univ. Press, Bloomington, 1959, pp. 115-127. See also Adler (in Ref. 42, below), pp. 348-349.

36. Russell, A.L.: Fluoride Domestic Water and Periodontal Disease. Am. J. Public Health, 47:688-694, 1957. (Reprinted in Fluoride Drinking Waters, 1962, pp. 427-430.)

37. Poulsen, S., and Møller, I.J.: Gingivitis and Dental Plaque in Relation to Dental Fluorosis in Man in Morocco. Arch. Oral Biol., 19:951-954, 1974.

38. E.g., Masaki, T.: Geographical Distribution of "Mottled Teeth" in Japan, Shikwa Gakuho, 36:875ff., 1931; Ainsworth, N.J.: Mottled Teeth. Br. Dent. J., 55:233-250, 1933; Lemmon, J.R.: Mottled Enamel of Teeth in Chil-

dren. Texas State J. Med., 30:332-336, 1934.

39. Feltman, R., and Kosel, G.: Prenatal and Postnatal Ingestion of Fluorides—Fourteen Years of Investigation—Final Report. J. Dent. Med., 16:190-199, 1961.

40. Garren, L., and Greep, R.: Effects of Thyroid Hormone and Propylthiouracil on Eruption Rate of Upper Incisor Teeth in Rats. Proc. Soc. Exp. Biol. Med., 90:652-655, 1955.

41. Short, E.M.: Domestic Water and Dental Caries. VI. The Relation of Fluoride Domestic Waters to Permanent Tooth Eruption. J. Dent. Res., 23: 247-255, 1944. (Reprinted in Fluoride Drinking Waters, 1962, pp. 137-141.)

42. Adler, P.: Fluorides and Dental Health, in WHO Monograph No. 59: Fluorides and Human Health. 1970, pp. 349-350.

43. Ast, D.B., Smith, D.J., Wachs, B., and Cantwell, K.T.: Newburgh-Kingston Caries-Fluorine Study. XIV. Combined Clinical and Roentgenographic Dental Findings After Ten Years of Fluoride Experience. J. Am. Dent. Assoc., 52:314-325. 1956;

44. Freitas, J.A.deS., Lopes, E.S., Alvares, L.C., and Tavano, O.: Influence of Fluoridation in the Chronology of Eruption of Permanent Teeth. Estomatol. Cult., 5:156-165, 1971.

45. Blayney, J.R., and Hill, I.N.: Fluorine and Dental Caries. J. Am. Dent. Assoc., 74(2):233-302, Jan. 1967.

46. Weaver, R.: Fluorine and Dental Caries. Further Investigations on Tyneside and in Sunderland. Br. Dent. J., 77:185-193, 1944.

47. Paluev, K.K., in Waldbott, G.L.: Medical Evidence Against Fluoridation of Public Water Supplies. Aust. J. Dent., 59:13-20, 1955. Cf. Appendix 3, in Exner, F.B., Waldbott, G.L., Rorty, J. (Ed.): The American Fluoridation Experiment, Revised ed., Devin-Adair, New York, 1961, pp. 244-248.

48. Ziegelbecker, R.: A Critical Review on the Fluorine Caries Problem. Fluoride, 3:71-79, 1970.

49. Dept. of Health and Social Security: Reports on Public Health and Medical Subjects No. 122: The Fluoridation Studies in the United Kingdom and the Results Achieved after Eleven Years. Her Majesty's Stationery Office, London, 1969, Table 7, p. 29.

50. Weaver, R.: Fluorine and Wartime Diet. Br. Dent. J., 88:231-239, 1950.

51. Klerer, M.: The Fluoridation Experiment. Contemp. Issues, 7:119-143, 1956.

52. Maxcy, K.F., Appleton, J.L.T., Bibby, B.G., Dean, H.T., Harvey, A. McG., Heyroth, F.F., Johnson, A.L., Whittaker, H.A., and Wolman, A.: Report of the Ad Hoc Committee on Fluoridation of Water Supplies. Nat. Res. Council–Nat. Acad. Sci. Med. Sci. Publ. No. 214, 1952; J. Am. Water Works Assoc., 44:1-9, 1952.

53. Scrivener, C.A.: Unfavorable Report from Kansas Community Using Artificial Fluoridation of City Water Supply for Three-Year Period. J. Dent. Res., 30:465, 1951.

54. Bellinger, W.R.: Preliminary Report on Ottawa, Kansas' Caries-Fluoridation Project. Division of Dental Hygiene, Kansas State Board of Health. December 1951. (Cited by Stadt, Z.M.: Résumé of Dental Benefits of Fluoride Ingestion, in J.H. Shaw, Ed.: Fluoridation as a Public Health Measure. Am. Assoc. Adv. Science, Washington, D.C., 1954, pp. 9 and 15.)

55. Bellinger, W.R., and Mankin, J.D.: Effect of Controlled Fluoridated Public Water Supplies on the Dental Caries Experience for Children Ages 9 through 12 in Three Kansas Cities. J. Kans. State Dent. Assoc., 49:117-120, 1965.

56. Adler (in Ref. 42, above), pp. 337-338; cf. Minoguchi, G.: Eleventh Year of Fluoridation Study at Yamashima in Kyoto. J. Dent. Res., 44:1153-1154, 1965 (Abstract).

57. Adler (in Ref. 42, above), pp. 338-340. See also Toth, K.: The Epidemiology of Dental Caries in Hungary. Akademiai Kiado, Budapest, 1970, Chapters 4 and 6.

58. Boyd, J.C., and Wessels, N.E.: Epidemiological Studies in Dental Caries. III. The Interpretation of Clinical Data Relating to Caries Advance. Am. J. Public Health, 41:967-986, 1951.

59. Radusch, D.F.: Variability of Diagnosis of Incidence of Dental Caries. J. Am. Dent. Assoc., 28:1959-1961, 1941. Cf. Ennis, LeR.R.: Oral Roentgenology and Its Possibilities. Ibid., 21:1367-1421, 1934.

60. Palfer-Sollier, M.: Étude comparative de plusieurs techniques d'évaluation de la carie dentaire sur un même groupe des infants. Odontol. Revy, 8:240-254, 1957.

61. Sutton, P.R.N.: Fluoridation: Errors and Omissions in Experimental Trials. Melbourne Univ. Press, Melbourne, Australia, 1959, p. 72. (Second Edition, enlarged, 1960.)

62. Dean, H.T., Jay, P., Arnold, F.A., Jr., McClure, F.J., and Elvove, E.: Domestic Water and Dental Caries, Including Certain Epidemiological Aspects of Oral *L. Acidophilus.* Public Health Rep., 54:862-888, 1939. (Reprinted in Fluoride Drinking Waters, 1962, pp. 90-101.)

63. Ludwig, T.G.: Recent Marine Soils and Resistance to Dental Caries. Aust. Dent. J., 8:109-113, 1963.

64. Adler, P., and Straub, J.: A Waterborne Caries Protective Agent Other Than Fluoride. Acta Med. Acad. Sci. Hung., 4:221-234, 1953.

65. Tank, G., and Storvick, C.A.: Effect of Naturally Occurring Selenium and Vanadium on Dental Caries. J. Dent. Res., 39:473-488, 1960.

66. Skougstad, M.W., and Horr, C.A.: Chemistry of Strontium in Natural Water. U.S. Geol. Surv. Water Supply Paper 1496. U.S. Geol. Survey, Wash-

ington, D.C., 1963.

67. Little, M.F., and Barrett, K.: Trace Element Content of Surface and Subsurface Enamel Relative to Caries Prevalence on the West Coast of the United States of America. Arch. Oral Biol., 21:651-657, 1976.

68. Hadjimarkos, D.M.: Effect of Selenium on Dental Caries. Arch. Environ. Health, 10:839-843, 1965.

69. Curzon, M.E.J., Kubota, S., and Bibby, B.G.: Environmental Effects of Molybdenum on Caries. J. Dent. Res., 50:74-77, 1971.

70. Losee, F.L., and Bibby, B.G.: Caries Inhibition by Trace Elements Other Than Fluorine. N.Y. State Dent. J., 36:15-19, 1970.

71. Ratcliff, J.D.: The Town Without a Toothache. Colliers, Dec. 19, 1942; Reader's Digest, February 1943.

72. Heard, G.W.: Letter to C.A. Barden, June 12, 1956. Copy in my possession.

73. Harris, R.S., and Nizel, A.E.: Caries-Producing Effect of Similar Food Grown in Different Soil Areas. N. Engl. J. Med., 244:361-362, 1951.

74. Russell, A.L.: Environment and Oral Disease. Science, 146:954-955, 1964.

75. Deatherage, C.F.: Mottled Enamel from the Standpoint of the Public Health Dentist (Including the Relation of Fluorine to Dental Caries in Illinois), in F.R. Moulton, Ed.: Fluorine and Dental Health. 1942, p. 83.

76. Editorial: Effect of Fluorine on Dental Caries. J. Am. Dent. Assoc., 31:1360-1363, 1944.

77. Editorial: Chronic Fluorine Intoxication. J. Am. Med. Assoc., 123:150, 1943.

78. Morris, J.W.: Skeletal Fluorosis Among Indians of the American Southwest. Am. J. Roentgenol. Radium Ther. Nucl. Med., 94:608-615, 1965.

79. Leone, N.C., Shimkin, M.B., Arnold, F.A., Jr., Stevenson, C.A., Zimmerman, E.R., Geiser, P.B., and Lieberman, J.E.: Medical Aspects of Excessive Fluoride in a Water Supply. A Ten-Year Study. Public Health Rep., 69:925-936, 1954. (Reprinted in Fluoride Drinking Waters, 1962, pp. 402-411.)

80. Jolly, S.S., Prasad, S., Sharma, R., and Rai, B.: Human Fluoride Intoxication in Punjab. Fluoride, 4:64-79, 1971. See also Ref. 29, above.

81. Lull, G.F.: Personal communication to the author, April 23, 1954.

82. Fletcher, D.C.: Editorial: Revised Statement on Fluoridation. J. Am. Med. Assoc., 231:1167, 1975.

83. Schumacher, H.R., Smolyo, A.P., Tse, R.L., and Maurer, K.: Arthritis Associated with Apatite Crystals. Ann. Intern. Med., 87:411-416, 1977.

84. Rich, C., and Ivanovich, P.: Response to Sodium Fluoride in Severe Primary Osteoporosis. Ann. Intern. Med., 63:1069-1074, 1965.

85. Hodge, H.C., and Smith, F.A.: Fluorides and Man. Ann. Rev. Pharmacol., 8:395-408, 1968.

86. Jowsey, J.: Fluoride Treatment in the Prevention of Osteoporosis. Fluoride, 2:125-127, 1969.

87. Inkovaara, J., Heikinheimo, R., Jarvinen, K., Kasurinen, U., Hanhijärvi, H., and Iisalo, E.: Prophylactic Treatment and Aged Bones. Br. Med. J., 3:73-74, 1975. For comment, see Jowsey, J., and Riggs, B.L.: ibid., 3:766, 1975; and reply by Inkovaara, J., and Heikinheimo, R.: ibid., 4:758, 1975.

88. Mills, C.A.: Letter to the Editor, J. Am. Med. Assoc., 114:179, 1940.

89. McClure, F.J.: Ingestion of Fluoride and Dental Caries. Quantitative Relations Based on Food and Water Requirements of Children One to Twelve Years Old. Am. J. Dis. Child., 66:362-369, 1943. (Reprinted in Fluoride Drinking Waters, 1962, pp. 283-286.)

90. Wilbur, C.G.: Water Requirements of Man. U.S. Armed Forces Med. J., 8:1121-1130, 1957.

91. McClure, F.J., Mitchell, H.H., Hamilton, T.S., and Kinser, C.A.: Balances of Fluorine Ingested from Various Sources in Food and Water by Five Young Men. Excretion of Fluorine Through the Skin. J. Ind. Hyg. Toxicol., 27:159-170, 1945. (Reprinted in Fluoride Drinking Waters, 1962, pp. 377-384.)

92. Auermann, E.: Fluoride Uptake in Humans. Fluoride, 6:78-83, 1973.

93. Greenberg, L.W., Nelson, C.A., and Kramer, N.: Nephrogenic Diabetes Insipidus with Fluorosis. Pediatrics, 54:320-322, 1974.

94. McCollum, E.V., Simmonds, N., Becker, J.E., and Bunting, R.W.: The Effect of Additions of Fluorine to the Diet of the Rat on the Quality of the Teeth. J. Biol. Chem., 63:553-562, 1925.

95. McClure, F.J.: Fluorine in Foods. Survey of Recent Data. Public Health Rep., 64:1061-1074, 1949. (Reprinted in Fluoride Drinking Waters, 1962, pp. 287-294.)

96. Farkas, C.S.: Total Fluoride Intake and Fluoride Content of Common Foods: A Review. Fluoride, 8:98-105, 1975.

97. Wiatrowski, B.S., Kramer, L., Osis, D., and Spencer, H.: Dietary Fluoride Intake of Infants. Pediatrics, 55:517-522, 1975.

98. Spencer, H., Kramer, L., Wiatrowski, E., and Osis, D.: Magnesium-Fluoride Interrelationships in Man. I. Effect of Fluoride on Magnesium Metabolism. Am. J. Physiol. 233:E165-E169, 1977. The average water consumption of two liters per day reported in this study is also used by the NAS-NRC Safe Drinking Water Committee in its Summary Report: Drinking Water and Health. National Academy of Sciences, Washington, D.C., 1977, p. 2.

99. Soriano, M.: Periostitis Deformans Due to Wine Fluorosis. Fluoride, 1:56-64, 1968.

100. Cook, H.A.: Crippling Arthritis Related to Fluoride Intake (Case Report). Fluoride, 5:209-212, 1972.

101. Waldbott, G.L.: Fluoride in Clinical Medicine. Int. Arch. Allergy

Appl. Immunol., 20, Suppl. 1, 1962.

102. Webb-Peploe, M.M., and Bradley, W.G.: Endemic Fluorosis with Neurological Complications in a Hampshire Man. J. Neurol. Neurosurg. Psychiatry, 29:577-583, 1966.

103. Analyses by R.J. Hall, Ministry of Agriculture, Fisheries and Food, National Agricultural Advisory Service (U.K.), sent to G.L. Waldbott, Feb. 27, 1963.

104. Taves, D.R., Fry, B.W., Freeman, R.B., and Gillies, A.J.: Toxicity Following Methoxyflurane Anesthesia. II. Fluoride Concentrations in Nephrotoxicity. J. Am. Med. Assoc., 214:91-95, 1970.

105. Hollenberg, N.K., McDonald, F.D., and Cotran, K.: Irreversible Acute Oliguric Renal Failure. A Complication of Methoxyflurane Anesthesia. N. Engl. J. Med., 286:877-879, 1972.

106. Cousins, M.J., Mazze, R.L., Kosek, J.C., Hitt, B.A., and Love, F.V.: The Etiology of Methoxyflurane Toxicity. J. Pharmacol. Exp. Ther., 190: 530-541, 1974.

CHAPTER 13

GENETIC DAMAGE, BIRTH DEFECTS, AND CANCER

ENVIRONMENTAL FACTORS play a major role in the production of genetic defects and tissue abnormalities, but identification of specific causes is usually quite difficult. Some known impediments are: the great number of agents involved, their general slowness of action, and the remarkable differences often found in their behavior toward test animals and humans.[1] Nevertheless, laboratory studies and large-scale statistical investigations on human populations have linked certain substances – tobacco smoke, coal-tar derivatives, nitrosamines, steroid hormones, and radioactive isotopes – to malignant diseases and congenital anomalies.

We now also know that carcinogens and mutagens have parallel effects. For example, about 90% of organic compounds found to be mutagenic in the Ames bacteria culture test[2] are also carcinogenic in mammals. Paradoxically, the degree of mutagenicity of a compound is not always comparable with its carcinogenic potency: a weak mutagen can be a strong carcinogen.[3] Certain types of inorganic carcinogens have also tested positively,[4] but Ames himself has stated that the procedure would require alteration for "fluoride to be adequately tested for mutagenicity."[5] An undocumented claim[6] that fluoride is not mutagenic in the Ames test must therefore be viewed with scepticism until the test is adequately modified.

CHROMOSOME DAMAGE

As early as 1958 the renowned geneticist H. J. Muller pointed out that an increasing number of substances in the environment, including fluoride, produce their primary damage by injuring the genetic material of the cells they enter.[7] Various investigations have subsequently confirmed the correctness of this assessment.

At concentrations too low to cause visible tissue injury, hydrogen fluoride induces significant mitotic and meiotic chromosome alterations in tomato plants[8] and in maize.[9] Although sodium fluoride interferes with the mutagenic activity of substances like Trenimon,[10] it enhances the production of recessive lethal mutations by X-radiation in *Drosophila* (fruit flies).[11] Hydrogen fluoride also increases lethal and sublethal genetic damage to *Drosophila.*[12, 13] In another experiment, female white rats exposed 6 hours daily for 5 months to small amounts of airborne cryolite (3 mg/m^3) or to a mixture of cryolite (0.5 mg/m^3) and HF (0.35 mg/m^3) showed significantly increased damage to bone marrow chromosomes.[14]

Chromosome studies on isolated cow, ewe, and mouse oocytes indicate that sodium fluoride "can be a potent meiotic mutagen" even at concentrations as low as 0.01 mg/ml (4.5 ppm F$^-$).[15] Another investigation showed that leucocytes in cattle suffering from environmental fluorosis displayed about the same number of chromatid gaps and breaks as those of non-exposed cattle, but the exposed cattle had more than twice as many chromosome gaps and fragmentations. Although the authors did not regard this difference as significant, they recognized that "lymphocytes bearing chromosome aberrations may have been eliminated since cattle lymphocytes have been shown to be extremely sensitive to such a selection process."[16]

Particularly relevant to water fluoridation are the results of *in vivo* studies on mouse cells by A. H. Mohamed and M. E. Chandler of the University of Missouri at Kansas City.[17] These workers found highly significant increases in the frequency of dose- and time-related chromosomal changes in bone marrow cells and spermatocytes of male adult mice given sodium fluoride in drinking water for periods of 3 weeks and 6 weeks at concentrations ranging from 0 to 200 ppm. The mice were maintained on a low-fluoride (0.263 ppm) diet, and separate control groups on fluoride-free deionized water were used in each of the two study periods. The results as summarized in Table 13-1 (opposite) indicated that the frequency of chromosomal aberrations was 1.3 to 2 times greater in the mice exposed to 1 or 5 ppm NaF in the drinking water than in the controls and 2 to 3 times greater in the mice ingesting the highest NaF concentrations. Statistical analysis of the differences showed that most of them were reliable to at least the 0.05 level of significance.

Table 13-1

Effect of NaF in Drinking Water on the Frequency of Chromosomal Aberrations in Two Types of Cells in Male Adult BALB/c Mice[17]

NaF (ppm)	% Aberrations — 3 Weeks		% Aberrations — 6 Weeks	
	Bone Marrow	Sperma-tocytes	Bone Marrow	Sperma-tocytes
0	18.4	16.0	19.3	15.8
1	25.7	21.4	32.1	21.1
5	29.9	23.2	41.3	22.8
10	35.5	30.5	46.0	29.7
50	44.6	34.3	47.1	41.3
100	47.5	40.3	47.9	48.2
200	45.6	45.5	49.2	50.3

Mohamed and Chandler also found "a high correlation between the amount of fluoride in the body ash and the frequency of chromosomal abnormalities."* In the bone marrow cells the latter consisted of "acentric fragments, ring chromosomes, translocations, dicentrics, and anaphase or telophase bridges with or without fragments." In the spermatocytes "abnormalities were mainly bridges, bridges plus fragments, and fragments alone." On the basis of these results, plus other evidence, they concluded that the increased frequency of aberrations was due primarily to enzymatic effects of fluoride that "might delay mitotic and meiotic cycles [thereby] causing chromosome breakage . . . and fragmentation." They further suggested that "fluoride could also act directly upon DNA [deoxyribonucleic acid], producing fragments and structural changes in either mitotic or meiotic chromosomes."[17]

These and other findings of fluoride damage to mammalian chromosomes have been the focus of considerable criticism, although no data disproving them have been published. Various allegations against them in a report prepared for the National Research Council[19] are speculative, and Mohamed has clearly shown that they are fallacious and totally without foundation.[20] Lack of chromosomal damage by fluoride in mice has also been claimed by

---

*Water consumption by the mice was slightly *greater* at the 1- and 5-ppm NaF levels than in the controls, just as has been observed in monkeys[18] and humans (see Chapter 9, above).

scientists at the National Institutes of Health.[6] Details of this work were promised to a Congressional investigating committee by December 1977[21] but were still not available in late March 1978. The abstract,[6] however, ignores some of the principal types of chromosomal aberrations found by Mohamed and Chandler.

Failure to find *any* deleterious effects would indeed be most surprising, for Mohamed has confirmed his results by re-examining the blind-coded slides made for the experiments. Furthermore, Dr. Beverly White, a mouse cytogeneticist at the National Institutes of Health, has also examined his slides and "agreed that what I [Mohamed] called 'ball metaphase' ['metaphase chromosome stickiness' or 'metaphase clumped chromosomes'] *was in fact different from the normal metaphase chromosomes.*"[20] [Emphasis added.]

BIRTH DEFECTS

As an agent capable of producing meiotic chromosome changes, fluoride also clearly has the potential for transmitting malformations to offspring – including man. One such birth defect, called mongolism or Down's syndrome, which arises from a trisomy of one of the G-group chromosomes, was the subject of a series of remarkable investigations by the late Ionel Rapaport, a French-trained endocrinologist at the Psychiatric Institute of the University of Wisconsin, Madison (Fig. 13-1, opposite). He had no prior interest in fluoride but was led to it by his investigations.

In searching for clues to the etiology of Down's syndrome, Rapaport was struck by the high prevalence of cataracts he encountered in mongoloids above age 20 – an incidence amounting to 70% (67 out of 95).[22] His curiosity was also aroused when he observed that nearly 40% of the mongoloids at one of the Wisconsin State colonies had been born in Green Bay, whereas only 17.5% of the epileptics in that institution had come from that city. He then discovered that the incidence of blindness due to senile cataracts in Green Bay among persons over age 65 was 44% higher (18.6% vs. 12.9%) than in other major cities of the state.[22]

Seeking an explanation for these remarkable coincidences, he considered the possibility that an environmental agent might be involved. He recalled that in 1853 Chatin had linked goiter and cretinism, another birth defect, with drinking water and had established a lack of iodine as the culprit. Rapaport also observed that

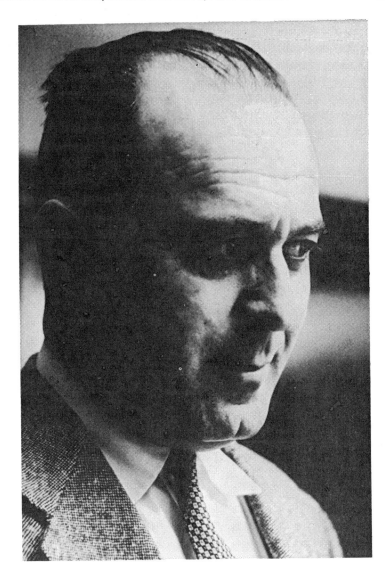

Fig. 13-1. Ionel F. Rapaport, M.D. (Paris), 1909-1972. School of Anthropology (France), 1946-1954; Psychiatric Institute, Univ. Wisconsin, 1954-1961; New School of Social Research, 1962-1968; Willowbrook State School, N.Y., 1968-1972.
(Courtesy Marjorie O'Brien Rapaport.)

many of the mongoloid children had mottled teeth and, apparently, an unusually low incidence of dental caries, a fact previously known and now well confirmed.[23] All these circumstances directed his attention to the fluoride content of the Green Bay water supply, which indeed turned out to have a comparatively high natural fluoride content: 1.2-2.8 ppm – much higher than in most other Wiconsin communities.

He then pursued this lead and ascertained the place of birth of all mongoloid children living in institutions as of July 1, 1956, in the four states of Wisconsin, North and South Dakota, and Illinois, and grouped them according to the published fluoride content of the municipal drinking water. In a tabulation of the 687 urban cases he found a statistically significant, two-fold greater prevalence or risk of mongoloid births in communities with 1 ppm or more fluoride than in those with little or none in the water.* He presented these findings to the French National Academy of Medicine in Paris in November 1956.[25]

How reliable are these discoveries? Application of Van Valen's formula[26] reveals a combined statistical probability of less than 1 in 125,000 that the entire set of correlations from all four states was due to chance.[27] The same parallelism between the prevalence of mongolism and the fluoride content of drinking water at the place of birth was subsequently corroborated by data supplied by 46 superintendents of institutions in other areas of the United States.[28]

Rapaport also correlated the age of the mothers of mongoloid children in Wisconsin with the fluoride content of the water supply. The mean maternal age was 34.26 years in the low (0.1-0.5 ppm) fluoride areas, whereas in the 1.0-ppm communities it was 33.17 years, and in the high (1.2-2.8 ppm) fluoride areas it was 29.81 years.[25,29] In other words, in the high-fluoride areas more mothers gave birth to mongoloid children at an earlier age than in the low-fluoride communities. This same trend can also be seen in

*In a frequently cited but unpublished analysis of the maternal residence and water histories of 125 cases selected from the 358 total tabulated cases in Illinois, A. L. Russell of the USPHS claimed that the difference in prevalence rate between some of the high-fluoride (1.0-1.9 ppm) and low-fluoride (0-0.3 ppm) cities decreased to a ratio of only 1.37 to 1.[24] Still, the same conclusion holds true: the incidence of mongolism increases with the fluoride content of the water supply.

Table 13-2

Maternal Age-Specific White Down's Syndrome Rates
in Metropolitan Atlanta, Georgia, 1960-1973[30]

Age	Fluoridated Areas 166,186 Births		Nonfluoridated Areas 101,639 Births	
	DS Births	Rate 10^5 Births	DS Births	Rate 10^5 Births
≤19	19	76.6	7	38.2
20-24	41	69.2	15	39.9
25-29	34	68.2	11	40.9
30-34	25	112.7	13	109.8
≥35	47	477.2	38	554.3
Total	166	99.9	86[a]	84.6

[a] Includes two cases of unknown maternal age.

a survey reported in 1976 by workers at the USPHS National Center for Disease Control.[30] As shown above in Table 13-2, distinctly higher age-specific rates of Down's syndrome births occurred among younger mothers in the fluoridated areas. Such an effect is exactly what would be expected from long-term exposure to increased levels of a widespread environmental mutagen.

Shortly after Rapaport's first report appeared, W. T. C. Berry of the British Ministry of Health published a 10-year study of the occurrence of 199 cases of Down's syndrome according to maternal residence in certain selected "high" (0.7–2.0 ppm) and "low" (≤0.2 ppm) fluoride cities of north-central England.[31] This survey, like two subsequent unpublished ones cited in a report by the Royal College of Physicians of London,[32] apparently contradicts the findings of Rapaport, since it revealed little difference in incidence between the two sets of cities. On the other hand, these studies did not provide maternal age data; without such data the major demographic and other differences between the small number of cities could easily lead to overall incidence findings that are not truly representative. This possibility becomes a reality when we discover that the 5-year pilot study in the county of Essex included by Berry in his paper actually showed a 38% higher incidence of mongolism in the high-fluoride areas than in the low-fluoride ones.

Rapaport also stated that the discrepancy between his findings and those of Berry can be attributed to the 10-fold greater drinking of tea in England, a habit that accounts for a substantial increase in fluoride consumption and therefore erases the narrow difference in fluoride intake between the "high" and "low" fluoride cities.[33] Furthermore, tea drinking in Britain has been linked with increased incidence of other birth defects, namely anencephalus (absence of brain) and stillbirths, especially in soft (low calcium) water areas.[34]

In a second investigation, Rapaport followed suggestions by Russell, whose *unpublished* criticisms of Rapaport's original study have been widely cited.[35] The new study included all officially recorded cases of mongoloid children in the State of Illinois who were born from 1950 through 1956 to mothers who lived in cities of 10,000 to 100,000 population. The data, reported in 1959[33] and later in amplified form,[36,37] indicated a highly significant association between the frequency of Down's syndrome and the fluoride content of the mother's drinking water (Table 13-3, below).

In 1961 Rapaport provided additional experimental evidence supporting fluoride involvement in mongolism. In the previous year the abnormal character of tryptophan metabolism in Down's

Table 13-3

Occurrence of Down's Syndrome by Maternal Residence in Illinois Cities of 10,000-100,000 Population 1950-1956 (Rapaport, 1959-1963)[33,36,37]

| | | | | Down's Syndrome Births | | |
No. of Cities	Total Births	Fluoride in water (ppm)	No.	Rate 10^5 Births	Mother >40 Years No.	Percent
15	63,521	0.0	15	23.6	3	20.0
24	132,665	0.1-0.2	52	39.2	13	25.0
17	70,111	0.3-0.7	33	47.1	4	12.1
12	67,053	1.0-2.6	48	71.6	5	10.4
Totals						
68	333,350	0.0-2.6	148	44.4	25	16.9

Statistical significance $\chi^2 = 16.29$ $P < 0.001$

syndrome had just been announced.[38] Rapaport then conducted studies on the previously known formation of melanotic tumors in fruit flies bred in a fluoridated medium and obtained evidence that these lesions were connected with a genetically altered metabolism of tryptophan as in Down's syndrome.[39] Other investigators have since confirmed the formation of these melanomas from fluoride in fruit flies[40] as well as the abnormal metabolism of tryptophan in mongoloid children.[41]

In connection with his studies on the occurrence of Down's syndrome in Illinois, Rapaport also showed that other known minerals in the water, with the possible exception of calcium, did not affect his results. Although not statistically significant, the incidence of mongolism *decreased* slightly with a *rise* in the calcium concentration, in agreement with the well-known antidotal effect of calcium on fluorine.[37] Furthermore, in the high-fluoride cities of Wisconsin he observed a significantly higher rate of premature stillbirths, which he attributed to fluoride-linked chromosomal anomalies or malformations incompatible with fetal life.[37]

Overall, his data from the second Illinois study indicated a probability of at least 1,000 to 1 that the association of waterborne fluoride with the incidence of mongolism is real and not a statistical illusion. This is the highest figure recognized by the chi-square treatment. Moreover, the combined probability against the results being due to chance in both the first and second series of studies has been calculated (by Van Valen's formula[26]) to be 62,500,000 to 1.[27] *No other comparable work on mongolism has achieved such a high degree of statistical reliability.*

Despite the impressive statistical significance of his findings, Rapaport himself recognized shortcomings inherent in any such retrospective study. For example, he explicitly stated that probably only about 41% of the actual number of cases are recorded at birth,[37] an estimate which has since been repeatedly confirmed.[42] In his investigations, however, death certificates and institutional records were also consulted, so that the same degree of ascertainment would be expected for both the fluoride and nonfluoride cities. As a matter of fact, his Illinois incidence figures are in the same range as those obtained by similar means in New York[43] and in Missouri.[44]

In 1974 Rapaport's findings were challenged by a study of Down's syndrome in the state of Massachusetts. This work covered the geographical distribution of 2,469 cases of mongolism born to resident mothers among a total of 1,833,452 live births from 1950 through 1966. These births occurred among residents of 321 non-fluoridated communities (less than 0.3 ppm fluoride in the water supply) and 30 fluoridated communities. In the latter group, nine towns ceased to fluoridate during the 17-year study period. In the nonfluoridating communities there were 1.34 mongoloid births per 1,000 live births and in the fluoridated ones 1.53 during periods of fluoridation.[45]

Although the higher rate in the fluoridated cities (14%) was attributed to a slightly higher maternal age in those cities – reported to be 34.0 years compared to 33.2 in the nonfluoridating ones – and to "a slight upward trend ['about 1 per cent per year overall'] in the rates of Down's syndrome" during the study period, no actual data were provided to support this claim; in fact, in *none* of the years did the overall statewide incidence exceed or even equal that of the fluoridated communities (highest = 1.51 in 1964).[46] Moreover, because the population exposed to fluoridated water was so extremely small, only 4.42% (81,017) of the total births and only 124 of the 2,469 cases of Down's syndrome, this difference of 1.53 versus 1.34 cases per 1,000 births was not formally significant statistically ($\chi^2 = 1.99; P < 0.12$). On the other hand, if the number of cases and total births in the fluoridated towns during this period had been exactly double (keeping the same rate of 1.53 per 1,000 births), the difference in rate between the fluoridated and nonfluoridated communities *would* then have become statistically significant ($\chi^2 = 3.99; P < 0.05$)!

In another report claiming "no association" between fluoridated water and Down's syndrome and other birth defects, the overall incidence of mongoloid births in the fluoridated counties of metropolitan Atlanta, Georgia, was actually higher than in the nonfluoridated ones by about the same amount as in Massachusetts (see Table 13–2 above, page 215).[30] Rapaport, too, had observed only a small increase in the incidence of mongolism after only five to ten years of fluoridation in Wisconsin.[25,29] The higher age-specific rate among younger mothers reported in the Atlanta study as well as the National Intelligence Surveillance survey,[30] also agrees with Rapaport's findings, although the authors were apparently unaware of the implications of this fact.

Finally, a recent analysis of data for over 2,000 cases of Down's syndrome available from an earlier USPHS investigation in lower Michigan has revealed that the occurrence of mongolism by local maternal residence reflected the same pattern and by about the same amount as in the Massachusetts and Atlanta studies. All incorporated cities of 2,500 population and over (1950 Census) were included and grouped according to either the natural or artificial fluoride content of the water supply. Not only were the overall incidence rates higher with fluoridation, but the proportion of mongoloid births among younger mothers in the fluoride communities was also greater.[47] The study also emphasized that many of the clinical and biochemical features regularly found in Down's syndrome are similar to various characteristics of the chronic toxic effects of fluoride.[48] A clear example of a fluoride-induced birth defect in rats is shown in Fig. 13-2 on the following page (220).

In summary, with the exception of the National Intelligence Surveillance survey,[30] which was based on admittedly incomplete ascertainment in only five major cities, all large-scale U.S. studies to date have shown higher incidence or prevalence rates of Down's syndrome births in communities with elevated levels of fluoride in the drinking water. Even if the actual increase has been only a conservative 10% with fluoridation, it would still amount to at least 150 *extra* cases per year among the nearly 100 million people currently supplied with artificially fluoridated water in the United States.* In this situation it is difficult to see how any conceivable dental benefit of fluoridation could outweigh such an increased risk; for the parents of a mongoloid child dental benefits provide little comfort.

CANCER

Certain inorganic compounds of chromium, arsenic, and nickel produce cancer in man, especially in the respiratory tract.[49] Can an even more physiologically active ion such as fluoride, with its

---

*Estimate based on an overall birth rate of 15 per 1,000 persons and the occurrence of one mongoloid birth per thousand live births.

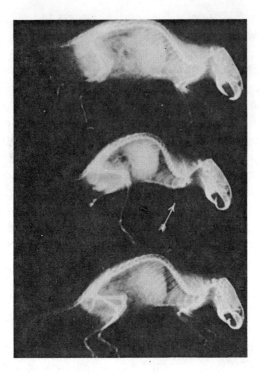

Fig. 13-2. X-Rays of rats (lower two animals) whose mothers were fed large doses (amounts unspecified) of sodium fluoride during pregnancy. Birth defects such as the absence of forepaws in the second animal have been recorded by Dr. A. Y. Charnot of Rabat, Morocco. The abnormal spinal curvature and the elongated, excessively curved upper incisors in the two lower animals are characteristic of fluorosis in rats. The animal at the top is a normal control. (Courtesy Dr. A. Y. Charnot.)

remarkable ability to penetrate and remain in many sensitive organs of the body, also be carcinogenic? The scientific evidence — circumstantial, experimental, clinical, and epidemiological — increasingly suggests that there is indeed a fluoride-cancer link.

Circumstantial Evidence. In areas where fluorspar (calcium fluoride) is mined, the incidence of lung cancer can be quite high. For instance, in St. Lawrence, Newfoundland, 21.8% of all mine employees and 36.2% of the underground miners died of lung cancer during the years 1933 to 1961.[50] The dust from this mine contained 62% fluorspar and 19% quartz, but it is not clear to what extent fluoride contributed to the carcinomas, since radioactivity was also present in the mine. The role of fluoride was not investigated.

Aluminum plant workers, particularly those in pot rooms where there is excessive exposure to fluoride fumes (see Table 10-1 above, page 129), also show elevated cancer mortality, especially from cancer of the lungs, pancreas, and lymph glands.[51] In the vicinity of two large aluminum plants, Soviet scientists encountered higher cancer death rates than in a control area seven to nine kilometers away, where the air was relatively unpolluted.[52] Although the major part of the carcinogenic activity was attributed to 3,4-benzpyrene (benzo[a]pyrene), which is one of the principal carcinogenic coal-tar products released in aluminum manufacture, the role of airborne fluoride was not excluded.

Other circumstantial evidence indicating that atmospheric fluoride may be carcinogenic comes from data gathered near steel foundries. In Hamilton, Ontario, the mortality from lung cancer in persons living near the steel mills was 65 per 100,000 inhabitants in 1966-1968 compared with a rate of only 12 per 100,000 inhabitants in the remote parts of the city and rates of 25 for the entire province of Ontario and 23 for Canada as a whole.[53] Although other toxic substances were also present, analyses showed a marked elevation in the fluoride content of vegetation in the areas of high cancer mortality around the mills. Higher neighborhood lung cancer mortality near a steel foundry in Scotland has also been reported.[54]

Circumstantial evidence of a different kind has been presented by Japanese scientists who found increased stomach cancer mortality in areas with high-fluoride levels in rice.[55] Another study showed a positive correlation of gastric cancer with the consumption of tea and ocean fish but a negative one with milk drinking.[56] In view of the generally high-fluoride content of both tea and whole ocean fish, plus the low-fluoride concentration and the known buffering and binding action of milk to reduce HF levels in the stomach, these findings again point to a possible carcinogenic role of fluoride.

Experimental Evidence. Various laboratory data also indicate a tumorigenic or at least a cancer-enhancing effect of fluoride. In long-term inhalation studies on rats, as little as 1.36 $\mu g/ft^3$ of

beryllium fluoride was carcinogenic, whereas 12 μg/ft^3 of beryllium sulfate or 100 μg/ft^3 of beryllium phosphate were required to
produce the same result.[57]   These differences, however, may also
reflect the fact that the latter two compounds are less soluble than
the fluoride. In fruit flies, exposure of the larvae to sodium
fluoride at concentrations as low as 0.001 molar (19 ppm) in the
nutrient medium has produced a dose- and time-dependent
increase in the incidence of melanotic tumors as well as lethal
mutations.[39,40]

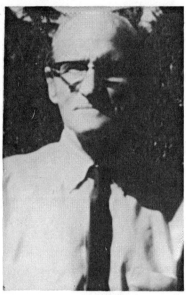

Fig. 13-3. Alfred Taylor, Ph.D.
(Oregon State College), 1896-1973.
Research Scientist, Clayton Founda-
tion Biochemical Institute, Univ. of
Texas, Austin, 1940-1965.
(Courtesy Dragi Milor.)

Much more pertinent, however, are the findings on mammals
such as those reported by the late Alfred Taylor (Fig 13-3, above).
In the early 1950s, while working at the Clayton Foundation Biochemical Institute of the University of Texas in Austin, this cancer
researcher discovered that female cancer-prone mice drinking distilled water "containing 1 ppm fluoride as sodium fluoride" developed mammary tumors at an earlier age in long-term studies than
control mice maintained on fluoride-free distilled water.[58] Although these results were immediately disputed on the grounds
that the high fluoride content of the ration (20-38 ppm) precluded
any significant effect from only 1-ppm sodium fluoride in the
drinking water, Taylor subsequently confirmed his findings by

including more than 360 female mice "fed a mixed grain diet containing a negligible fraction of fluoride."[59]

In these expanded studies he discovered a slightly higher percentage of tumors at death in the fluoridated mice than in the nonfluoridated controls (59% vs. 54% and, in the 10-ppm fluoride group, 63% vs. 50%). He also observed a statistically significant 9 to 10% decrease in the average life span in the experimental groups, and urinary calculi developed in the mice drinking fluoridated water whereas none were detected in the controls.

At variance with these findings are those reported by J. J. Bittner and W. D. Armstrong of the University of Minnesota. Using one-fourth as many mice of a *different* strain receiving either 0, 5, 10, or 20 ppm fluoride in the drinking water, these observers reported no significant difference in life span or the age at which tumors appeared.[60] Commenting on the apparent disparity between these results and his own, Taylor stated: "Since our data indicate that fluoridated water does not affect every mouse in a group but only certain susceptible individuals, it becomes necessary to have large numbers of animals in order to obtain results which are not due to chance segregation. Accordingly, a control group of 31 mice is entirely inadequate."[61]

Other studies by H. A. Schroeder and co-workers at Dartmouth also apparently showed no differences in life span or cancer incidence in both female and male mice (54 in each group) drinking either fluoride-free or 10-ppm fluoridated water.[62] In this work the males in the experimental group slightly outlived the controls, but the females exhibited an initially higher mortality at three to nine months and a significantly greater average body weight as they grew older.[63] Because of the use of a different strain of mice and the special nature of the diet and particularly the addition of chromium, cobalt, copper, manganese, molybdenum, and zinc to the water, the failure of these studies to confirm Taylor's findings is not surprising, especially since manganese has been shown to counteract the toxic effects of fluoride in rodents.[64] It is also striking that, contrary to what has been repeatedly observed for such organs as the aorta, Schroeder and co-workers claimed: "No fluorine was detected in the [soft] tissues of mice fed this element, even when the mice were two years old."[63]

Investigations on the growth rate of tumor transplants in rodents have also given conflicting results. With potassium fluoride in the drinking water at concentrations ranging from 170 to 500 ppm, one study showed no effect on the rate of growth of sarcoma implants in rats.[65] In another study – unfortunately only a preliminary abstract has appeared – the growth rate of sarcomas transplanted into mice and guinea pigs was reported to be retarded by 20 ppm of sodium fluoride in the drinking water or by injection of sodium fluoride at the tumor site.[66] Untreated animals were claimed to have shortened life spans and larger tumor masses.

Studies by Taylor and Taylor, published in 1965, showed that fluoride can either accelerate or suppress tumor growth, depending on the amount reaching the affected cells.[67] This work focused on the size of tumor growths in 991 mice and 1,817 embryonated chicken eggs containing mouse cancer tissue transplants (RC mammary adenocarcinoma). At low concentrations sodium fluoride gave highly significant but nearly dose-independent increases in the growth of the cancer implants in mice (DBA strain), whether the halide was added to the drinking water, injected subdermally at the tumor site, or added to the saline suspensions of the cancer cells before implantation. In the eggs tumor growth was also significantly accelerated, whether NaF was added to the suspensions before inoculation into the yolk sac or introduced over the chick embryo membrane.

On the other hand, as much higher levels of sodium fluoride were added to the tumor suspensions, a marked dose-dependent decrease in the rate of tumor growth that also paralleled the increase in NaF concentrations was observed. The apparent lack of a discernible dose-response relation to the degree of tumor growth acceleration in the low-fluoride-level experiments has been a source of criticism,[68] but a similar situation has been encountered in the inhibition of succinic dehydrogenase in the kidneys of golden hamsters after nine months of exposure to NaF in the drinking water at concentrations ranging from 1 to 100 ppm.[69] Furthermore, Taylor and Taylor also found that the addition of minute amounts of both sodium iodide[67] and sodium bromide[70] to their tumor suspensions increased the tumor growth rate after implantation. The concentrations, however, had to be at least 10 to 100 times greater than those at which sodium fluoride was still effective. But the very fact that these other two halides also accelerated the growth of tumor implants prepared from 0.85% saline suspension of tumor tissue provides impressive additional support for the validity of the results with sodium fluoride.

Clinical Evidence. Observations on persons undergoing fluoride therapy for osteoporosis strongly suggest that fluoride may, under certain conditions, contribute to the development of malignancies. In three elderly patients who received 16 to 150 mg of NaF daily for 1 to 36 months, "giant monocytoid cells, suggestive of reticuloendothelial malignancy," were discovered in the bone marrow in connection with symptoms of anemia. After discontinuation of the therapy these abnormal cell growths gradually disappeared.[71]

Although the amounts of fluoride used in such bone therapy are larger than those normally ingested from fluoridated water, there is a related clinical aspect of the Newburgh-Kingston study that "has never been followed up."[72] After 10 years of fluoridation the incidence of cortical bone defects in the children in Newburgh was 13.5%, but in nonfluoridated Kingston it was only 7.5% – a "statistically significant" difference. The original authors thought these defects were merely "benign lesions of childhood."[73] Taves, however, has drawn attention to the fact that "the age and sex of the afflicted persons and the anatomical distribution of these bone defects are 'strikingly' similar to . . . osteogenic sarcoma" and that "while progression of cortical defects to malignancies has not been observed clinically, it would be important to have direct evidence that osteogenic sarcoma rates in males under 30 have not increased with fluoridation."[72]

Epidemiological Evidence. Considering the many difficulties and uncertainties involved in the extrapolation of laboratory data to humans, it is not surprising that statistical studies on the relation of fluoride to cancer in man have also produced apparently contradictory findings. In Chapters 3 and 4 we saw that fluoride is very widely distributed in the environment and that there are many sources of intake even in low-fluoride water areas. Despite these handicaps, there is statistical evidence that fluoridation is associated with an increased incidence of cancer mortality in exposed populations.

With respect to naturally occurring fluoride in water, a USPHS survey of cancer mortality in 32 selected pairs of cities in 16 states indicated no significant differences among cities of 0.7 ppm or more fluoride and those with less than 0.25 ppm.[74] On the other hand, a later British study revealed higher stomach cancer mortality in high-fluoride areas of northern but not southern England.[75] An Italian survey of four volcanic districts near Rome disclosed a higher percentage of deaths from cancer in the fluoride areas (14.9%) than in the neighboring nonfluoride ones (10.9%), but the difference was not considered significant.[76] In Japan higher cancer death rates have been correlated with elevated levels of fluoride in the diet, especially in tea, seafood, and chemically fertilized rice and other crops.[55,56]

None of these studies, however, dealt with the effects of artificial fluoridation. In 1975 L. Kinlen of Oxford reported he could find no significant differences in the age-adjusted incidence of cancer in artificially or naturally fluoridated areas as compared with nonfluoridated or low-fluoride ones.[77] Although populations of several million were represented in this investigation, there were no comparisons of rates before and after fluoridation. Moreover, it is not known how the particular selection of many of the cities and areas, especially those abroad, may have affected the results.

It is of interest, therefore, that in the United Kingdom, where the fluoridated cities of Anglesey, Watford, and Birmingham-Solihull were compared with "nearby unfloridated areas," age-adjusted cancer incidences were appreciably higher in six of nine categories in the fluoridated areas than in the nonfluoridated ones (Table 13-4, opposite.) Indeed, the weighted average ratios of found to expected numbers of cancers in the fluoridated areas was 5.3% higher than in the nonfluoridated ones ($1.027 \div 0.975 = 1.053$). These results certainly do not support the author's assertion that "there is no significant excess of cancer of any site in fluoridated areas as compared with nearby nonfluoridated areas."[77]

About the time Kinlen's paper appeared, J. Yiamouyiannis, Science Director of the National Health Federation, and Dean Burk, retired Head of Cytochemistry at the National Cancer Institute, presented the first in a series of reports showing that the crude cancer death rates in the 10 largest fluoridated U.S. cities were higher and had risen faster since fluoridation than those in

Table 13-4

Ratio of Observed to Expected Cancers in Fluoridated and
Nearby Nonfluoridated Areas in the United Kingdom [77]

Site of Cancer	Fluoridated Areas[a]		Nonfluoridated Areas[a]	
Thyroid	1.09	(100)	0.91	(81)
Kidney	1.04	(223)	0.96	(201)
Stomach	0.98	(678)	1.02	(684)
Esophagus	0.99	(141)	1.01	(140)
Colon	1.03	(634)	0.97	(572)
Rectum	1.06	(480)	0.94	(416)
Bladder	1.04	(730)	0.96	(658)
Bone	0.88	(20)	1.18	(28)
Breast	1.03	(1099)	0.97	(986)
Total population (Av. 1961-1971)	1,295,212		1,304,676	

[a] Numbers in parentheses indicate total number of cancers observed.

the 10 largest nonfluoridated U.S. cities that had essentially the same crude cancer death rates during the decade before fluoridation. By the year 1969 the overall (unweighted) cancer death rate of the nearly 11 million inhabitants of the fluoridated cities was approximately 15% higher than that of the more than 7 million residents of the nonfluoridated cities. Data for major cancer sites and for regional comparisons of the cities also showed higher cancer mortality for the fluoridated than the nonfluoridated cities.[78]

Following the release of these preliminary findings, critics took sharp issue with the conclusion that these differences in cancer death rates were in any way connected with fluoridation. In particular, scientists at the National Cancer Institute argued that when appropriate corrections were made for disparities in age, race, sex, and cancer site distribution, the cancer death rates (CDRs = cancer deaths per 100,000 population) for the two sets of cities are almost identical. A formal study by R. N. Hoover and his colleagues at the NCI considered cancer mortality during the years 1950-1969 but did not deal with the same cities. Using data for age, sex, and cancer site for white populations at 5-year intervals in selected nonfluoridated, artificially fluoridated, and natural low- and high-fluoride counties, they concluded that there was no significant difference in cancer mortality ascribable to either artificially or naturally fluoridated water.[79]

In their study the task of relating community fluoridation to total county populations is complicated by the varying definitions of "community," the small size of many of the water districts, and the inclination of many communities to purchase their water from others, making it difficult to obtain an accurate identification of "exposed" and "unexposed" populations throughout the country. Moreover, their comparison of Birmingham, Alabama (nonfluoridated but heavily industrialized), with Denver, Colorado (fluoridated since March 1954), is severely flawed by the fact that lung cancer was much greater in Birmingham than in Denver, especially among the males. When lung as well as skin cancer are both excluded, then the increase in age-adjusted relative risk for all other types of cancer was *not* the same, as claimed, but *higher* in Denver than in Birmingham for both white males and females (Table 13-5, below).[80]

Other variables having a considerable effect on mortality data that were not taken into account by either the NCI or the Yiamouyiannis-Burk survey are the hardness of water (mineral content other than fluoride), increased consumption of fluoride from food as well as inhalation from polluted air, and the intercity and interstate shipment of foods and beverages prepared with fluoridated water.

In a critical analysis prepared for the Safe Drinking Water Committee of the National Academy of Sciences, Taves argued that the

Table 13-5

Age-Adjusted Relative Risk of Cancer
(All sites except lung and skin)[80]

Group	Denver/Birmingham		Change
	1947-1948	1969-1971	
White males	1.015	1.120	+10.3%
White females	1.005	1.085	+8.0%

standardized mortality ratios (SMRs = observed/expected cancer deaths) in the 20 largest fluoridated and 15 largest nonfluoridated U.S. cities show that the differences in CDRs were not real and that the observed increases were limited primarily to a particular group of fluoridated cities. Furthermore, he claimed that the adjusted CDRs in the fluoridated cities were already higher before fluoridation. He also noted that only one of the fluoridated cities had gained in population between 1950 and 1970, in contrast to seven of the nonfluoridated cities.[81]

In rebuttal, Yiamouyiannis demonstrated that SMRs can be completely misleading and can actually give a reverse of the true difference in CDRs, depending on the composition of the reference population used for the standardization. In his view, actual age-group data (direct method) are needed to make reliable comparisons.[82] Accordingly, he and Burk collected the cancer death figures for four age groups in each of their 20 cities; they found that while the CDRs differed only slightly up to age 44, *the rates for the age groups 45-64 and 65+ were significantly higher in the fluoridated cities* (Table 13-6, below).[83]

No appreciable sex-ratio differences were found in any age group, and the unweighted age distribution trends within the two older age groups, which had the significant CDR differences, were

Table 13-6

Increase in the Difference in Cancer Death Rate (per 100,000 population) of Ten Largest Fluoridated and Nonfluoridated U.S. Cities by Age Groups from 1952 to 1969 by Three Different Standard Statistical Procedures[83]

Method[a]	Age Group			
	0-24	25-44	45-64	65+
A	-0.09	+0.15	+13.1	+33.9
B	-0.06	+0.99	+16.4	+36.7
C	+0.04	+0.38	+15.2	+35.4
	(NS)[b]	(NS)[b]	($P < 0.02$)	($P < 0.05$)

[a] Given in Tables 6a, 6b, and 7 of Ref. 83.

[b] Not significant.

virtually identical in the two sets of cities. Furthermore, even though the nonwhite population of the fluoridated cities increased faster than that of the nonfluoridated cities, the CDR of nonwhites in the central cities was not increasing as rapidly as that of the whites. Overall, the age-adjusted CDR (unweighted) was still 4% to 5% higher (a rate of 8 to 9 per 100,000 population, or expressed in another way, 8,000 to 9,000 per 100 million population) in the fluoridated cities than in the nonfluoridated ones.

In papers published shortly before the detailed report of Yiamouyiannis and Burk appeared, two groups of British scientists argued, like Taves, that SMR calculations do not show any significant differences in CDRs between the two sets of cities.[84,85] In these papers, however, an incorrect figure (supplied by the NCI but not acknowledged by the authors) was used for the 1970 cancer death total in the nonfluoridated cities. Furthermore, only the data for the census years (1950, 1960, and 1970) were used, and one of the papers[84] based its calculations on a *shifting* reference population! As Yiamouyiannis has pointed out, when the correct 1970 figure for the nonfluoridated cities is used, and linear regression of all the available 1950-1968 data is employed, then even the SMR method shows a 4.5% higher CDR in the fluoridated cities than in the nonfluoridated ones.[86]

In an inquiry into the Yiamouyiannis-Burk findings and the manner in which the NCI had responded to them, a Congressional Committee held formal hearings on September 21 and October 12, 1977, at which time a full airing of the arguments and presentation of further evidence took place. Among the new data supporting the Yiamouyiannis-Burk results were those of V. A. Cecilioni, a Hamilton (Ontario) physician, showing a 17% higher crude CDR in fluoridated cities of Ontario during the period 1966-1974 as compared with nonfluoridated ones of the same size (15,000 or more population, 1971 census).[87] Similar findings were also reported for the year 1970 by Yiamouyiannis and Burk for all cities east of the Mississippi River having a population of 10,000 and over.[83]

On the other hand, an abstract of another NIH–USPHS study was also presented at these Congressional hearings that claimed no increase in cancer mortality between 1950 and 1970 in U.S. cities of 25,000 population and over.[88] This investigation involved comparison of age-adjusted CDRs from 187 low-fluoride (<0.7 ppm) nonfluoridated cities with 140 cities fluoridated in the period 1945-1959 and 87 cities fluoridated in the period 1960-1969. Among the latter were Atlanta, Dallas, Detroit, New York, Seattle, and several other major cities fluoridated *after* 1965. Although no increase in cancer mortality was found for cities of 200,000 population and over, the increase in mortality ratio was 1% to 3% higher in the three categories of fluoridated cities of 25,000 to 199,999 inhabitants.[89] (For further discussion, see Chapter 19, pp. 381-382.)

Also at these hearings the NCI scientists conceded that they had made and communicated an error to others in their reanalysis of the Yiamouyiannis-Burk findings. But they maintained that the cancer mortality differences between the fluoridated and nonfluoridated cities have demographic origins (mainly in age and race) rather than any connection with the introduction of fluoridation. Their data, as reported by one of the British groups (Table 13-7, next page), give a slightly greater increase in SMR for the nonfluoridated cities. On the other hand, when the statistically more accurate values derived from the best-fit line trend of the year-by-year average (weighted) CDR data are used, then the fluoridated cities show a greater overall increase in SMR, which agrees with the direct method results reported by Yiamouyiannis and Burk.

*

Can fluoride be linked to genetic abnormalities, including birth defects, as well as cancer? A wealth of scientific evidence discussed in this chapter clearly reveals the fluoride connection. Why then has fluoride not received sufficient emphasis in investigations of environmental contaminants? Why have scientists time and time again donned their armor to defend the virtue of fluoridation and increased fluoride ingestion despite mounting evidence of grave dangers to life? Why especially since: Rapaport's research on mongolism has *never* been refuted by redoing his work; Mohamed's studies on the deleterious effects of fluoride on chromosomes still stand; Taylor's experimental discoveries about cancer have successfully weathered intense criticism; and the conclusions of Yiamouyiannis and Burk on cancer mortality have not been invalidated? These fundamental discoveries, and others related to them, belie the supposed safety of fluoridation and have an ominous message for the human race.

Table 13-7

1950-1970 Cancer Death Rate Changes in Ten Largest Fluoridated and Nonfluoridated U.S. Cities by Two Standardized Mortality Ratio Calculations

A. By Weighted Average of Individual Census-Year CDR Data[85]

	Fluoridated		Nonfluoridated[a]	
	1950	1970	1950	1970
Observed (O)	180.8	217.4	179.0	194.3[b]
Expected (E)	146.9	174.7	155.5	166.0
O/E (SMR)	1.231	1.244	1.151	1.170
SMR Increase		+0.013		+0.019

B. By Best-Fit Line Trend of 1944-1972 Annual Weighted Average CDRs

	Fluoridated		Nonfluoridated[a]	
	1950	1970	1950	1970
Observed (O)	180	220	179	191
Expected (E)	146.9	174.7	155.5	166.0
O/E (SMR)	1.225	1.259	1.151	1.151
SMR Increase		+0.034		0.000

[a] Two of these cities (Atlanta and Seattle) began fluoridating their water supplies in 1969.

[b] Corrected from the erroneous value of 197.16 reported in Ref. 85.

REFERENCES

1. Epstein, S.S.: Environmental Determinants of Human Cancer. Cancer Res., 34:2425-2435, 1974.

2. McCann, J., Choi, E., Yamasaki, E., and Ames, B.N.: Detection of Carcinogens as Mutagens in the *Salmonella*/Microsome Test: Assay of 300 Chemicals. Proc. Natl. Acad. Sci. U.S.A., 72:5135-5139, 1975. For comment and reply, see Rubin, H., and Ames, B.N.: Carcinogenicity Tests. Science, 191: 241-245, 1976.

3. Ashby, J., and Styles, J.A.: Does Carcinogenic Potency Correlate with Mutagenic Potency in the Ames Assay? Nature (Lond.), 271: 452-455, 1978.

4. De Flora, S.: Metabolic Deactivation of Mutagens in the *Salmonella* Microsome Test. Nature(Lond.), 271:455-456, 1978.

5. Ames, B.N.: Letter to Dr. Arthur C. Upton, Director, National Cancer Institute, Bethesda, Md., October 19, 1977. Reproduced in: The National Cancer Program (Part 2.–Fluoridation of Public Drinking Water). Hearings before the Subcommittee on Intergovernmental Relations and Human Resources of the Committee on Government Operations, U.S. House of Representatives, 95th Congress, First Session, Sept. 21 and Oct. 12, 1977. Washington, D.C., 1977, p. 243.

6. Munn, J.I., and Kraybill, H.F.: Fluorides: Mutagenicity Studies Summary. National Cancer Institute, 12 October 1977. Reproduced in hearing record cited above in Ref. 5, pp. 484-486. See also Brown, K.S., Martin, G.R., Matheson, D.W., Lebowitz, H., Singer, L., and Ophaug, R.: Chromosome Studies in Fluoride Treated Mice. IADR Abstracts, 1978, No. 1052.

7. Muller, H.J.: Do Air Pollutants Act as Mutagens? In Symposium on Emphysema and Chronic Bronchitis Syndrome (Aspen, Colorado, June 13-15, 1958). Am. Rev. Respir. Dis., 83:571-572, 1961. (Quoted by A. H. Mohamed in Ref. 17, below.)

8. Mohamed, A.H., Smith, J.D., and Applegate, H.G.: Cytological Effects of Hydrogen Fluoride on Tomato Chromosomes. Can. J. Genet. Cytol., 8:575-583, 1966; Mohamed, A.H.: Cytogenetic Effects of Hydrogen Fluoride Treatment in Tomato Plants. J. Air. Pollut. Control Assoc., 18:395-398, 1968.

9. Mohamed, A.H.: Chromosomal Changes in Maize Induced by Hydrogen Fluoride Gas. Can. J. Gent. Cytol., 12:614-620, 1970; Mohamed, A.H.: Cytogenetic Effects of Hydrogen Fluoride Gas on Maize. Fluoride, 10:157-164, 1977.

10. Vogel, E.: Strong Antimutagenetic Effects of Fluoride on Mutation Induction by Trenimon and 1-Phenyl-3,3-Dimethyltriazene in *Drosophila Melanogaster*. Mutat. Res., 20:339-352, 1973.

11. Mukherjee, R.N., and Sobels, F.H.: The Effects of Sodium Fluoride and Iodoacetamide on Mutation Induction by X-Irradiation in Mature Spermatozoa of *Drosophila*. Mutat. Res., 6:217-225, 1968

12. Mohamed, A.H., and Kemner, P.A.: Genetic Effects of Hydrogen Fluoride on *Drosophila Melanogaster*. Fluoride, 3:192-200, 1970.

13. Gerdes, R.A.: The Influence of Atmospheric Hydrogen Fluoride on the Frequency of Sex-Linked Recessive Lethals and Sterility in *Drosophila Melanogaster*. Fluoride, 4:25-29, 1971.

14. Gileva, E.A., Plotko, E.G., and Gatiyatullina, E.E.: The Mutagenic Activity of Inorganic Fluorine Compounds. Gig. Sanit., 37:9-12, Jan. 1972. (Condensed translation in Fluoride, 8:47-50, 1975.)

15. Jagiello, G., and Lin, J.-S.: Sodium Fluoride as Potential Mutagen in Mammalian Eggs. Arch. Environ. Health, 29:230-235, 1974.

16. Leonard, A., Deknudt, Gh., Decat, G., and Leonard, E.D.: Cytogenetic Investigations on Leucocytes of Cattle Intoxicated with Fluoride. Toxicology, 7:239-242, 1977.

17. Mohamed, A.H., and Chandler, M.E.: Cytological Effects of Sodium Fluoride on Mice, in American Chemical Society Symposium on Fluoride Compounds in the Environment. San Francisco, Calif., Aug. 29-Sept. 3, 1976. (Reproduced in source cited above in Ref. 5, pp. 42-60.)

18. Manocha, S.L., Warner, H., and Olkowski, Z.L.: Cytochemical Response of Kidney, Liver and Nervous System to Fluoride Ions in Drinking Water. Histochem. J., 7:343-355, 1975.

19. Taves, D.R.: Fluoride, in Drinking Water and Health. Safe Drinking Water Committee, National Research Council–National Academy of Sciences, Washington, D.C., 1977, pp. 389-395.

20 Mohamed, A.H.: Letter, commenting on draft copy of work cited in Taves (Ref. 19, above), to Dr. Philip Handler, President, National Academy of Sciences, Washington, D.C., August 29, 1977. Copy in my possession.

21. Hearing record cited in Ref. 5 above, p. 243.

22. Rapaport, Y.[I.]: Les opacifications du cristallin mongolisme et cataracte sénile (Données statistiques récentes). Rev. Anthropol. (Paris), 2(3):133-135, 1957. See also Refs. 29 and 36, below.

23. Orner, G.: Dental Caries Experience Among Children With Down's Syndrome and Their Sibs. Arch. Oral. Biol., 20:627-634, 1975.

24. Hodge, H.C., and Smith, F.A.: Chronic Effects of Inorganic Fluorides, in J.H. Simons, Ed.: Fluorine Chemistry, Vol. IV. 1965, pp. 135-136.

25. Rapaport, I.: Contribution à l'étude du mongolisme. Rôle pathogénique du fluor. Bull. Acad. Natl. Med. (Paris), 140:529-531, 1956.

26. Van Valen, L.: Combining the Probabilities from Significance Tests. Nature (Lond.), 201: 642, 1964.

27. Douglas of Barloch, Lord: Mongolism and Fluoride Water. National Pure Water Assoc., Huddersfield, Yorks., England, 1964.

28. Rapaport, I.: Letter to A.L. Russell, D.D.S., Chief, Epidemiology and Biometry Branch, National Institute of Dental Research, Bethesda, Md., May 7, 1957. Copy in my possession.

29. Rapaport, I.: Contribution à l'étude étiologique du mongolisme. Rôle des inhibiteurs enzymatiques. Encephale, 46:468-481, 1957.

30. Erickson, J.D., Oakley, G.P., Jr., Flynt, J.W., Jr., and Hay, S.: Water Fluoridation and Congenital Malformations: No Association. J. Am. Dent. Assoc., 93:981-984, 1976; correction of tables, ibid., 95:476, 1977.

31. Berry, W.T.C.: A Study of the Incidence of Mongolism in Relation to the Fluoride Content of Water. Am. J. Ment. Defic., 62:634-636, 1958.

32. Report from the Royal College of Physicians of London: Fluoride, Teeth and Health. Pitman Medical, London, 1976, pp. 51-53.

33. Rapaport I.: Nouvelles recherches sur le mongolisme. A propos du rôle pathogénique du fluor. Bull. Acad. Nat. Med. (Paris), 143:367-370, 1959. See also Refs. 36 and 37 below.

34. Fedrick, J.: Anencephalus and Maternal Tea Drinking: Evidence for a Possible Association. Proc. R. Soc. Med., 67:356-360, 1974.

35. E.g., Dunning, J.M.: Current Status of Fluoridation. N. Engl. J. Med., 272:30-34, 84-88, 1965. See also Ref. 24 above.

36. Rapaport, I.: Oligophrénie mongolienne et ectodermoses congénitales. Ann. Dermatol. Syphiligr., 87:263-278, 1960.

37. Rapaport, I.: Oligophrénie mongolienne et caries dentaires. Rev. Stomatol. 64:207-218, 1963.

38. Jérôme, H., Lejeune, J., and Turpin, R.: Étude de l'excrétion urinaire de certains métabolites du tryptophane chez les enfants mongoliens. C. R. Hebd. Acad. Sci., 251:474-476, 1960.

39. Rapaport, I.: A propos du mongolisme infantile. Une déviation du métabolisme de tryptophane provoquée par le fluor chez la drosophile. Bull. Acad. Natl. Med. (Paris), 145:450-453, 1961.

40. Herskowitz, I.H., and Norton, I.L.: Increased Incidence of Melanotic Tumors in Two Strains of Drosophila Melanogaster Following Treatment with Sodium Fluoride. Genetics, 48:307-310, 1963.

41. Coleman, M., Ed.: Serotonin in Down's Syndrome. North-Holland, Amsterdam-London; American Elsevier, New York, 1973.

42. Hook, E.B.: Estimates of Maternal Age-Specific Risks of Down-Syndrome Birth in Women Aged 34-41. Lancet, 2:33-34, 1976.

43. Gentry, J.T., Parkhurst, E., and Bulin, G.V., Jr.: An Epidemiological Study of Congenital Malformations in New York State. Am. J. Public Health, 49:497-513, 1959.

44. Silberg, S.L., Marienfeld, C.J., Wright, H., and Arnold, R.C.: Surveillance of Congenital Anomalies in Missouri, 1953-1964. Arch. Environ. Health, 13:641-644, 1966.

45. Needleman, H.L., Pueschel, S.M., and Rothman, K.J.: Fluoridation and the Occurrence of Down's Syndrome. N. Engl. J. Med., 291:821-823, 1974.

46. Fabia, J.J.: Down's Syndrome (Mongolism): A Study of 2421 Cases Born Alive to Massachusetts Residents 1950-1966. D.Sc. Thesis, Harvard School of Public Health, 1970, Table 1.

47. Burgstahler, A.W.: Fluoride in Drinking Water and the Occurrence of Down's Syndrome. Paper presented at the Eighth Conference of the International Society for Fluoride Research, Oxford, England, May 29-31, 1977, and at the 13th Midwest Regional Meeting of the American Chemical Society,

Rolla, Mo., Nov. 3-4, 1977.

48. Burgstahler, A.W.: Editorial Review: Fluoride and Down's Syndrome (Mongolism). Fluoride, 8:1-11, 120, 1975.

49. Fraumeni, J.F., Jr.: Guest Editorial: Respiratory Carcinogens: An Epidemiological Appraisal. J. Natl. Cancer Inst., 55:1039-1046, 1975.

50. deVilliers, A.J., and Windish, J.P.: Lung Cancer in a Fluorspar Mining Community. Radiation, Dust, and Mortality Experience. Br. J. Ind. Med., 21: 94-109, 1964.

51. Milham, S., Jr.: Cancer Mortality Patterns Associated with Exposure to Metals. Ann. N.Y. Acad. Sci., 271:243-249, 1976.

52. Litvinov, N.N., Goldberg, M.S., Kimina, S.N.: Morbidity and Mortality in Man Caused by Pulmonary Cancer and Its Relation to the Pollution of the Atmosphere in the Areas of Aluminum Plants. Acta Unio Int. Contra Cancrum, 19:742-645, 1963.

53. Cecilioni, V.A.: Lung Cancer in a Steel City — Its Possible Relation to Fluoride Emissions. Fluoride, 5:172-181, 1972. Cecilioni, V.A.: Further Observations on Cancer in a Steel City. Fluoride, 7:153-165, 1974.

54. Lloyd, O. Ll.: Respiratory-Cancer Clustering Associated with Localised Industrial Air Pollution. Lancet, 1:318-320, 1978.

55. Okamura, T., Matsuhisa, T.: The Fluorine Content in Favorite Foods of Japanese. Jpn. J. Public Health, 14:41-47, 1968.

56. Hirayama, T.: Epidemiology of Cancer of the Stomach with Special Reference to Its Recent Decrease in Japan. Cancer Res., 35:3460-3463, 1975. For comment on the possible relationship of these findings to fluoride, see Taves (in Ref. 19, above), pp. 387-388.

57. Schepers, G.W.H.: Neoplasia Experimentally Induced by Beryllium Compounds. Prog. Exp. Tumor Res., 2:203-244, 1961. Cf. Schepers, G.W.H.: Lung Tumors of Primates and Rodents. Ind. Med. Surg., 40:48-53 (April), 23-31 (May), 8-26 (June), 1971.

58. Taylor, A.: Statement before House Select Committee to Investigate the Use of Chemicals in Foods and Cosmetics, U.S. House of Representatives, 82nd Congress, H. Res. 74 and H. Res. 447, 1952, pp. 1529-1543.

59. Taylor, A.: Sodium Fluoride in the Drinking Water of Mice. Dent. Digest, 60:170-172, 1954.

60. Bittner, J.J., and Armstrong, W.D.: Lack of Effects of Fluoride Ingestion on Longevity of Mice. J. Dent. Res., 31:495, 1952 (Abstract). Cf. Armstrong, W.D.: Statement before the Committee on Interstate and Foreign Commerce, U.S. House of Representatives, 83rd Congress, H.R. 2341, 1954, pp. 306-310.

61. Taylor, A.: Letter to the Science Editor: Fluoride and Cancer. Saturday Review, Oct. 2, 1965, p. 73.

62. Kanisawa, M., and Schroeder, H.A.: Life Term Studies on the Effect of Trace Elements on Spontaneous Tumors in Mice and Rats. Cancer Res., 29: 892-895, 1969.

63. Schroeder, H.A., Mitchener, M., Balassa, J.J., Kanisawa, M., and Nason, A.P.: Zirconium, Niobium, Antimony and Fluorine in Mice: Effects on Growth, Survival and Tissue Levels. J. Nutr., 95:95-101, 1969.

64. Tusl, J.: Effect of Fluoride and Manganese in Large Doses on Minerals and Trace Elements in Rats. Fluoride, 3:49-53, 1970.

65. Finerty, J.C., and Grace, J.D.: Effect of Fluoride on Tumor Growth. Tex. Rep. Biol. Med., 10:501-503, 1952.

66. Fleming, H.S.: Effect of Fluorides on the Tumor S 37 After Transplantation to Selected Locations in Mice and Guinea Pigs. J. Dent. Res., 32:646, 1953 (Abstract).

67. Taylor, A., and Taylor, N.C.: Effect of Sodium Fluoride on Tumor Growth. Proc. Soc. Exp. Biol. Med., 119:252-255, 1965.

68. Taves (in Ref. 19, above), p. 389.

69. Sullivan, W.D.: The In Vitro and In Vivo Effects of Fluoride on Succinic Dehydrogenase Activity. Fluoride, 2:168-175, 1969.

70. Taylor, A.: Effect of Sodium Bromide on Cancer Growth. Cancer Res., 24:751-753, 1964.

71. Duffey, P.H., Tretbar, H.C., and Jarkowski, T.L.: Giant Cells in Bone Marrows of Patients on High-Dose Fluoride Treatment. Ann. Intern. Med., 75:745-747, 1971.

72. Taves (in Ref. 19, above), pp. 388-389.

73. Schlesinger, E.R., Overton, D.E., Chase, H.C., and Cantwell, K.T.: Newburgh-Kingston Caries-Fluorine Study. XIII. Pediatric Findings After Ten Years. J. Am. Dent. Assoc., 52:296-306, 1956.

74. Hagan, T.L., Pasternack, M., and Scholz, G.C.: Waterborne Fluorides and Mortality. Public Health Rep., 69:450-454, 1954.

75. Heasman, M.A., and Martin, A.E.: Mortality in Areas Containing Natural Fluoride in Their Water Supplies. Mon. Bull. Minist. Health, 21:150-160, 1964. Cf. Nixon, J.M., and Carpenter, R.G.: Mortality in Areas Containing Natural Fluoride in Their Water Supplies, Taking Account of Socioenvironmental Factors and Water Hardness. Lancet, 2:1068-1071, 1974.

76. Mirisola, F., and Cruciani, A.: Indagine statistica sulla mortalità in alcuni paresi del Lazio con acque naturalmente fluorate. Ann. Stomatol., 13: 559-569, 1964.

77. Kinlen, L.: Cancer Incidence in Relation to Fluoride Level in Water Supplies. Br. Dent. J., 138:221-224, 1975.

78. Burk, D., and Yiamouyiannis, J.: Fluoridation and Cancer. Congressional Record, U.S. House of Representatives, 94th Congress, First Session, July 21, 1975, pp. H 1773-H 7176; Yiamouyiannis, J., and Burk, D.: Cancer From Our Drinking Water? Ibid., Dec. 16, 1975, pp. H 12731-H 12734; Yiamouyiannis, J., and Burk, D.: Fluoridation of Public Water Systems and Cancer Death Rates (CDRs) in Humans. (Paper presented before the American Society of Biological Chemists, San Francisco, Cal., June 6-10, 1976.) Fed. Proc., 35:1707, 1976.

79. Hoover, R.N., McKay, F.W., and Fraumeni, J.F., Jr.: Fluoridated Drinking Water and the Occurrence of Cancer. J. Natl. Cancer Inst., 57:757-768, 1976.

80. Data obtained from R.N. Hoover, NCI, by J. Yiamouyiannis, Personal communication, March 28, 1978. Calculations by Dr. Yiamouyiannis.

81. Taves, D.R., (in Ref. 19, above), pp. 381-389; also pp. 121-140 of hearing record cited in Ref. 5, above).

82. Yiamouyiannis, J.: Fluoridation and Cancer. Presented at the 143rd Natl. Meeting, Am. Assoc. Adv. Sci., Boulder, Col., Feb. 1977; cf. pp. 10-11 and 317-318 in hearing record cited in Ref. 5, above.

83. Yiamouyiannis, J., and Burk, D.: Fluoridation and Cancer. Age-Dependence of Cancer Mortality Related to Artificial Fluoridation. Fluoride, 10: 102-123, 1977.

84. Doll, R., and Kinlen, L.: Fluoridation of Water and Cancer Mortality in the U.S.A. Lancet, 1:1300-1302, 1977.

85. Oldham, P.D., and Newell, D.J.: Fluoridation of Water Supplies and Cancer—A Possible Association? J. Roy. Statist. Soc. Series C (Applied Statistics), 26(2):125-135, 1977.

86. Yiamouyiannis, J.: Letter to the Editor: Cancer Mortality and Fluoridation. Lancet, 1:150, 1978. For comment, see Doll, R., and Kinlen, L., and Oldham, P.D., Ibid., 1:150-151, 1978.

87. Cecilioni, V.A.: Letter to Gilbert S. Goldhammer, House Subcommittee on Intergovernmental Relations, Washington, D.C., August 27, 1977. Reproduced in hearing record cited in Ref. 5 above, pp. 258-261.

88. Rogot, E., Sharrett, A.R., Feinlein, M., and Fabsitz, R.R.: Trends in Urban Mortality in Relation to Fluoridation Status (Abstract). Reproduced in hearing record cited in Ref. 5 above, p. 183. Cf. Erickson, J.D.: Mortality in Fluoridated and Non-Fluoridated Cities (Abstract). Ibid., p. 182.

89. Rogot, E., Sharrett, A.R., Feinlein, M., and Fabsitz, R.R.: Trends in Urban Mortality in Relation to Fluoridation Status. Am. J. Epidemiol., 107: 104-112, 1978. Cf. Erickson, J.D.: Mortality in Selected Cities with Fluoridated and Non-Fluoridated Water Supplies. N. Engl. J. Med., 298:1112-1116, 1978.

CHAPTER 14

CRITICISMS OF POISONING REPORTS

IMPORTANT DISCOVERIES in science that run counter to orthodox beliefs often meet strong opposition or are accepted very slowly. Copernican astronomical ideas, for example, emerged victorious only after a bitter fight lasting over a century. For decades, William Harvey's brilliant arguments for the circulation of the blood met vigorous resistance from traditional biologists.

The history of medicine also has many instances where new theories and data, as well as reinterpretations of existing data, have been strongly opposed. In 1847, for example, the Hungarian obstetrician Ignaz Semmelweis found that childbed fever was caused by septic matter inadvertently picked up by doctors and medical students in operating and dissecting rooms. By initiating the simple procedure of washing hands with chlorinated lime (calcium hypochlorite) before making pelvic examinations of expectant mothers, he established the basis for the conquest of the disease, which had a staggering death toll rising to 25% among mothers and infants in European maternity hospitals. Unfortunately, many women and children were still doomed to die because the medical profession refused to accept his conclusions for another generation and adamantly maintained their "old [orthodox] ways" of treating maternity patients.

For over thirty years, proponents of fluoridation have steadfastly ignored or rejected all data showing adverse effects of fluoridated drinking water. Their attitude on this subject is typified by the following remark: "The author never ceases to marvel at those opponents of fluoridation who when faced with this mass of data [supporting fluoridation] fanatically continue their opposition, basing it on a mass of speculation."[1] Another writer has attempted by innuendo to cast all forms of opposition to fluoridation – scientific, ideological, political, ethical, etc. – into the same mold with little or no regard for their obvious differences.[2]

Equally common, however, is the practice by scientists of ignoring or slighting scientific evidence of harm from fluoridation. A recent report of the National Academy of Sciences discussed "Sensitivity to Fluoride" in precisely this manner. Although my numerous investigations (over 50 publications, many of which are cited in this book) on this subject are well known to the author of the fluoride section of the report, he nevertheless cited *only* my monograph published in 1962[3] and dismissed it on two grounds: that I "was the only one to report such effects, and that sensitivity of this type has not been reported among the billions of tea drinkers in the world who would be ingesting extra fluoride (WHO, 1970, p. 15)."[4] He tacitly admitted, nevertheless, that my cases have been scientifically substantiated by many others. Moreover, the sensitivity of some tea drinkers to fluoride[3,5-7] should be well known to scholars -- indeed, I had discussed in detail a clear example in the 1962 article[3] cited by the author of the NAS report in the very paragraph in which the above quotation appears!

Proponents of fluoridation have gone to extraordinary lengths in criticizing my work. They attribute the wide-ranging reactions that I have reported in my patients to psychosomatic origins or to disorders that occur "irrespective of the fluoride content of water supplies." They maintain that there is no consistent, uniform pattern to the symptomatology and that my double-blind tests are inadequate or inconclusive. They ask why I do not consider a "placebo effect" when my patients are switched to drinking distilled water. They believe that persons in India with skeletal fluorosis should exhibit symptoms of the type I and others have found in America and Europe. Finally, they ask why other physicians have not confirmed my observations. Let us, then, examine these objections to see if they do in fact hold water.

DIAGNOSIS

Like most other kinds of chronic poisoning, intoxication from long-term fluoride intake is difficult to diagnose because it develops slowly and unobtrusively with a wide variety of symptoms of the kind that are common to many other ailments. Dwelling on this point, W. D. Armstrong wrote in the *American Journal of Public Health:*

He [Waldbott] describes patients who complained of a variety of bizarre symptoms affecting a large number of organ systems. These symptoms, attributed by Dr. Waldbott to the use of fluoridated water, were present with few or no objective signs of specific disease and included gastric distress, pain in the spine, paresthesias, flatulence, polydipsia, mental aberrations, tinnitus, muscular weakness, etc. Rapid symptomatic cures were reported on withdrawal of fluoridated water, and Dr. Waldbott attempts to discount the suggestion that his patients' complaints had a psychogenic basis.[8]

E. R. Schlesinger elaborated further on this seemingly plausible criticism in a publication of the World Health Organization:

Of a selected group of 123 allergic patients tested, five developed a wide variety of symptoms and signs which developed five minutes to three hours after the test dose and lasted from twelve hours to ten days. Of the 21 symptoms and signs reported, only six occurred in more than one patient, and these were mainly of a nondescript nature, such as headache, nausea, vomiting, and epigastric pain. Physical findings such as muscular fibrillation, "cystitis", "spastic colitis", and facial edema were each found in not more than one patient.

The absence of any suggestion of a clinical syndrome leads to the conclusion that a variety of unrelated conditions were presented as cases of so-called "fluoride intolerance".[9]

This statement creates the false impression that only a limited number of patients experienced chronic poisoning. Actually, the five cases mentioned were only a part of a larger group of allergic patients without symptoms of fluoride intolerance. They were subjected to a special fluoride loading test for the purpose of recording any unusual reactions following the test dose. My experience with the disease now includes approximately 500 cases.

With respect to the wide spectrum of symptoms, I have already shown in Chapter 11 that there is solid experimental evidence to link every one of the above-named manifestations with fluoride intake. This nonskeletal phase of chronic fluoride poisoning was first discussed by Roholm,[10] one of the foremost authorities on the subject, in conjunction with advanced skeletal fluorosis and has been well confirmed by other investigators.[11-13] Furthermore, any experienced physician can usually recognize whether or not he is dealing with a real disease or psychosomatic complaints. Having had a lifetime of experience in the practice of allergic diseases — a medical specialty that concentrates, more than any other, on the detection of the causes of a disease — I have learned to distinguish readily between imaginary and real complaints. Moreover, a careful appraisal of the combination of the unusual symptoms which I described suggests a distinct syndrome that does not occur in any other disease: an attenuated phase of the acute stage of fluoride poisoning.

DOCUMENTATION

Another frequently reiterated comment has appeared in the *Journal of Asthma Research* by L. F. Menczer, a dental health officer of Hartford, Connecticut: "At no time has an authenticated case of 'fluoride intoxication' or 'fluoride poisoning' been reported. The word 'authenticated' is carefully chosen because Hartford like most cities has its share of anti-fluoridationists who have attributed their 'vague' symptoms to fluoridation."[14] But what constitutes "documentation" or "authentication" of a case of poisoning? There are at least three ways in which the cause of an illness such as fluorosis can be determined: (1) clinical observations, (2) laboratory procedures, and (3) epidemiological statistics.

1. Clinical Observations. In this respect the medical history of the individual is undoubtedly the most important element, particularly in chronic poisoning. Many patients retrospectively identified the onset of their disease with the beginning of fluoridation or with taking up residence in a fluoridated community, although usually they had been unaware of fluoride or fluoridation at the time. Most patients, before they came under my care, had undergone intensive diagnostic studies and a diversity of treatments, all to no avail. Critics must remember that diseases with symptoms similar to preskeletal fluorosis, such as diabetes, have always been considered and rejected when appropriate. Nearly all patients were under close observation before and after fluoridated water was eliminated, either at my advice or that of consultants who ruled out other diseases. Moreover, the presence of "Chizzola" maculae among persons consuming fluoridated water and their disappearance upon its elimination provides a tangible, objective sign verified by biopsies, which could not have been induced by a psychogenic factor.

2. Laboratory Procedures. In my work on fluorosis I have utilized various analytical data. Whenever possible, the fluoride content of the water consumed by patients has been verified. The 24-hour urinary fluoride excretion has been recorded on most cases with adequate controls. In the urine, the amount of the halogen rarely exceeded substantially the expected levels, an indication that the amount of fluoride in water at the "optimal" concentration is sufficient to induce the disease. It is true that I have not been able to obtain fluoride assays of blood and of bone tissue in my patients. Although such data might be desirable, they are not essential determinants for the diagnosis because there is considerable overlapping of these values in "normal" and fluorosed individuals.[3] The degree of poisoning does not necessarily parallel the amount of a toxic agent stored in organs or present in the blood stream;[15] merely the flow of a toxic agent through the organism can damage its health.

Unfortunately, at the moment no other direct laboratory tests for patients are available that might be regarded as specific for the diagnosis of fluoride intoxication, even in its advanced stage. Attempts have been made repeatedly to link changes in calcium and phosphorus levels of the blood and urine as well as certain enzyme activities, especially that of alkaline and acid phosphatase, with fluoride intake. I have been engaged in investigations on this question by determining these parameters before and after giving test doses of fluoride to patients suspected of poisoning.[16] Although these levels are occasionally elevated or lower than normal, lack of consistency does not permit the use of these tests as absolute diagnostic criteria for fluoride poisoning.

3. Epidemiological Statistics. Hard data on fluorosis from population studies in places like the United States and Canada are very difficult to obtain for the following reasons: (a) Few persons can escape the widespread fluoride contamination of food and drink because these products are often shipped great distances from the point of processing. Living in a nonfluoridated community therefore is not adequate protection from fluoridated products. (b) Population mobility diminishes or increases the impact of any one substance on a particular population in an unpredictable manner. (c) Widespread ignorance by the medical profession obscures the broad range of symptoms, especially since misdiagnosis is probably very common. (d) Pinpointing death from fluorosis in mortality statistics is difficult because apparent common causes are usually selected, even though they may not be fundamental causes. (e) Many variables must be considered when discussing the etiology of the disease—general health of the patient, his or her nutritional condition, environmental factors, etc.

Schlesinger demanded still another concept of "documentation" when he stated in the WHO monograph: "The several original case reports in the paper were not documented by any independent observer."[9] On the contrary, as many as nine specialists were consulted in evaluating some of my cases in order to rule out any other disease that could account for the patients' complaints (see Chapter 9, above). To eliminate possible bias, I took care not to select any physician who had taken a position on the fluoridation controversy, and, for reasons which will become apparent, I refrained from turning my cases of poisoning over to the supervision of health officials who had been engaged in the promotion of fluoridation. On June 2, 1955, however, I asked Governor G. M. Williams of Michigan to appoint a bipartisan committee to study my cases.[17] Unfortunately, for reasons unknown to me, it failed to materialize.

FLUORIDE INTAKE

Several critics have stated that I have not distinguished clearly between the effect of large doses of fluoride and repeated minute ones consumed by drinking fluoridated water. Referring to my work Schlesinger stated:

> Publications regarding adverse systemic effects from fluoridated water have often drawn analogies with the acute effects of toxic doses of fluorides or with the chronic effects of high levels of fluoride, particularly in hot climates. The latter observations have been further complicated by the effects of chronic malnutrition and by a high intake of dietary fluoride other than from drinking water. In citing the actual or stated systemic effects of high fluoride intake, the all-important factor of dosage has often been neglected. Many substances essential to life are toxic at excessively high levels, and this applies to oxygen and even to water itself.[18]

This statement raises several important questions: (1) What are "toxic" doses of fluoride? (2) Can the long-term effect of *minute* doses of fluoride be adequately assessed without reference to high intakes? (3) Is the toxicity of water and of oxygen comparable to that of fluoride?

1. The Toxic Dose. Until the mid-1950s, the American Medical Association carried a significant note on its stationery letterhead: "People differ.... no two living things are alike. . . . There is no standard dosage for drugs applicable to all patients under all circumstances." Indeed, every physician is aware that some individuals are intolerant to even extremely small amounts of a drug, and that it is impossible to establish a standard dose which is harmless for everyone.

As far as fluoride is concerned, numerous scientific reports of skeletal and dental changes have clearly demonstrated long-term toxic effects from the halogen at levels considered safe. In one case the concentration of fluoride in water naturally ranged from 0.8 to 3.45 ppm,[19] in another between 0.4 and 2.6, in a third it was 1.7 ppm.[20] Recent data from India have associated fluorotic bone disease with a concentration as low as 0.73 ppm,[21] which is considered "optimal" for fluoridation in hot climates. The death of a newborn infant in Ames, Iowa, reported by J. F. Bacon, was almost certainly related to the consumption of artificially fluoridated water by his parents (Chapters 8 and 11, above). Even at 0.3 ppm fluoride in water naturally, Webb-Peploe's middle-aged heavy tea-drinking patient developed skeletal fluorosis.[5] In combination with other sources, therefore, even low concentrations of the halogen in drinking water can be hazardous.

2. Acute vs. Chronic Fluoride Effect. Can the effects of large doses of fluorides be disregarded in discussing fluoride poisoning from drinking water? Of course not. Schlesinger himself referred to such poisoning when he stated: "With regard to acute fluoride poisoning there is at least a 2,500-fold factor of safety in water fluoridation. The mechanics of water fluoridation are such that it is impossible to produce acute fluoride poisoning either by accident or intent."[22]

This statement is false. Two episodes of mass poisoning from excess fluoridation of water were described in Chapter 7. Moreover, the manifestations of acute intoxication from large doses of fluoride—especially the excruciating stomach pain, gastric hemorrhages and diarrhea combined with muscular pains, extreme exhaustion, and the neurological symptoms culminating in convulsions—do in fact set the pattern for the less conspicuous and more subtle cardinal signs of chronic intoxication following intake of minute amounts. They likewise involve primarily the gastrointestinal tract (nausea, vomiting, gastric pain, diarrhea) and the central nervous system (headache, paresthesias, beginning retinitis) and increasingly severe general debility termed by early writers "fluoride cachexia."[23]

3. Toxicity of Water. Schlesinger's comparison of the toxicity of water and oxygen—two agents on which life depends—with that of fluoride is completely fallacious. In evaluating the toxic properties of an agent "at excessively high levels," we must consider its toxic threshold. McClure, one of the foremost advocates of fluoridation, considered a daily fluoride intake above 4.0 to 5.0 mg to be hazardous: "The data suggest that these [4.0 to 5.0 mg daily] may be limits of fluorine which may be ingested daily [by healthy adults] without an appreciable hazard of body storage of fluorine."[24] If we are to believe McClure, there is *no* latitude between the harmless and the toxic dose of fluoride, since in a fluoridated community a total intake of 4.0 to 5.0 mg/day is now common, as a result of the increase of the fluoride content in many food items. In hot climates or working environments, far more water than the adult average of two liters per day must be consumed to maintain health. But anyone who drinks two to three times more than the average amount of water for whatever reason is definitely at risk because fluoride intake will be increased significantly above what is considered safe. The toxicity of water *per se* simply cannot be placed in the same category with fluoride toxicity.

EXCESSIVE ABSORPTION OF FLUORIDE

In addition to the question of intake, H. M. Leicester has raised a point concerning the mode of absorption of fluoride. After commenting on my description of health effects from large doses of fluoride, he stated in a review:

He [Waldbott] is equally uncritical in describing the form of absorption of the fluorides. His only excuse for bringing in the corrosive action of hydrofluoric acid is his description of the case of a boy who, after taking a fluoride tablet containing 0.4823 mg of fluoride, suffered from stomach hemorrhage. Waldbott, who admits he is not a biochemist, believes that this occurred because the hydrochloric acid of the gastric juice (pH 1 to 2.5) liberated enough hydrofluoric acid to corrode the stomach lining.[25]

That small amounts or low concentrations of fluoride ion in contact with gastric juice generate enough undissociated hydrofluoric acid to irritate or damage the lining of the stomach is not a new suggestion by me. As pointed out years ago by Roholm, Wieland and Kurtzahn observed that both fluoride and silicofluoride salts react with gastric hydrochloric acid to produce hydrofluoric acid that penetrates the stomach mucosa in a nondissociated state (HF) causing corrosive changes: "For absorption of fluoride from low-solubility compounds such as calcium fluoride, fluoroapatite, and cryolite, the acidity of the stomach plays a decisive role."[26]

Roholm further elaborated his view on this question as follows: "The corrosive action of fluoride upon the skin and mucous membranes is not likely to be mediated by the acidity [per se] but by the fact that the undissociated HF molecule penetrates the epidermis and the mucosa and thus damages the underlying tissue. Therefore, not only hydrogen fluoride and silicofluoride have a corrosive action but all other acid solutions of fluorides as well, particularly bifluorides and silicofluorides."[27] Other studies have also demonstrated the formation of hydrogen fluoride in an acid urine and its penetration into soft tissue (the bladder) at a pH range of 1.85 to 5.5.[28]

DOUBLE BLIND TEST

G. N. Jenkins of the Dental School, University of Newcastle upon Tyne, in England, has taken issue with the technique of the double blind test that I have employed to prove the relationship of the disease to fluoride. He doubted that the "observer was unaware of whether the dose or the placebo was given."[29] As a matter of fact, in my blind studies neither the patient nor the observer (double-blind) could have known which of the three bottles contained fluoride. In several instances the test was performed by other physicians without my being in any way involved. The patients were free to choose the sequence in which they consumed the contents of each bottle. The pharmacist who numbered the bottles 1, 2, and 3 was the only person who knew which bottle contained fluoride. An even more meticulous approach was followed by Grimbergen in 1974 in conjunction with other clinicians who confirmed my observations; a notary public was the sole individual who knew which bottle contained fluoride.[30]

Concerning the concentrations of the dose used in my tests, Jenkins stated:

> In three cases, the dose given was 6.8 mg, but in one case only 0.9 mg of sodium fluoride in 300 ml of water, in another case the fluoride was injected intradermally and, in two others applied as a 1% solution of sodium fluoride under the tongue. It is unfortunate that no supervised blind tests appear to have been carried out with water containing 1 *p.p.m.* of fluoride. In the one 'double-blind' test described the dose was 1 mg of fluoride in one tablespoonful of water for seven days (i.e. 30 times the concentration in fluoridated water). A reaction occurred after the third daily dose. FELTMAN (1956) reported three cases of eczema resulting from the daily ingestion of tablets containing 1 mg of fluoride. It is quite conceivable that a reaction might occur in some subjects to these doses administered in these ways and yet they would not be affected by the much lower concentrations which are present in the tissue when water containing 1 *p.p.m.* is taken.[29]

We must ask: Does the toxic action of a poisonous agent depend on a total specified dose or on its concentration? Whereas a highly concentrated solution may indeed inflict damage to organ tissues with which it comes into contact, total organism toxicity studies are usually based on overall dose, rather than on concentration. Originally I performed the test as described by Jenkins because I wanted to determine whether or not one patient is less tolerant to fluoride than another. Subsequently, however, I utilized many modifications with different concentrations and varying doses. Finally, I gave patients three bottles of water and instructed them to use the water in each bottle sequentially for an entire week for all drinking and cooking needs – one of the three was fluoridated at 1 ppm, the others were fluoride-free distilled water. *In none of the cases thus tested did I fail to reproduce the symptoms,* usually within 24 to 48 hours following consumption of the fluoridated water.

In many instances, the purpose of the double-blind test was fulfilled by the course of events since both the patient and his physicians were completely unaware that they had been consuming fluoride in their drinking water. The following case report furnishes a striking example of this fact:

Mr. N.K.T., age 45, consulted me in early April 1976 because of a variety of complaints that his physician had not been able to diagnose. He had been in perfect health until 1954 when he moved to Milwaukee (fluoridated August of 1953).* He then developed increasingly severe headaches, low back pain, frequent nausea, and abdominal pains that forced him to seek lighter work as a salesman in 1956. In the fall of 1957 he had two episodes of convulsions for which his physicians could find no explanation. Shortly thereafter he moved to Okauchee, Wisconsin (own well water†) where, unexpectedly, all his symptoms cleared up completely. Upon resuming residence in Milwaukee in late 1959 he found that his illness immediately recurred. Again in 1961 he took another job in Antioch, Illinois, and he remained in good health while living there until 1968. He had consumed water from a shallow private well, the composition of which could not be ascertained because it was abandoned after he left. In 1968 he again returned to Milwaukee and worked as a salesman. He soon experienced persistent backaches, headaches, extreme fatigue, and excessive thirst. He became forgetful and unable to comprehend. He also experienced weakness in his muscles, tinnitus (ringing) in both ears, pain and edema (swelling) in hands and ankles, and bleeding of the gums. After five months he was forced to stop working because of this progressive illness. During his illness he received a variety of treatments, including traction of the spine, muscle relaxing drugs, and analgesics, all to no avail. According to his physician's record, diagnostic studies revealed only a minor hearing loss in his left ear. Another attempt at working on a job operating heavy equipment had to be terminated because of his gradually worsening backaches.

In October 1969 he moved to Woodruff, Wisconsin (nonfluoridated‡), where his illness again cleared up without medication.

---

*Milwaukee water then contained 0.95 ppm F^-, 16.1 ppm Ca^{++}, 9.6 ppm Mg^{++}, and 80 ppm total hardness.

†Okauchee (own well) water contained 0.15 ppm F^-, 37 ppm Ca^{++}, 8 ppm Mg^{++}, and 164 ppm total hardness.

‡Woodruff water contained 0.10 ppm F^-, 42 ppm Ca^{++}, 17 ppm Mg^{++}, and 176 ppm total hardness.

When on December 1, 1972, he once more took up residence in Milwaukee the backaches returned promptly, this time with pains and swelling in most other joints, paresthesias in the fingers, and muscular fibrillation. Because of the muscular weakness, it became difficult for him to open doors; he had to sleep for at least 12 out of 24 hours. There was a slight, temporary rise in blood pressure (160/90). His condition improved somewhat by taking large amounts of vitamin C (1500 mg daily) and bone meal tablets, but during October 1973 the arthritis gradually became much more pronounced, especially in his knees, and failed to yield to salicylates prescribed by his physician. He also showed evidence of allergic nasal disease. Because of several episodes of acute abdominal pains, his gall bladder and appendix were removed, but the abdominal symptoms (pains, bloating, diarrhea) persisted. The records obtained from his physician, however, showed no unusual physical or laboratory findings.

In late 1974, while his health continued to deteriorate, his attention was directed to fluoridated water when a generalized skin rash on his infant son cleared up promptly and completely as soon as distilled water was substituted for Milwaukee's water in the baby's formula, a measure suggested to him by a friend. Although skeptical about this apparent cure, the father, upon further urging by his friend, decided likewise to substitute distilled water for himself. The bowel disturbances, especially the abdominal pains, were promptly alleviated. Within ten days all other symptoms had disappeared. Since using distilled, fluoride-free water he has remained in perfect health, operating heavy construction equipment and performing difficult physical work without any of the previous adverse reactions.

In August 1976 his symptoms recurred while he was using a filter which, it was claimed, would remove fluoride. He learned that the filtered water he had been drinking for three days contained 1.3 ppm fluoride.

This is but one of many similar cases which eliminate any doubt that the individual involved could have imagined his disease. No double-blind nor any other test could more conclusively document fluoridated water as the cause of this disease than the fact that neither the patient nor his physician had any previous knowledge of the presence of fluoride in drinking water. Because of the ease and rapidity with which the patient recovered simply by changing to nonfluoridated water, as well as the failure to respond to any other treatment, and because of the prompt recurrence of the disease upon renewed consumption of fluoride in water or from other sources, no additional tests were either necessary or would have provided any better proof. Nevertheless, about one-third of my patients were willing to undergo double-blind tests that fully confirmed the correctness of the diagnosis.

Jenkins has also doubted the reality of "allergy [intolerance] to fluoride" on the grounds that "allergy to tea [rich in fluoride] has not been described" – at least in Britain, which "should be the ideal country to study it because, as a tea drinking nation, almost the whole population has been at risk for centuries!"[29] As we have seen in the beginning of this chapter, intolerance ("allergy") to tea in Britain has been unequivocally established. Administration of tea by nasogastric tube to eliminate taste repeatedly elicited symptoms characteristic of fluorosis – including abdominal pain, headache, tachycardia, nausea, and vomiting – whereas plain water did not.[7] Although reactions to the caffeine and xanthines in tea might be expected sometimes, those reported in these cases probably are due to fluoride.

PLACEBO EFFECT

It is also claimed that in my work "no mention was made of any symptoms experienced while taking distilled water alone, such as are commonly noted in trials using a placebo."[31] Presumably this means that I should find that some patients *become ill* or are made *more ill* when they are tested with distilled water. I have never observed this to occur, nor would I expect to unless the illness *is* psychosomatic. It is one thing to see a positive "placebo" effect in a patient who thinks he or she is made better by taking only a blank or "placebo" in place of a real drug or medication. It is quite another matter to expect that the removal or absence of a known toxic agent like fluoride might actually precipitate the toxic effects of that agent!

If indeed there are any better explanations for the various nonskeletal ill effects that I have shown are caused by fluoridated water, then critics would do well to point out what they might be. To date they have not done so, and their efforts to discredit the truth of my discoveries on the basis of such objections and criticisms as reviewed above are no more compelling than the arguments that were used to reject the revelations of Semmelweis on the cause of childbed fever.

CONFIRMATION OF MY REPORTS

To what extent have others in the last thirty years discovered nonskeletal fluorosis from artificially fluoridated water or in areas of endemic skeletal fluorosis? A report by English physicians discounts such a possibility: "It may be noted that studies in parts of the U.S.A. where the fluoride concentration is 8 mg/litre [Bartlett, Texas] have produced no evidence of this symptom described by Waldbott."[31] But how could such an incredibly small sample — under 120 persons, only 11 of whom were born in the community — produce conclusive results, universally applicable, especially since the examining physicians were not trained to detect the nonskeletal symptoms of the disease? The episodic, fleeting character of these symptoms also obscures diagnosis of fluoride poisoning, as Roholm observed.[10]

The same English report has also claimed that scientists in India have not described these symptoms among patients with skeletal fluorosis.[31] Work by J. W. Suttie has shown that new generations of cells damaged by fluoride have a tendency to build up resistance to it,[32] and populations subjected to long-term fluoride exposure — as in India or in Bartlett, Texas — may to some extent adapt to the toxicity. However, the claims made by the English report are simply incorrect. Arthritis-like symptoms, without skeletal fluorosis, have been observed in endemic areas of India.[33] Moreover, in high-fluoride regions of Sicily, gastrointestinal distress and liver damage from fluoride have been detected.[11] A wide spectrum of these nonskeletal features among industrial workers has also been described.[34]

Fortunately, clinicians are now recognizing the preskeletal symptoms of chronic fluoride poisoning. In addition to confirmations in reputable scientific reports,[30,35-37] I have received numerous communications from practicing physicians who have corroborated my clinical observations. For instance, W. P. Murphy of Boston, a 1934 Nobel Prize winner in medicine, diagnosed fluoride poisoning from drinking water (Fig. 14–1, opposite). Unfortunately,

WILLIAM P. MURPHY, M. D.
1101 BEACON STREET
BROOKLINE 46. MASSACHUSETTS

LONgwood 6-4445

May 4, 1965

Dr. George L. Waldbott
2930 West Grand Boulevard
Detroit 2, Michigan

Dear Dr. Waldbott:

I was glad to receive your letter of April 1st
on the subject of fluoride treatment. I shall look up your
monographs as suggested in the first paragraph. I did see
and read your letter in the May 1st issue of Saturday Review.
This is very well stated and should help to dispel the idea
that fluorides are entirely safe.

I regret to say that I have not had sufficient
knowledge of fluoride effects so that I would know whether or
not the thrombocytes are increased after its use. It is possible
that this is an early manifestation of a bone marrow irritation
which might later show in the production of the erythrocytes
and leukocytes. One of the early manifestations of poisoning
with benzol,and some of its relatives, is a rise in all of the
bone marrow produced cells.

The patient to whom I referred while living in a
community in which the water was fluoridated had rather continuous swelling of the lower legs and face,aggravated by certain
foods or medications to which she was allergic. After moving
from this community to a non-fluoridated one this swelling largely
disappeared and only appears now after exposure to fairly large
amounts of allergens. After moving she started using a fluoride
tooth paste at which time she developed a rash on her cheeks
and mouth with swelling of the face. After stopping this toothpaste this condition cleared up completely.

I doubt very much that it would be possible to
carry out further studies on this patient, although if you would
give me an outline of what you might like, perhaps it could be
arranged.

Sincerely,

William P. Murphy, M. D.

WPM:j

Fig. 14-1. Facsimile of letter from William P. Murphy, M.D., 1934 Nobel
Laureate in Medicine, concerning a patient sensitive to fluoridated water and
toothpaste.

physicians appear to be reluctant to present such cases to the scientific community. The absence of conclusive laboratory data, the slow and insidious onset of the disease, the wide spectrum of symptoms, the general ignorance of the medical profession about possible side effects from fluoridated water and airborne fluoride —all these things undoubtedly account, to some extent, for the paucity of reports in the medical literature. Furthermore, physicians are constantly being assured that fluoridation is safe, which is bound to influence an objective appraisal of their findings. For the same reasons the untoward effects of many other environmental pollutants have escaped our recognition for many decades. As will be seen in Chapter 18, physicians would also lose referrals and suffer other forms of recrimination.

OTHER COMMENTS: CHIZZOLA MACULAE

Proponents of fluoridation have long demanded more objective symptoms of nonskeletal fluorosis. Yet when precisely this kind of evidence is presented, they invariably deny it. For example, Hodge and Smith [38] question the relationship of fluoride to Chizzola maculae, the suffusion-like skin lesions found near fluoride-emitting factories and, less frequently, in artificially fluoridated communities (see Chapters 10 and 11 above, pages 141-145 and 166-167). They base their views on an incomplete summary of the literature with emphasis on the work of Cavagna and Bobbio, [39] whose research, I learned from Dr. Cavagna himself, was sponsored by one of the companies involved in litigation from fluoride pollution in Italy. Who can truthfully say that the interpretations of these Italian scientists were unbiased?

Hodge and Smith claim that other Italian scientists "cast doubt on the accepted etiology by pointing out that in the village of Pilcante, 7 km from Chizzola, 23% of the children were affected [in 1967] although fluoride contamination *must have been* less than in Chizzola." [38] [Emphasis added.] This statement is misleading, since the article cited made no such claim. In fact, the opposite conclusion should be drawn: villages farther than Chizzola from the polluting factory should have had *fewer* cases of the lesions, which is indeed the case. [39-41]

That the scientists cited by Hodge and Smith thought the maculae were caused by fluorides is certainly a reasonable inference: "For many years, women and children have complained of skin lesions similar to suffusions in an area of Trentino, near an aluminum plant. These lesions first were observed in the same place about 30 years ago. *The symptomatology is related to damage to the vegetation due to emission of fluorine compounds.*"[40] [Emphasis added.] When fluoride pollution abated between 1937 and 1965 (the factory had installed anti-pollution devices), so also did damage to vegetation – and Chizzola maculae did not appear.

Hodge and Smith also claim a lack of increased fluoride levels in urine when Chizzola maculae are present is proof that these lesions have other causes. This opinion is false: there are records of persons with Chizzola maculae exhibiting increased fluoride levels in their urine, just as there are cases with normal levels.[41] Elevated urinary fluoride is not a prerequisite for nonskeletal fluoride intoxication.

*

If fluoridation is the long-awaited universal panacea which will eliminate the ravages of tooth decay with no harm to anyone, why have my critics responded to my work by distorting scientific facts? Why have false statements been made about numerous reports of adverse effects? Why have proponents of fluoridation failed to offer viable alternative medical explanations of my discoveries rather than falsely claiming that they have "not been confirmed?" Why have these proponents not admitted that in Europe and elsewhere fluoridation is diminishing, not growing? Why has the majority of the world rejected this particular brand of American "wisdom"? Perhaps scientists, who are after all human beings, find it difficult to abandon ideas supported for three decades. This Great Dilemma has apparently become a political, not a scientific health issue.

REFERENCES

1. Largent, E.J.: Fluorosis: The Health Aspects of Fluorine Compounds. 1961, p. 73.

2. McClure, F.J.: Water Fluoridation: The Search and the Victory. 1970, pp. 263-284.

3. Waldbott, G.L.: Fluoride in Clinical Medicine. Int. Arch. Allergy Appl. Immunol., 20, Suppl. 1, 1962.

4. Taves, D.R.: Sensitivity to Fluoride, in Drinking Water and Health. 1977, pp. 378-379.

5. Webb-Peploe, M.M., and Bradley, W.G.: Endemic Fluorosis with Neurological Complications in a Hampshire Man. J. Neurol. Neurosurg. Psychiatry, 29:577-583, 1966.

6. Cook, H.A.: Crippling Arthritis Related to Fluoride Intake (Case Report). Fluoride, 5:209-213, 1972; cf. Lancet, 2:817, 1971.

7. Cf. Finn, R., and Cohen, H.N.: "Food Allergy": Fact or Fiction? Lancet, 1:426-428, 1978.

8. Armstrong, W.D.: Books and Reports: Review of *The American Fluoridation Experiment*. Am. J. Public Health, 47:1022, 1957.

9. Schlesinger, E.R.: Statements on Adverse Systemic Effects from Fluoridated Water, in Fluorides and Human Health. WHO Monograph Series No. 59. 1970, p. 309.

10. Roholm, K.: Fluorine Intoxication: A Clinical-Hygienic Study. 1937, pp. 137-138.

11. Fradà, G., Mentesana, G., and Nalbone, G.: Ricerche sull'idrofluorosi. Minerva Med., 54:45-59, 1963.

12. Schmidt, C.W.: Auftreten von Nachbarshaftsfluorose unter der Bevölkerung einer Säshsischen Kleinstadt. Dtsch. Gesundheitswes., 31:1271-1274, 1976.

13. Murray, M.M., and Wilson, D.C.: Fluorine Hazards with Special Reference to Some Social Consequences of Industrial Processes. Lancet, 2:821-824, 1946.

14. Menczer, L.F.: Fluoridation and the Allergist. J. Asthma Res., 3:121-131, 1965 (at p. 128). For reply, see Waldbott, G.L.: Dr. Waldbott's Reply *re* Fluoride Allergy. Ibid., 3:249-251, 1965.

15. Gettler, A.O., and Ellerbrook, L.: Toxicology of Fluorides. Am. J. Med. Sci. 197:625-638, 1939.

16. Waldbott, G.L.: A Clinical Test for Determination of Tolerance to Fluoride. Bull. Henry Ford Hosp. Med. Soc., 5:259-268, Dec. 1957.

17. Waldbott, G.L.: Letter to Dr. A.E. Heustis, Commissioner, Michigan Department of Health, and G.M. Williams, Governor of Michigan, June 2, 1955.

18. Schlesinger (in Ref. 9, above), p. 308.

19. Sauerbrunn, B.J., Ryan, C.M., and Shaw, J.F.: Chronic Fluoride Intoxication with Fluorotic Radiculomyelopathy. Ann. Intern. Med., 63:1074-1078, 1965.

20. Juncos, L.I., and Donadio, J.V., Jr.: Renal Failure and Fluorosis. J. Am. Med. Assoc., 222:783-785, 1972.

21. Jolly, S.S., Prasad, S., Sharma, R., and Chander, R.: Endemic Fluorosis in Punjab. I. Skeletal Aspect. Fluoride, 6:4-18, 1973.

22. Ast., D.B., and Schlesinger, E.R.: The Conclusion of a Ten-Year Study of Water Fluoridation. Am. J. Public Health, 46:265-271, 1956.

23. Cristiani, H., and Chausse, P.: Nouvelles expériences sur le temps nécessaire à l'apparition de la cachexie fluorique chez cobayes à la suite d'ingestion de divers sels de fluor. C. R. Séances Soc. Biol. Fil., 95:15-16, 1926.

24. McClure, F.J., Mitchell, H.H., Hamilton, T.S., and Kinser, C.A.: Balances of Fluorine Ingested from Various Sources in Food and Water by Five Young Men. Excretion of Fluorine Through the Skin. J. Ind. Hyg. Toxicol., 27:159-170, 1945. (Reprinted in Fluoride Drinking Waters. 1962, pp. 377-384.)

25. Leicester, H.M.: Library at Large: Review of *A Struggle With Titans.* Chemistry, 40(3):33-38, March 1967.

26. Roholm, K.: Fluor and Fluorverbindungen, in W. Heubner and J. Schüller, Eds.: Handbuch der experimentellen Pharmacologie, Ergängzungswerk, Vol. 7. 1938, p. 38.

27. Preceding Reference, p. 20.

28. Whitford, G.M., Pashley, D.H., and Stringer, G.I.: Fluoride Renal Clearance: A pH–Dependent Event. Am. J. Physiol., 230:527-532, 1976.

29. Jenkins, G.N.: Fluoride. World Rev. Nutr. Diet., 7:138-203, 1967 (at pp. 194-195).

30. Grimbergen, G.W.: A Double Blind Test for Determination of Intolerance to Fluoridated Water (Preliminary Report). Fluoride, 7:146-152, 1974.

31. Report of the Royal College of Physicians of London: Fluoride, Teeth and Health. 1976, p. 63.

32. Suttie, J.W., cited in Special Report: AAAS Fluoride Symposium in Denver. Fluoride, 10:141-144, 1977. Suttie, J.W.: Fluoride Resistance in Cell Cultures, in E. Johansen and D.R. Taves, Eds.: Continuing Evaluation of the Use of Fluorides. Westview Press, Boulder, Col., in press, 1978.

33. Teotia, S.P.S., Teotia, M., and Teotia, N.P.S.: The Joints, in Symposium on the Non-Skeletal Phase of Chronic Fluorosis. Fluoride, 9:19-24, 1976.

34. Czerwinski, E. and Lankosz, W.: Fluoride-Induced Changes in a Group of 60 Retired Workers from an Aluminum Factory. Fluoride, 10:125-136, 1977.

35. Kailin, E.: Letters of the International Society of Allergists, 34:150, December 10, 1971; Lee, C.H.: ibid., 35:9, January 1972.

36. Petraborg, H.T.: Chronic Fluoride Intoxication from Drinking Water (Preliminary Report). Fluoride, 7:47-52, 1974; Hydrofluorosis in the Fluoridated Milwaukee Area. ibid., 10:165-169, 1977.

37. Zanfagna, P.E.: Allergy to Fluoride, in Symposium on the Non-Skeletal Phase of Chronic Fluorosis. Fluoride, 9:36-41, 1976.

38. Hodge, H.C., and Smith, F.A.: Occupational Fluoride Exposure. J. Occup. Med., 19:12-39, 1977.

39. Cavagna, G., and Bobbio, G.: Contributo allo studio delle caratteristiche chimico-fisiche e degli effetti biologici degli effluenti di una fabbrica di alluminio. Med. Lav., 61:69-101, 1970.

40. Colombini, M., Mauri, C., Olivo, R. and Vivoli, G.: Observations on Fluorine Pollution due to Emissions from an Aluminum Plant in Trentino. Fluoride, 2:40-48, 1969.

41. See Refs. 3, 4, and 34 in Chapter 10, above.

CHAPTER 15

SETTING THE STAGE

THE STORY of water fluoridation in the United States would be incomplete without a brief account of the curious history describing how scientists and laymen learned about the process. Friction, strife, and furious debates characterize these episodes. Indeed, The Great Dilemma — the problem of how to eradicate tooth decay by adding fluoride to water supplies without at the same time harming the human body — divided the scientific community into two opposing camps. There were those who wanted to make the measure available to everyone immediately, believing that there were no adverse health effects, whereas others — particularly scientists in the U.S. Public Health Service — maintained a conservative attitude and were reluctant to commit themselves to a blanket approval of fluoridation before much more research had yielded conclusive proof of its safety.

The position of the first group was spearheaded by a Wisconsin dentist, J. J. Frisch. Inspired by the original suggestion of G.J.Cox (Chapter 5, above), Frisch mounted a vigorous promotional campaign for fluoridation. In his book, *The Fight for Fluoridation,* the historian D.R. McNeil described Frisch as "a man possessed." In fact, "Fluoridation became practically a religion with him."[1] Frisch enlisted many supporters, including the state dental health officer, Francis A. Bull, who organized political campaigns in order to persuade local officials to approve the measure. Their attempts to fluoridate Frisch's home town of Madison in 1946 were frustrated because the city council's expert advisory group, including several outstanding University of Wisconsin scientists, recommended against approval. Eventually, however, Frisch's lobbying effort convinced the city fathers to disregard the recommendation of the expert panel. Events in Wisconsin set the pace for a drive on a much broader scale throughout the nation.

Scientists in the USPHS, on the other hand, were much more reserved and had urged many additional years of research before implementing fluoridation on a broad basis. "This means that experiments must be made whereby fluorine is added to the water supply of some large group of people. Such a study may take 12 to 15 years before the final answer is clearly delineated." Until the experiment was completed, two procedures were suggested: "topical applications of fluoride solutions to the teeth" and "supplementing individual diets with fluoride in drinking water, fruit juice, or milk."[2]

To learn more about the effects of fluoride, Washington scientists organized a number of conferences early in the 1940s. December 29, 1941, marks the date of the first symposium in Dallas, Texas, where the nation's leading authorities on fluoride presented their findings. In a review of the background to water fluoridation, F.S. McKay pointed to "the rapidly accumulating evidence that fluorine in some way exerts an inhibitory influence on the inauguration of dental caries."[3] H.T. Dean summarized his extensive studies on mottled teeth in the United States: in several communities surveyed, dental fluorosis in the classification of "mild" – white, opaque areas (often later becoming stained) on not more than half the surfaces of the teeth involved (see Fig. 5–6 above, p. 67) – were observed in Marion, Ohio; Pueblo, Colorado; and Elgin, Kewanee, Aurora, and Joliet, Illinois (fluoride concentrations of 0.4 to 1.3 ppm).[4] Thus, even at about the fluoride level recommended for fluoridation, a substantial number of children would probably develop mottled teeth. Cox, the originator of the fluoridation idea, and his co-worker Margaret M. Levin, also warned that in our enthusiasm about the decay-reducing potential of fluoride we should not lose sight of other factors that affect resistance to dental caries:

Fluorine is the only element thus far proved to have a definite relationship to dental caries. It is not unlikely that other factors are required for the caries-resistant structure. We have ourselves observed much improved teeth in rats coming from diets in which the mother had a high-fat diet, half being butter fat, suggesting that vitamin D may play a part if present during the period of the formation of the teeth.[5]

H. V. Smith, who had made extensive studies on endemic fluorosis in southern Arizona, sounded an outright warning on artificial fluoridation:

> If extremely rigid control of the fluorine ingested could be had, if absolute control is not maintained or if an individual secures some fluorine from water, an additional amount from foods, and still more from spray residues, it is not beyond the realm of possibility that the toxic limit may be exceeded, when mottled enamel would result.[6]

Smith questioned the benefits of fluoridation in later life. In St. David, Arizona, where the water was naturally fluoridated (1.6 to 4 ppm), he had found among 12- to 40-year-old residents that "more than seventy per cent of the individuals over 24 years of age had lost some teeth by extraction after unsuccessful attempts at repair. Fifty per cent of all individuals over 24 years of age had lost all of their teeth and are now wearing plates." He emphatically added: "In St. David, fluorine has not eliminated caries."[6] M.C. Smith (H.V. Smith's wife and co-worker) collaborated with Isaac Schour of Chicago on experimental work with dental fluorosis. They reported: "Any plan to build caries-resistance into teeth by addition of fluorides to public water supplies as a public health procedure is extremely hazardous. The range between toxic and non-toxic levels of fluorine is of such small order as to make even the continuous use of fluoride dentifrices a probable danger."[7] Thus, the spirit of this first American Association for the Advancement of Science conference on fluoridation in Dallas was one of a search for the truth, and both the advantages and disadvantages of the measure were freely debated. The conferees were fully aware of The Great Dilemma confronting them.

A second symposium followed in September 1944 in Cleveland, Ohio, and a third one in New York City on October 30th of the same year. In Cleveland, Dean suggested "the disclosure of the relationship of minute amounts of fluorine to dental health constitutes probably the outstanding dental research finding of the present century."[8] Unfortunately, his belief did not eliminate The Great Dilemma. Two scientists from foreign countries related their experiences with dental fluorosis in natural fluoride areas. R. Weaver had found 21.2% mottling in South Shields, England (1.4 ppm), as compared with 0.4% in North Shields (<0.25 ppm).[9] On the other hand, T. Ockerse referred to studies conducted in 843 South African endemic areas since 1935 which revealed that "the caries-experience rate among children with mottled enamel is considerably lower (29%) than among those with no mottling (69%)."[10] Also at this conference, B. G. Bibby of the Dental School, University of Rochester, New York, gave the following sound advice:

> There is no reason to believe that fluorine therapy alone can produce a tooth which will resist decay regardless of the strength of the attack. It would therefore be unwise in our enthusiasm over the possibilities of fluorine therapy to lose sight of the necessity of continuing to seek improved methods of weakening the power of the caries attack.[11]

The New York City conference, which was held about six months prior to the start of pilot studies in Newburgh, seemed to be directed toward informing and arousing the support of the rank and file of the dental profession. Five leading sponsors of fluoridation addressed more than 1,000 dentists, physicians, and laymen at the New York Institute of Clinical Oral Pathology, and the edited transactions of the symposium were published and widely disseminated to the dental profession.[12] This conference, like the two previous ones, reflected the uncertainty about the outcome of the proposed measure, particularly with respect to its long-term effects upon the health of the Newburgh population. McKay characterized fluoridation as "another 'biological experiment station,'" in which the rationale is applied directly to humans without previous laboratory experiments on animals."[13] Although many unproved assumptions and unanswered questions were in evidence throughout the session, he thought there was "ample reason to believe that the project at Newburgh will justify itself; and if so, the same method could be applied anywhere: there would be no limit."[13]

Most authorities of the PHS shared his certainty that their experiment would turn out successfully; nevertheless, they hesitated to approve its general use. Initially, as McNeil observed: "David Ast, like H. Trendley Dean, wanted no part of wholesale fluoridation. Grand Rapids and Newburgh were to be large-scale experimental laboratories. Both Ast and Dean urged that other communities considering fluoridation do it on a study basis only, not as an accepted public health measure."[14]

From 1945 to 1950 PHS officials were able to hold the Wisconsin promoters "at bay," and when local city officials in Wisconsin requested a formal opinion from the PHS, they received word that mass fluoridation "cannot be recommended."[15] This "cautious attitude" greatly disturbed the Wisconsin dentists and thwarted their campaign to fluoridate Oshkosh, Wisconsin. In 1948 Frisch and Bull applied political pressure through Congressman Frank Keefe, a member of the House Appropriations Subcommittee, who urged PHS officials to approve the measure, but they persisted in their refusal to fluoridate the nation's water supplies prematurely.[16]

By 1949 preliminary data began to leak out of Grand Rapids and Brantford, indicating that after four years of artificial fluoridation 4- and 5-year-old children had a lower incidence of tooth decay than the control groups. This evidence induced Bull and Frisch to renew and intensify their nationwide lobbying campaign, particularly among professional leaders at medical and dental society meetings.

Eventually, in May of 1950, at a conference of state dental directors, Bull, Ast (who obviously reversed his earlier position), and two other state dental health officers were able to weaken the resistance of Dean, Arnold, and Bruce Forsyth, the assistant surgeon general. The late M. Wollan, lawyer and historian, gave this account of the meeting as described to him in an interview with Frank Bull:

> Dr. Bull once again buttonholed every major Public Health Service official attending the conference. In particular, he concentrated on Dr. Bruce Forsyth, assistant surgeon general and chief dental officer for the PHS. Bull drew Forsyth aside and told him he was "being made a sap out of," because before long the PHS would be the only major health organization refusing to endorse fluoridation.[17]

Within the PHS, however, the debate continued. Wollan stated:

> Although Dean stuck to his original position, Forsyth and Surgeon General Leonard Scheele were becoming convinced that it was time for the PHS to back fluoridation. Finally, Forsyth and Scheele, as the nation's top-ranking public health officers, either formally overruled Dean or informed him that they were about to endorse fluoridation, with or without him.[17]

A few days later, on June 1, 1950, came a major turning point in the campaign with the announcement by the PHS that, "Communities desiring to fluoridate their communal water supplies should be strongly encouraged to do so."[18] From then on the cautious policy of the PHS gave way to an enthusiastic political campaign rarely witnessed in the scientific community; significantly, at all subsequent government-supported scientific gatherings the health hazards of the measure were given little consideration. This turn of events was particularly evident at another symposium held in the late 1950s at the University of Indiana, Indianapolis, in which only strong advocates of fluoridation participated. The Great Dilemma seemed to have been "solved" until February 25, 1977, when for the first time in two decades, a symposium of the American Association for the Advancement of Science permitted debate on the possible relationship of fluoride to cancer, as well as other deleterious effects.[19]

THE CRUCIAL CONFERENCE: 1951

Early in June 1951, dental health representatives from various American states and territories met with federal health authorities to discuss the promotion and implementation of fluoridation. In emphatic and candid language the PHS spokesmen outlined a program calculated to introduce fluoridation as widely as possible. Attending the conference were the nation's state dental health directors as well as dental officials from Costa Rica, Puerto Rico, and the Virgin Islands. The World Health Organization was represented by Phil Blackerby of the Kellogg Foundation; the ADA had delegated Philip Phair, a former dental health officer of the State of Washington, as their representative. J.W. Knutson, at the time Assistant Surgeon General and Chief of the Dental Division of the PHS, chaired the conference.[20]

Katherine Bain, the first speaker and also a member of the technical service committee for the Kingston-Newburgh fluoridation study, explained that the fluoridation experiment in Newburgh, New York, initiated on May 2, 1945, was to have been kept "under wraps for 10 years." At the end of that period, the experiment was to provide an answer on the benefits of fluoridation and on any possible harm it might have on human health. But so much "pressure" developed — she did not indicate the source — that health authorities were obliged to "go ahead with these programs," i.e. fluoridation and topical applications, before the experimental period had been completed.

Dr. Bain's introductory speech was followed by remarks by Leonard Scheele, PHS Surgeon General, who had just returned from the World Health Assembly where he was elected president and where a resolution in support of fluoridation by the U.S. delegation had passed. Scheele spoke of the obstacles to the program, particularly among officials of the District of Columbia who objected to its experimental nature. The Washington D.C. commissioners had wondered "whether glass might turn white, plastics might dissolve, bread might taste different," and about similar problems that might arise. Scheele, however, felt confident that the "communities that do move ahead will make the ones who don't decide they had better get on the band wagon."

Scheele then turned to what he called the "pièce de résistance" of the program — a presentation entitled "Promotion and Application of Water Fluoridation," by F. A. Bull. Through his close association with Frisch in Wisconsin, Bull had gained considerable experience in the technique of putting across the case for fluoridation. His campaign had been so successful that in 1950 fifty communities in Wisconsin had already approved fluoridation of communal water supplies; this was more than triple the number of *all* other communities then fluoridated in the entire United States. Still, there were many unresolved problems impeding his promotional efforts, and appropriate answers had to be found. Would diabetics and people with kidney diseases be harmed? What significance does mottling, a permanent and irreparable tooth defect, have on general health? Could the kind of bone changes and spontaneous fractures that were reported from high fluoride areas in India, North Africa, and Italy also be produced by artificially fluoridated water? Moreover, could the concentration of 1 ppm be maintained throughout the water mains of a large city?

Terminology in the Campaign. One of the foremost promotional hurdles to overcome was the problem of dental fluorosis resulting from fluoridation. Bull instructed his colleagues to describe mottled teeth to the public and to the profession as "egg-shell white" and "the most beautiful looking teeth that anyone ever had," even though these teeth are known to turn brown and brittle in later years. Acting upon his advice, some of his listeners subsequently called such teeth "pearly white" to impart a dramatic image of their attractiveness.

In fact, a new terminology, requiring George Orwell's "doublethink," was proposed for many other concepts related to fluoridation. The term "artificial fluoridation" was to be avoided. "There is something about the term," he advised, "that means a phoney.... We call it 'controlled fluoridation.'" The word "experiment" should never be used. "To take a city of 100,000 and say, 'We are going to experiment on you, and if you survive, we will learn something' — is kind of rough treatment on the public. In Wisconsin, we set up demonstrations. They weren't experiments." Bull even objected to the name "sodium fluoride" since this compound, which was at that time being used for fluoridation, was also widely known as rat poison. The term "fluoride" would be less objectionable, he advised.[21]

The "Reverse Technique" and Cancer. An even more serious problem had to be dealt with. At the Clayton Foundation Biochemical Institute of the University of Texas, A. Taylor had just presented experimental evidence that fluoride causes earlier tumor formation and shortens the lifespan of cancer-prone mice (Chapter 13, above). Bull commented on this important scientific finding: "When this thing came out we never mentioned it in Wisconsin. All we did was to get some publicity on the fact [!] that there is less cancer and less polio in high-fluoride areas. We got that kind of information out to the public so that if the opposition did bring up this rumor they would be on the defensive rather than have us on the defensive." "The best technique is the reverse technique, not to refute the thing but to show where the opposite is true."[22]

This promotional approach of calling bad, *good*, and sour, *sweet* has been used repeatedly in the campaign for fluoridation. Again, in Orwell's *1984* this process is called "Newspeak," where what is true becomes "false," and the false becomes "true." Promotion of fluoridation was to be pushed vigorously, even if accounts about health hazards were grossly distorted or ignored most of the time. The truth of the matter is that no studies were then available on the relationship of fluoride to the incidence of cancer or poliomyelitis.

During the question-and-answer session following his talk, Bull again evaded the scientific issues when he responded to a question on fluorides and cancer. "You know it was a technique in advertising years ago to take the weakest point and stress it as the best part of the thing that you were trying to sell." Fluoridation didn't really cause cancer: "There are data that definitely show that our fluoride areas are the healthiest places in the United States."[22]

Fluoridation Surveys. Nor were there adequate statistical data to support the claim that tooth decay can be prevented by the addition of fluoride to drinking water. To overcome this handicap, Bull exhorted his fellow health officers to speak of fluoridation as a great success and recommended that pre-fluoridation surveys be made at the state level by representatives of the state board of health and of the state dental society but not really to find out if fluoridation works: "No, we have told the public that it works, so we cannot go back on that." The early surveys would have to be followed up by subsequent ones to "prove to the public and to the dental community that fluoridation is effective. You want your pre-fluoridation data so [that] 3, 5 or any year[s] from now you can go back into these same areas and do the same type of survey, and show the people what they got for their money."[23]

Meetings and Lobbying. Much of Bull's speech was devoted to how the press, the dental societies, and the citizens of a community should be swayed. He recommended public hearings to which the press was to be invited: opposition speakers were to be excluded or, at least, given limited time. A dentist should always be looked upon as "The Authority" on the subject. Before such meetings, members of the press should be contacted and be given articles on fluoridation of the kind published in the *Cleveland Press* for which the Lasker Foundation paid $500 and gave a gold cup — "a terrific piece of publicity." "You tell them [the press] how fluoridation helps the poor devil who can't afford proper dental care and all that."[24]

Sponsors. Public meetings should also be sponsored by lay groups and service clubs. The PTA (Parent-Teacher Association) was singled out as a "honey when it comes to fluoridation. Give them all you've got." Public officials, aldermen, mayors, "anybody you can get," should be contacted — a "sort of lobbying procedure you are carrying out."[25]

Bull particularly urged that physicians be enlisted in the cause. "The medical audience is the easiest audience in the world to present this thing to," and a resolution by the county medical society would be easy to obtain. "You build a fire under somebody at the local level"[26] in medical and dental societies, he instructed his fellow conferees. Chemists and engineers might also be needed for the campaign. Bull predicted the ease by which the press was to be won for the cause. Reporters undoubtedly would rely on what they were told by the new "authorities" on the subject, namely the local promoting dentists. Unfortunately, they had only fragmentary knowledge of the available scientific research and usually relied entirely upon the promotional material received from the Public Health Service and the American Dental Association.

Bull summarily cast aside all possible hazards to health. Fluorosed teeth were "the most beautiful looking teeth that anyone ever had," not clear evidence of physical harm. He also realized that most physicians in 1951 knew as little about the toxicity of fluoride as they knew about the health effects of cadmium, selenium, and many other toxic substances, and he conceded that he had no solution for this dilemma. "This toxicity question is a difficult one. I can't give you the answer on it. So when you get the answer on the question of toxicity please write to me at once, because I would like to know."[21] Later in his talk he referred again to this vexing problem:

> If it is a fact that some individuals are against fluoridation, you have just got to knock their objections down. The question of toxicity is on the same order. Lay off it altogether. Just pass it over, "We know there is absolutely no effect other than reducing tooth decay," you say, and go on. If it becomes an issue then you will have to take it over, but don't bring it up yourself.[27]

Except for a brief allusion to the claimed remote possibility that workers at the water works might inhale sodium fluoride dust, the above-quoted remarks represent Bull's *only* comments on the possible ill effects of fluorides. The rest of his words focused entirely on selling and promotion in the same way that many advertisers sell their products. Whether Bull's long-range intentions were "noble" is beside the point, for his disregard for the known toxic effects of fluoride can neither be justified nor defended.

Significance of the 1951 Conference. Bull's keynote speech reveals the heart of early fluoridation efforts and the key emphasis on Madison-Avenue promotion, not on scientific evidence. The significance of this meeting cannot be overestimated for two important reasons. In the first place, fluoridation was to be promoted on the basis of authority: "We have told the public it works, so we can't go back on that." Marshall influential supporters—mayors, PTAs, waterworks operators, aldermen, public officials, *et al.* —in the "lobbying procedure." Evade purely scientific issues; play down costs; tout benefits, which must—and therefore *will*—result. In the second place, strategically placed health officials from states and territories had been presented the time-tested strategies that had been used to persuade the inhabitants of Wisconsin to fluoridate. Their power over the Nation's health was enormous.

The sponsors of this meeting, particularly Surgeon General Scheele and his deputy Knutson, were also exceedingly influential in the scientific community. They were in a position to distribute or withhold research grants and other public funds to universities, which depend on PHS support. They could manipulate scientific thinking by rewarding cooperating scientists with research funds and positions of higher rank. They could blacklist and impose penalties on those who failed to fall in line. Even dental schools in foreign countries were dependent on PHS grants. Since the World Health Organization is liberally supported by U.S. tax funds, the voice of Washington officials was also influential in establishing its policies. This fact, combined with their ability to win the cooperation of leading scientists abroad by means of research grants, gave USPHS officials entry into many countries outside the United States and made it extremely difficult for top officials in such countries as Ireland, The Netherlands, and Great Britain to reject fluoridation.

PROMOTION BY THE ADA

The promotional design evolved by Bull at the Fourth Annual Conference was promptly taken up by the American Dental Association whose representative, Philip Phair, had attended the conference. In February 1953, the ADA issued a brochure that is a masterpiece in the art of engineering consent.[28] It was distributed to local and state dental societies and thus reached every corner of the U.S.A. In this pamphlet, Bull's directives were embellished with new and more powerful promotional tools, unique in the history of scientific organizations. It outlined the fine points in the technique of lobbying and of molding public opinion without giving the citizenry a chance to hear the other side of what had become one of the most vehement scientific controversies in the history of the Nation.

Downgrade Opponents. A major addition of this brochure to Bull's approach pertained to downgrading the public image of opponents. The pamphlet categorized the opposition as follows:

- — "Drugless healers of all types."
- — "Members of religious groups who believe that fluoridation constitutes medication."
- — "Those who oppose—because it is advocated by an opposing political party."
- — "Those who fear an economic threat to the sale of such things as vitamin and mineral preparations."
- — And finally, so-called "obscure 'scientists' and self-appointed protectors of the public who object to *every* public health measure."[29]

Besmirching the public image of opponents in advance effectively prevented anyone from presenting any significant opposition.

Citizens Committees. The ADA pamphlet elaborated on the method for winning community leaders to the cause. Representatives on every level in the community were to be approached. Members of labor groups, teachers, health leaders, business people, Chambers of Commerce, church, civic and social groups were to be chosen to man so-called "citizen's committees." Their chairman was to be selected on the basis of aggressiveness and of determination to see the job through to a successful conclusion. "Important names are not enough—members of the committees must be willing to assist in local fluoridation efforts," the pamphlet stated. The committee members had to be dedicated to promoting the local fluoridation efforts.

The first task of these committees was to obtain written endorsements of fluoridation from the local dental society, the medical society, and other influential community organizations.

Dentists were asked to display and distribute leaflets and to write letters to newspapers praising the merits of fluoridation. Suggested speeches for presentation to groups were available from the ADA.

Out-of-town "experts" were to be recruited, thus providing countless "newspegs" for purely local news releases. The presence of the state dental director or other representatives of the state health department was imperative in order to impress the audiences with the significance of the new health measure.

The pamphlet also gave explicit instructions on how dentists should conduct themselves at such hearings with decorum and restraint: "At no time should the dentist be placed in the position of defending himself or his profession or the fluoridation process." Special care should be taken that the legislation on fluoridation "not be submitted to the voters, who cannot possibly sift through and comprehend the scientific evidence."[30]

How to Refute Objections. Objections to fluoridation should be refuted in the following manner:

— The (objections) are "documented from out-of-date materials written by well-known persons."

— They are obtained "from little-known lay magazines, newspaper articles, letters to the editor, or health faddist periodicals."

— They are "based on incorrect and ill-chosen terminology used by well-known persons."

— They are "partial quotes from authoritative sources" and "misinterpretations based upon an incomplete knowledge of the subject."

— They are "unwarranted and hasty conclusions drawn from research work."

— They are "completely unsubstantiated and undocumented statements from obscure 'scientists.'"

— They are quoted from "little-known, and out-of-date or unrecognized medical dictionaries and encyclopedias."[31]

Do's and Don'ts. The balance of the brochure provided additional helpful hints on what to do and what not to do. The promoting dentist should not attempt to rebut every assertion made by opponents. As a matter of fact, he need not have a personal technical knowledge of the subject. He could simply refer to the fact that health authorities in the United States have approved fluoridation and, therefore, objections need not be answered. This advice merely reiterated that given in the 1951 conference.

The ADA interpretation of the term fluoridation, however, went much further than that of Dr. Bull. Fluoridation should be labelled "nutritional," "tooth-building," or a "public health measure." Such terms as "therapeutic," "medicative," "artificial," and "experimental" should be avoided. On the contrary, emphasis should be placed on such expressions as "adding fluoride to water [which is] deficient in this mineral" or "supplementing water with fluoride," "fortifying our water with fluoride," "controlled fluoridation." The procedure should be compared with the addition of such genuine tooth-building elements as calcium, as well as with "fortifying milk with sunlight vitamin D." "Dentists are 'urging' and 'requesting' consideration of fluoridation," the pamphlet asserted, "they are not 'insisting' or 'demanding' it."[32]

The ADA pamphlet and especially Bull's statements at the Washington Conference show the fluoridation movement in its true light. *Neither the pamphlet nor Bull's talk presented any scientific data on fluoride and its effect on human health,* which should have been of primary concern. Neither of them referred to the two features of the campaign for fluoridation that have characterized nearly every major drive in the U.S. and abroad. One is the incessant attacks on the competence and intellectual honesty of opposing scientists. These onslaughts did not originate – as one might think – with a few zealous proponents, but were officially instituted by the ADA through a brochure[33] that was widely circulated and subsequently published in its journal.[34]

The other feature that characterized most fluoridation drives was a systematic infiltration of groups opposing fluoridation by individuals secretly allied with promoters. The infiltrators' purpose was to downgrade the image of opponents, to sow discord among them, and ultimately to silence them. These false allies appeared at public hearings claiming that they represented opponents and conducted themselves in such a manner as to make the opposition cause appear ridiculous.[35]

*

When scientists resort to the tactics described in this chapter, they abandon their primary quest for truth and provoke a serious question: why would anyone employ such devious methods if fluoridation were really a sound, safe, and effective procedure? Scientific data can hardly be evaluated rationally and objectively if truth is intentionally obscured by falsehoods and distortions. Under these circumstances, do the various endorsements touted by proponents of fluoridation have any real value?

REFERENCES

1. McNeil, D.R.: The Fight for Fluoridation. Oxford Univ. Press, 1957, p. 50.

2. Arnold, F.A., Jr.: The Possibility of Reducing Dental Caries by Increasing Fluoride Ingestion, in F.R. Moulton, Ed.: Dental Caries and Fluorine. 1946, pp. 105-106.

3. McKay, F.S.: Mottled Enamel: Early History and Its Unique Features, in F.R. Moulton, Ed.: Fluorine and Dental Health. 1942, p. 4.

4. Dean, H.T.: Geographical Distribution of Endemic Dental Fluorosis (Mottled Enamel), in Moulton (Ref. 3, above), p. 29.

5. Cox, G.J., and Levin, M.M.: Resume of the Fluorine-Caries Relationship, in Moulton (Ref. 3, above), p. 73.

6. Smith, H.V.: The Chemistry of Fluorine as Related to Fluorosis, in Moulton (Ref. 3, above), pp. 19-20.

7. Schour, I., and Smith, M.C.: Experimental Dental Fluorosis, in Moulton (Ref. 3, above), p. 47.

8. Dean, H.T.: Some General Epidemiological Considerations, in Moulton (Ref. 2, above), p. 2.

9. Weaver, R.: Epidemiological studies in the British Isles and India, in Moulton (Ref. 2, above), pp. 32-35.

10. Ockerse, T.: Fluorine and Dental Caries in South Africa, in Moulton (Ref. 2, above), pp. 36-42.

11. Bibby, B.G.: Topical Applications of Fluorides as a Method of Combatting Dental Caries, in Moulton (Ref. 2, above), p. 97.

12. Merritt, A.H. (Chairman), and Gies, W.J., Ed.: Fluorine in Dental Public Health (Symposium, Oct. 30, 1944). New York Institute of Clinical Oral Pathology, New York, 1945.

13. McKay, F.S.: Fluorine and Mottled Enamel; Historical Survey, in Ref. 12, above, p. 18.

14. McNeil (Ref. 1, above), p. 43.

15. McNeil (Ref. 1, above), p. 66.

16. McNeil (Ref. 1, above), p. 67.

17. Wollan, M.: Controlling the Potential Hazards of Government-Sponsored Technology. The George Washington Law Review, 36:1105-1137, 1968.

18. Am. Dent. Assoc. Newsletter, June 1, 1950.

19. Waldbott, G.L., and Yiamouyiannis, J.: (Special Report) AAAS Fluoride Symposium in Denver. Fluoride, 10:141-144, 1977. Cf. Johansen, E., and Taves, D.R., Eds.: Continuing Evaluation of the Use of Fluorides. In press, 1978.

20. Proceedings of the Fourth Annual Conference of State Dental Directors With the Public Health Service and the Children's Bureau, Federal Security Building, Washington, D.C., June 6-8, 1951. The original transcript was made available through the courtesy of Congressman T.M. Pelley of the State of Washington. A slightly different version is in the Library of Congress (RK 21.C55, 1951) and has been privately reprinted (R.J. Mick, D.D.S., 915 Stone Road, Laurel Springs, N.J., 08021, and National Fluoridation News, Route One, Gravette, Arkansas 72736). The pagination of this printed version differs from the original typescript which is quoted here.

21. Ibid., pp. 24-25 and 104.

22. Ibid., pp. 54, 55, and 59.

23. Ibid., pp. 35-36.

24. Ibid., pp. 37-38.

25. Ibid., p. 45.

26. Ibid., pp. 39-41.

27. Ibid., pp. 42-43.

28. How to Obtain Fluoridation for Your Community Through a Citizens Committee. Am. Dent. Assoc., Chicago, Ill., Feb. 1953; revised, 1963.

29. Ibid., p. 10.

30. Ibid., pp. 1, 3, 6, 8.

31. Ibid., pp. 10-11.

32. Ibid., pp. 11-12.

33. Comments on Opponents of Fluoridation Compiled by Bureau of Public Information. Am. Dent. Assoc., Chicago, Ill., July 1956.

34. Comments on Opponents of Fluoridation. J. Am. Dent. Assoc., 65: 694-710, 1962; ibid., 71:1155-1183, 1965.

35. Waldbott, G.L.: A Struggle With Titans. Carlton Press, New York, 1965, p. 277.

CHAPTER 16

ENDORSEMENTS

BEFORE 1950 scientists generally regarded fluoride as dangerous; it was definitely known to be hazardous and toxic as well as the cause of dental mottling and skeletal deformities. Such an evil reputation had to be overcome if fluorides were to be added to the drinking waters in America. But how might proponents effect this extraordinary reversal of opinion? The answer was that fluoridation could be widely implemented *only* if the nation's scientific organizations endorsed it enthusiastically. Normally, endorsements arise from careful analyses of evidence at scientific meetings, in journals, or in monographs. Fluoridation, however, has rarely received the objective appraisal demanded by science, nor have the sentiments of national societies usually been determined. I do not recall a single example where an endorsement by a scientific organization has been obtained by polling the entire membership for opinions on fluoridation. Can a statement on fluoridation, issued to the public by small appointed committees, truly represent the consensus of an entire group?

THE GROUNDWORK

Shortly after the infamous 1951 conference discussed in the previous chapter, several symposia undoubtedly strengthened the foundations for endorsements by numerous scientific organizations. For instance, the American Association for the Advancement of Science (AAAS) held two important symposia devoted exclusively to fluoridation — one in Philadelphia, Pennsylvania (1951) and the other in St. Louis, Missouri (1952). In the preface of the proceedings, Harvard dental researcher J.H. Shaw stated: "The eminent qualifications of each of the chapter authors should be sufficient evidence as to the high caliber and *unbiased* authenticity of the contents."[1] [Emphasis added.]

Unfortunately, the excellent credentials of these distinguished authors were not matched by a passion for rigorous objectivity. All participants were dedicated proponents, either members of or consultants to the PHS, or scientists associated with industries having problems with fluoride emissions. No scientist with data adverse to fluoridation took part in the program; the papers presented at the conferences, as finally published, leave the clear impression that they were a direct outcome of Bull's advice at the 1951 conference in Washington, D.C.: "We have told the public it works, so we can't go back on that."

One of the early endorsements came in 1954 from the Commission on Chronic Illness, an independent national agency founded by the American Hospital Association and the American Public Welfare Association to study "problems of chronic disease, illness and disability." The Commission's members, professional and lay persons, included such notables as the president of Vassar College, the president of a drug company, a former and future U.S. Surgeon General, Walter Reuther (representing labor), and other civic leaders. Little time was available for these busy executives to study the involved literature on fluoride; they had to rely on the findings of a committee. The Commission itself acknowledged in its report that it had not carried out an independent investigation.[2]

THE NATIONAL RESEARCH COUNCIL

The composition of this committee of scientists is significant because it established the pattern for most subsequent fluoridation study committees created to obtain endorsements on the national, state or local level. The three committee members, headed by K.F. Maxcy, Professor of Public Health, John Hopkins University, were charged with studying the subject but, instead, they merely adopted the opinion of another committee, the Ad Hoc Committee of the National Research Council (NRC), whose chairman was – the *same* Professor Maxcy![3]

The NRC, a subgroup of the National Academy of Sciences, consists of leaders in specialized fields of science. Organized in 1916 with the cooperation of major scientific and technical societies as a research arm of The Academy, it provides a close liaison between the PHS and industry, both of which are sponsors of fluoridation.

   The nine members of the NRC committee were guided in their deliberations by three scientists, two of whom were closely associated with fluoride-promoting industries: B.G. Bibby, Director of the Eastman Dental Dispensary, Rochester, New York, had been carrying out research for the Sugar Research Foundation, Inc. Another, F.F. Heyroth, was Cincinnati's Health Commissioner and Assistant Director of the Kettering Laboratory, University of Cincinnati, which was supported financially by ALCOA and eight other corporations confronted with serious fluoride pollution problems. The third scientist was H.T. Dean of the USPHS, often called the "father of fluoridation." It was therefore most unlikely that any "neutral" members of the NRC's Ad Hoc Committee would become aware of adverse health effects without personally reviewing the extensive and complex literature on fluoride at great cost in time and effort. The committee's Final Report, issued on November 29, 1951, contained references to papers by about 30 authors; all except two, the late Danish scientist Dr. Kaj Roholm and Dr. P.C. Hodges, were closely linked with a promotional agency such as the PHS or industry.[3]

   The report suggested that fluoridation is harmless because more than three million people have been drinking naturally fluoridated water for generations. This assertion is tantamount to claiming, as many have, that smoking is harmless because millions of people have been smoking for hundreds of years without proven adverse effects. When physicians are not aware of the cause of an illness, they can rarely identify its source no matter how often they encounter the disease in their practice. This has been true with respect to smoking, chronic fluoride poisoning, and chronic poisoning from numerous other environmental agents such as asbestos, cadmium, and mercury.

   Another item in the NRC report is important. Concurrently with the reported decline of tooth decay in Grand Rapids, Michigan, there had also been a slight decrease in tooth decay in Muskegon, Michigan, the nonfluoridated control city: 22% in the six-year olds and 28% in the seven-year olds. In other words, some factor other than fluoride was apparently reducing the incidence of tooth decay both in fluoridated Grand Rapids and in nonfluoridated Muskegon. The Committee offered no explanation for this curious fact.[4]

SOME DUBIOUS ENDORSEMENTS

In the early 1950s, the NRC Report and the 1954 Newsletter of the Commission on Chronic Illness won the support of many scientists. Because readers naturally assumed that the subject had been thoroughly examined, they were not inclined to question statements by prestigious members of the two learned organizations. An endorsement of fluoridation, however, clearly does not reflect the position of the members at large of the endorsing organization if their views have not been solicited. For instance, J. P. Cooney, M.D., Vice-President for Medical Affairs of the American Cancer Society, whose "endorsement" had been widely quoted in PHS news releases, wrote to my secretary, E.L. Myler, on February 1, 1965: "I would point out that the Society has never been on record either pro or con regarding fluoridation." Other health organizations were compelled to issue denials that they had endorsed fluoridation (see Table 16-1, next page).

The American Water Works Association, through its president, Mr. F.C. Amsbary, Jr., in a letter to me on August 5, 1955, merely repeated the resolution adopted by his Board of Directors in 1949: "You will note that this position neither approves nor disapproves fluoridation. The matter is entirely left up to those qualified to judge its benefits or deleterious effects."

If the proponents expected support from practicing physicians, they needed endorsements from universities, medical schools, and medical societies. Medical personnel were therefore subjected to constant prodding, as shown in a letter dated October 31, 1956, and written by Dr. S. P. Lucia, Chairman of the Department of Preventive Medicine, University of California Medical Center, School of Medicine, San Francisco, to Mrs. A. H. Cordwell of Glenridge, New Jersey. The letter stated that Dr. Gordon Bates of the Health League of Canada had been canvassing officials of medical schools in North American universities in the summer of 1954 for their opinions on fluoridation. As Dr. Lucia had no first-hand information on the subject, he ignored Dr. Bates' first letter, but a second request (June 25, 1954) "was accompanied by quotations from many professors, whose opinions I respect, in 71 University departments of Preventive Medicine." In response to Dr. Bates' third letter (July 8, 1954), Dr. Lucia stated to Mrs. Cordwell

Table 16-1

Organizations and Institutions Wrongly Listed as Endorsing Fluoridation

Organization	Person	Date	Statement
American Water Works Association, Inc.	F.C. Amsbary, Jr. President	8/5/55	"This position neither approves nor disapproves fluoridation."
Heads of departments of Prevent. Med. of 68 U.S. Medical Colleges. N.Y. Times		6/14/56	21 stated definitely they had not officially endorsed; 15 statements issued from a professor or a dept. head speaking as an individual and not for the department.
American Psychiatric Association	A.M. Davies, Exec. Asst.	7/5/56	"We did not, in fact, give authorization for endorsement in any way and have subsequently contacted the proper persons and corrected this error."
American Heart Association	R.E. Rothermel, M.D. Asst. Director Comm. Serv. and Education	7/10/56	"The American Heart Association, as far as I know, has not endorsed fluoridation."
National Foundation for Infantile Paralysis, Inc.	M.A. Glasser, Asst. Exec. Director	7/10/56	"National Foundation has taken no position in this matter. It was listed in error as an organization endorsing fluoridation."
American Chemical Society	R.M. Warren	8/20/56	"American Chemical Society has not conducted studies upon nor evaluated fluoridation."
University of California Medical Center	S.P. Lucia, M.D. Dept. Chairman	10/31/56	"There has never been any official sanction of fluoridation of water by this department."
Howard University	R.S. Jason, M.D., Dean	11/1/56	"There has been no approval nor disapproval coming from this office."
Harvard Medical School	G.P. Berry, M.D. Dean	1/21/57	"Harvard Medical School has not authorized use of its name in any statement on the question of fluoridation."
American Cancer Society	J.P. Cooney, M.D. Vice-Pres. for Medical Affairs	7/27/62	"The Society is taking no position whatever on the question of the desirability or undesirability of fluoridation. . . . This question is outside the Society's area of concern."
Assoc. Casualty Surety Companies	J.D. Dorsett, General Manager	10/1/62	"Our Association has not taken a public position on the subject of fluoridation . . ."
Texas Medical Association	J.D. Nichols, M.D.	5/22/63	"T.M.A. refuses to endorse, guarantee or recommend fluoridated or unfluoridated water."
American Legion	W.J. Caldwell, Asst. Dir. Americanism, Children & Youth Div.	9/19/77	"We as a national organization did not take a stand for or against the issue (fluoridation). . . ."

that he had sent the following reply (July 20, 1954): "The anatomical and histopathological evidence presented in the support of the thesis seems to bear out the conclusion that not only is controlled fluoridation of water harmless but actually beneficial." He added, however: "There has never been any official sanction of fluoridation of water by this department."

G.P. Berry, Dean of the Harvard Medical School, was even more emphatic in denying an endorsement. He wrote to Mrs. Cordwell on January 21, 1957: "The Harvard Medical School has not authorized the use of its name in any statement on the question of fluoridation. . . . The inclusion of its name in any list of institutions either endorsing or opposing fluoridation is fully unjustified."

In some instances, members of the staff had taken it upon themselves to issue an endorsing statement that subsequently caused much embarrassment to the university. The Dean of the College of Medicine at Howard University in Washington, D.C., Dr. R. S. Jason, stated in a letter to E. L. Myler (Feb. 19, 1965) that Dr. P. B. Cornely, the Head of the Department of Preventive Medicine and Public Health, had adopted an affirmative position "based upon the data available to him as published by the United States Public Health Service and the fact that the fluoridation of water has been instituted in the District of Columbia without any difficulty whatsoever." Dr. Jason thus acknowledged that the faculties of his school had received only one-sided information. "Insofar as I know," Dean Jason wrote, "Howard as a University has not endorsed fluoridation."

THE AMERICAN MEDICAL ASSOCIATION

To a physician the voice of his medical society may be even more authoritative than that of his medical school. An endorsement by the American Medical Association was therefore mandatory if the fluoridation bandwagon was to keep rolling. Because research on fluoride was a virgin field in medicine at that time, no experienced clinician was available to convince the top echelon of the AMA that fluoridation was not hazardous, and the PHS sent F. J. McClure, a biochemist, to do that job.

In 1951 McClure appeared before the AMA's Councils on Pharmacy and Chemistry and on Foods and Nutrition and assured them that the addition of fluorides to drinking water was not harmful. The two AMA Councils were, therefore, "unaware of any evidence" that fluoridation was hazardous. They warned, however, that the "use of products which are naturally high in fluoride content such as bone meal tablets or of lozenges, dentifrices, or chewing gum to which fluoride has been added, should be avoided where the drinking water has been fluoridated."[5]

Surprisingly few leaders of the AMA seemed to have realized that its 1951 endorsement was obtained without presentation of data on the clinical aspect of long-term fluoride intake. The lack of such data and the political aspect of the AMA endorsement, however, were clearly perceived by Dr. C. L. Farrell of Providence. R.I., then chairman of the AMA's Public Health Committee. In a letter to me (dated October 16, 1954), he explained that at the Los Angeles meeting of the AMA's political body, the House of Delegates, two state health commissioners, one from Connecticut, the other from Wisconsin, submitted resolutions that "would have made the AMA strongly support, completely endorse, and go on record as extolling the virtues and benefits of fluoridation."[6]

"I fully recognized," Dr. Farrell explained, "that in the House of Delegates there would be no opposition – at least no organized opposition – and no one well informed or thoroughly enough informed to stand up on the floor and lead the fight against the adoption of fluoridation proposals." As the lesser of two evils, Dr. Farrell proposed a mildly worded substitute to endorse fluoridation "in principle." "It did not commit the AMA to full endorsement," he added.

Once fluoridation was endorsed "in principle," however, staff officials – particularly Dr. G. F. Lull, the AMA's executive secretary, and Dr. W. W. Bauer, editor of *Today's Health* – engaged in a vigorous promotional campaign. Dr. Austin Smith, editor of the *JAMA,* wrote me on July 9, 1954, that he could not accept any publications unfavorable to fluoridation unless first approved by the "policy-making body" of the society. Of the few articles containing data adverse to fluoridation that have appeared in that journal during the past 20 years, *all* have asserted that, in spite of the evidence presented, fluoridation is safe. The general membership of the AMA, therefore, has been exposed to an extremely biased interpretation of the value as well as the safety of fluoridation.

At my request the AMA Councils on Foods and Nutrition and on Pharmacy and Chemistry reviewed fluoridation at a hearing in Chicago August 7, 1957. Drs. H. T. Dean and W. D. Armstrong presented the proponent side; I was invited to represent the opposing view together with Dr. F. B. Exner, a radiologist who had become one of the most knowledgeable experts on the health effects of fluoride. Only two of the Council members present, Dr. C. A. Elvehjem, a biochemist, and Dr. M. H. Seevers, a pharmacologist, had carried out research on fluoride, although neither of them were practicing clinicians. Some of the members, e.g., Dr. A. C. Curtis of the University of Michigan, Ann Arbor, had been engaged in promotion of fluoridation; others were PHS consultants.

Dr. Exner gave a scholarly presentation, highlighting major fallacies of the PHS statistical studies. He also discussed the case of the 21-year-old Texas soldier whose exposure to natural fluoride water (1.2-5.7 ppm) most of his life had induced extensive skeletal fluorosis and undoubtedly contributed to a fatal kidney disease. I presented a brief account of research in which I was engaged at that time on the effect of fluoride on the phosphorus and calcium metabolism (see Chapter 14). Previously, I had submitted to the Councils reprints of my reports on poisoning from fluoridated water, but this crucial subject was virtually ignored. I also showed photographs of mottled teeth that I had encountered in nonfluoridated (0.1 ppm) Detroit, and Dr. Dean himself confirmed that they were fluoride-related (cf. Figs. 12-1 and 12-2 above, pp. 180 and 181). He briefly outlined his experience with mottled teeth but had no answer to my query regarding the role of minerals other than fluoride in protecting teeth in natural fluoride areas. Dr. Armstrong spoke mainly of his new method of analyzing fluoride in blood. By acknowledging that he had not anticipated speaking, he inadvertently disclosed the purpose of the hearing—that it was not a *bona fide* examination of both sides of the problem, but that, on the contrary, it was merely a gesture intended to convince the medical profession that both sides of the controversy had been carefully examined.

I began to detect a hostile atmosphere when my own and Dr. Exner's presentations were being continuously interrupted by three members, one of whom—Dr. Perrin Long—appeared to be quite emotional. Even prior to the meeting another panelist, C. A.

Elvehjem, attempted to downgrade my work in the eyes of his colleagues.

In the Report of the two Councils, my case reports—including seemingly irrefutable medical evidence against fluoridation—were curtly dismissed by a single sentence: "These [Dr. Waldbott's] reports [of chronic poisoning] fail to demonstrate enough consistency to justify impartial acceptance as showing a symptom complex due to fluoridated water."[7] Since one of the most characteristic features of the beginning stage of chronic fluoride poisoning is the wide variation and intermittent appearance of its manifestations (see Chapter 9), this comment actually supported my evidence, and certainly did not invalidate it!

Although the AMA Report endorses fluoridation, a careful examination of its 20 pages reveals as much adverse as favorable data. For example, mottling of teeth is described as "the most delicate criterion of harm from fluoride ingestion."[8] The Report also pointed to the unpredictable variation from individual to individual in the physiological effect of fluoridated water, depending on the nature and concentration of the other ions present. The need for considering the total daily amount of fluoride rather than "the number of parts per million in the liquid or food consumed" was also emphasized. It warned that "intakes of different people with different habits under different temperature conditions may vary widely." The Report contained the significant admission that "it is practically impossible to measure the fluid-fluoride or food-fluoride intake of large enough groups of people over long enough periods of time to secure sufficient data to show safe limits."[9] Thus, in the fine print of the AMA statement, The Great Dilemma is once more spotlighted, and no amount of filtering its brightness by endorsements could obscure it.

In the AMA House of Delegates, The Report was supported by a formidable array of health officials who testified in favor of fluoridation. Some opposing members attempted to side-step the explosive issue. Dr. J. A. DeTar, one of four Michigan delegates, candidly described the situation in a letter to me (December 11, 1957): "To oppose fluoridation openly is political suicide." Nevertheless, after a stormy debate, about one third of the delegates voted against fluoridation.[10]

Support of fluoridation by the PHS, AMA, ADA, and other

prestigious groups prompted additional endorsements in the U.S. and abroad. Interlocking memberships on executive boards and on committees of scientific societies, as well as the paucity of free discussion of the subject in scientific organizations, contributed materially to the adoption of these endorsements. The long list of endorsing organizations (Table 16-2, next page) includes many with close ties to the PHS, such as the American Public Health Association, as well as some of the independent professional societies such as the American Academy of Pediatrics.

With these respected organizations leading the way, many lay groups in the U.S., including the Junior Chamber of Commerce, labor unions, the League of Women Voters, PTA groups, service agencies, and even charitable organizations followed suit without personally investigating the subject. Numerous outstanding citizens, science writers, politicians, government officials, and even United States presidents also lent their names to the cause. Snowballing endorsements were therefore obtained at both the national and local levels through the many so-called fluoridation "study committees" that closely followed the PHS and ADA instructions.

THE WORLD HEALTH ORGANIZATION

Despite extraordinary success in obtaining endorsements in the U.S.A., fluoridation received only limited acceptance abroad, the Fédération Dentaire Internationale being one of the few exceptions, and advocates decided to push for endorsements at the international level. In 1958, the year following the AMA Report, the World Health Organization (WHO) established an Expert Committee in Geneva to study fluoridation. At least five of the seven committee members had promoted fluoridation in their respective countries. Two well-known American proponents, Dr. J. W. Knutson and Professor H. C. Hodge, presented the case to the committee. Some of Hodge's research had been financed by the Ozark Mahoning Chemical Company and some by the now defunct Atomic Energy Commission, both of which were confronted with serious fluoride disposal problems. Another member of the Expert Committee, Professor Yngve Ericsson of the Dental School, Karolinska Institute, University of Stockholm, one of Europe's most prominent advocates of fluoridation, had been a recipient of USPHS

Table 16-2

Approving American Organizations (According to the USPHS, 1970)[a]

American Academy of Pediatrics
American Association for the Advancement of Science
American Association of Dental Schools
American Association of Industrial Dentists
American Association of Public Health Dentists
American Cancer Society
American College of Dentists
American Commission on Community Health Services
American Dental Association
American Dental Health Society
American Dental Hygienists' Association
American Federation of Labor and Congress of Industrial Organizations
American Heart Association
American Hospital Association
American Institute of Nutrition
American Legion
American Medical Association
American Nurses Association
American Osteopathic Association
American Pharmaceutical Association
American Public Health Association
American Public Welfare Association
American School Health Association
American Society of Dentistry for Children
American Veterinary Medical Association
American Water Works Association
Association of Public Health Veterinarians
Association of State and Territorial Health Officers
Commission on Chronic Illness
College of American Pathologists
Federation of American Societies for Experimental Biology
Conference of State Sanitary Engineers
Industrial Medical Association
Child Study Association of America
National Congress of Parents and Teachers
United States Junior Chamber of Commerce
Heads of Departments of Preventive Medicine at 68 accredited medical
    colleges
Inter-Association Committee on Health
National Education Association
National Institute of Municipal Law Officers

[a]From McClure, F.J.: *Water Fluoridation: The Search and the Victory.* National
Institute of Dental Research, Bethesda, Maryland, 1970, pp. 249-251; but see Table
16-1 (above, p. 278) for exceptions.

research grants and subsequently received royalties from Sweden's toothpaste industry. My offer to furnish reports on poisoning from fluoridated water was rejected. To the credit of WHO, their 1958 document stated: "This report contains the collective views of an international group of experts and does not necessarily represent the decisions of the stated policy of the World Health Organization."[11] The official endorsement followed 11 years later.

On July 23, 1969, fluoridation was brought up again at the 22nd World Health Organization Assembly in Boston. The resolution recommending the measure appeared on the agenda daily but was strongly opposed and blocked by delegates from Italy, Senegal, the Congo, and elsewhere. G. Penso, head of the Italian delegation, expressed his concern regarding "this mania of our century to add additives to anything." He pointed out that there are unknown amounts of fluoride in the air we breathe and in the food we eat. He cautioned particularly about possible damage to future generations.[12] Nevertheless, during the final hours of the session, when only 55 to 60 of the 1,000 delegates from 131 countries were still present, all bills that had not been accepted were collected into one and voted upon, including a statement on fluoridation. The mildly-worded resolution urged that member states examine the possibility of introducing fluoridation in those communities where fluoride intake from water and other sources "is below the optimal levels." It also requested the Director General "to continue to encourage research into the etiology of dental caries, the fluoride content of diets, the mechanism of action of fluoride at optimal levels in drinking water, and into the effects of greatly excessive intake of fluoride from natural sources, and to report thereon to the World Health Assembly. . . ."[13]

ENDORSEMENTS IN OTHER COUNTRIES

Foreign scientific organizations and health ministries also created study committees. During February through April 1952, the United Kingdom Mission, headed by J. R. Forrest, Dental Officer, Ministry of Health, London,[14] visited Grand Rapids, Michigan; Newburgh, New York; Brantford, Ontario; and Bartlett, Texas; the National Institute of Dental Health, Bethesda, Maryland; and the American Dental Association headquarters in Chicago. Their hosts were Surgeon General Scheele, Assistant Surgeon General Knutson,

Dr. Dean, and Dr. Arnold. This visit and the warm reception by their American colleagues sparked much enthusiasm for fluoridation among the four members of the British committee, each of whom became a strong advocate of the measure.

Following official endorsement of fluoridation in England, PHS health officials—primarily Arnold, Dean and McClure concentrated their efforts on introducing fluoridation into Australia and New Zealand, where a visit by one of the PHS scientists and the formation of a three-member "Commission of Inquiry"—one scientist and two lay persons—initiated the campaign, à la American style.

In Canada, Ontario's Minister of Health, Dr. M. B. Dymond, created "The Committee Appointed to Inquire into and Report upon the Fluoridation of Municipal Water Supplies," also composed of two lay members, Justice K. G. Morden (chairman), Mrs. E. L. Frankel, and a physician, Dr. G. E. Hall, president of the University of Western Ontario, London (Ontario). The scientist, Dr. Hall, who guided the committee's deliberations at the hearing in Toronto on May 2 to 13, 1960, had a threefold conflict of interest. His daughter was employed by an aluminum corporation with fluoride pollution problems; he himself was serving as Honorary Advisory Director to a leading Canadian promotional organization, the Health League of Canada; and his university was recipient of research grants from the PHS, the key U.S. promotional organization. Prior to the hearing the committee had distributed briefs by six Canadian dental researchers—all in favor of fluoridation. Of course, fluoridation throughout Canada was advocated.

In other foreign countries, however, the going was not so easy, since many scientists were reluctant to endorse fluoridation. In France, skeletal fluorosis in residents and workers at the French-owned phosphate mines of North Africa had been reported. In Italy, illness had been encountered from high-fluoride food and water near volcanic areas such as those north of Rome and in Sicily. In Iceland, repeated eruptions of the volcano Hekla had caused serious economic loss through fluoride damage to sheep, cattle, and vegetation, and had driven home the hazards of fluoride. In India, with its vast areas of endemic fluorosis, health authorities were mainly concerned with the *removal* of fluoride from water supplies.

THE AMERICAN ACADEMY OF ALLERGY

At the very time when scientists abroad, especially in Sweden and Holland, were becoming aware of the hazards of fluoridation, the PHS requested the officers of the American Academy of Allergy to add the weight of their voices to the promotion. In June 1971, the 11-member Executive Board of this body declared unequivocally and unanimously: "There is no evidence of allergy or intolerance to fluorides as used in the fluoridation of communal water supplies."[15] By acknowledging that the PHS had requested their statement, the officers attempted to neutralize the impact of reports of fluoride poisoning, especially since allergic persons are notably more susceptible to poisoning from drugs than normal individuals.

Curiously, none of these prominent scientists had carried out research on the health effects of fluoride; no hearings were held on the subject, and no inquiries were made of the members of the Academy regarding fluoride poisoning among their patients. The statement was accompanied by seven references to the literature and could not pretend to cover the subject in depth. One paper described *severe cases of allergy to fluoride in toothpaste and drops;* another recorded *atopic dermatitis and urticaria from fluoride tablets.*[16,17] The bibliography did not include any of my original publications on chronic fluoride poisoning; instead, it referred to pages in a book that I had written primarily for lay readers *A Struggle With Titans* (1965). My various other reports in the scientific literature,[18-30] which reveal harm from fluoridated drinking water, evidently had not been consulted.

About the time when the statement by the 11 scientists was released, the PHS announced research grants for 1971 to four of the 11-member Executive Board of The Academy amounting to a total of $780,621 (see Table 16-3, next page).[31] Most other members of the Board had previously been recipients of such grants for research on various phases of allergy. It is no secret that PHS research grants play an important role in the political arena as they are often awarded to individual scientists "with strings attached."[32] The resolution by the eleven allergists may therefore be interpreted as a gesture of good will and appreciation toward their federal benefactors.

Table 16-3

PHS Grants to Members of the Executive
Board of the American Academy of Allergy (1971)[31]

Recipient	Location	Amount
K.F. Austin	Boston, Mass.	$486,112
R.S. Farr	Denver, Col.	101,682
E. Middleton, Jr.	Denver, Col.	88,149
C.E. Reed	Madison, Wis.	104,678

Unfortunately their statement has been accepted widely at face value as though it had genuine scientific merit. For instance, in 1976 a committee of the British Royal College of Physicians (RCP) of London cited the Academy's statement in order to deny the validity of my case reports of fluoride poisoning from drinking water:

> As a result of reports of allergy and intolerance the U.S. Public Health Service asked the American Academy of Allergy to evaluate available clinical reports in terms of the main types of allergic response; and also to examine the possibility that certain cases might belong to less well understood types of drug reaction. A statement was later issued by the Academy that there was no evidence of allergy or intolerance to fluorides as used in the fluoridation of community water supplies.[33]

This RCP statement—which ignored my unrefuted rebuttal of the Academy's report[34] —is not unlike that of the American Academy of Allergy, in that it was also requested by a proponent organization, the "dental profession." The RCP report was based largely on outdated, highly biased references gleaned mainly from the monographs of the World Health Organization[13] and the National Research Council;[3] for the most part it merely reiterates the many controversial statements of the U.S. proponent literature. No scientists with data unfavorable to fluoridation were consulted, nor was there any objective evidence that an independent study was made.

Curiously enough, a 1977 report by the National Research Council[35] refers to the conclusions of the RCP that in turn had obtained much of their information from the National Research Council. Here we can see a common story: the same promotional message that originated from the PHS in Washington has been carried from one scientific organization to another and eventually returned home to the PHS in Washington where it is used to reinforce that agency's position!

Why did so many learned organizations climb on the bandwagon in response to a small group of individuals without seriously deliberating the full impact of fluoridation? There are many answers. Among them certainly are: the ardent desire of dentists to prevent tooth decay; the prestige of the sponsors of the program; the ability of public health officials to impress others with their special knowledge of the subject in the face of a general lack of knowledge concerning the long-term effects of fluoride; the easy access of the promoting scientist to research funds that could be withheld from opponents; the great appeal of the project to humanitarians—all these factors combined to promote fluoridation. But we must never forget the Dental Division of the PHS, for its influence upon the medical, dental, and news professions has been profound.

THE PUBLIC HEALTH SERVICE

The PHS, which endorsed fluoridation on June 1, 1950,[36] is a part of the Department of Health, Education, and Welfare. The National Institute of Dental Research (NIDR) at Bethesda, Maryland, one of its divisions, probably is the best equipped and staffed dental research center in the world. Many scientists and dental schools here and abroad rely on the PHS for research information and for monetary assistance.[37] Because of its high standing in the scientific community, congressional leaders and U.S. presidents accept the advice of the PHS scientists without seriously questioning whether the judgment of their advisors is actually in the best interest of the country.

Top officers of the Dental Division of the PHS are intimately associated with those in the American Dental Association and hold interlocking memberships on its boards, committees, and councils as well as in numerous other organizations.[38] They are also represented on policy-making bodies of the American Medical Association. For instance, an official of the PHS has a permanent position at AMA headquarters in Chicago, and PHS officers are members of important committees and councils in the AMA and in county and state medical societies.

Thus, the PHS reaches into every state and into every scientific organization. It maintains close liaison with Congress, the Army, the Navy, and the Air Force, with the Food and Drug Administration and, more recently, the Environmental Protection Agency (EPA). It is linked with industry through the National Research Council of the National Academy of Sciences, a venerable organization of top scientists that is called upon to furnish scientific data to government agencies. Significantly, PHS officials are also represented on editorial boards of every important medical and dental journal in the U.S.A., and their public relations men are in constant contact with press, radio, television, medical writers, and news commentators. Who can doubt that PHS officers and scientists can easily sway the thinking of scientists and lay persons by virtue of the prestige of their position and particularly by their ability to distribute – or withhold – research grants?

No one knows precisely how many millions of dollars have been allocated to fluoride research. According to S. J. Kreshover, Director of the National Institute of Dental Research, the Office of Management and Budget in the U.S. Government "advises that a breakdown of budgeted funds spent specifically on such programs or portions of projects dealing with fluorides is not available."[37] We do know, however, that from 1957 to 1973 the ADA received a total of $6,453,816.[38] How much of this money was allotted to fluoridation cannot be ascertained. It is safe to say, though, that it has run into several millions of dollars.

Two former giants in Congress, the late Representative J. A. Fogarty, Chairman of the House Subcommittee on Appropriations for the Department of Health, Education, and Welfare, and Senator Lister Hill, the former member of the Senate Appropriations Committee, were in continuous contact with the PHS. They strongly supported this agency in Congress regardless of the size of its financial requests. For this yeoman service, these two congressional leaders received Lasker Awards in 1959 upon the recommendation of the Surgeon General.[39]

What caused PHS dental scientists in Washington to plunge so vigorously into the promotion of fluoridation, a measure which before 1950 they themselves had labeled a "calculated risk"?

Their organization was established originally to protect society from the spread of contagious diseases and has been remarkably successful, whereas preventive dentistry had made relatively little progress before World War II. For years, PHS dental researchers had fought tooth decay, their most serious health problem. Fluoridation, therefore, had a natural appeal to these officials: it seemed to be the answer to their prayers. In their enthusiasm, they rushed to promote it without adequately investigating its potential harm.

Other considerations also contributed to their eagerness to promote fluoridation. Like most public agencies with unlimited resources, officials constantly endeavor to enlarge their sphere of influence. Indeed, in 1953 PHS Surgeon General Leonard Scheele, addressing a conference of state and territorial health directors, called fluoridation but one example of "mass application methods for controlling non-infectious diseases."[40] Fluoridation was but another means of achieving their ambitious goals.

*

From 1950 onward, endorsements of fluoridation grew from the tip of an inverted pyramid to a veritable mushroom cloud. Scientific organization after organization followed the pied piper lead of the Public Health Service and climbed aboard the fluoridation bandwagon. The reader can judge for himself: whether scientific objectivity was really a guiding light for the "select" committees which evaluated fluoridation; and what *scientific* value can be attached to statements of approval by the American Water Works Association, the Consumer Federation of America, the Health Insurance Association of America, the National Congress of Parents and Teachers, the Office of Civil Defense, the U.S. Department of Agriculture, the U.S. Department of Defense, the U.S. Junior Chamber of Commerce, and various presidents of the United States?

Everyone understands the effect of "mob psychology," however, and recent medical history should stimulate our memories about the consequences of supporting public health procedures before all the facts are known. The swine flu vaccination program of the USPHS, for example, was also endorsed by numerous health authorities throughout the land. As a consequence, President Gerald Ford committed his administration to mass inoculation of millions of Americans at a cost of $135,000,000.

On December 16, 1976, however, the program was abruptly suspended because the flu shots were apparently causing a form of paralysis which can lead to death (Guillain-Barré syndrome), and the public abandoned the program like the plague. To the chagrin of the PHS, negligence claims against the U.S. Government are approaching the billion dollar mark. *Significantly, the PHS has never publicly admitted the serious mistake made by promoting an ill-advised program leading to paralysis and even death.* Fortunately, in this case the bandwagon became derailed after more than 40 million persons were inoculated.

Of course, the dental division of the PHS was not solely responsible for the widespread eagerness to participate in the great American fluoridation experiment. The public, including many scientists, wanted to believe in a kind of dental utopia. And from the very beginning, certain industries working closely with the PHS played an important role in the promotional activities that will probably never be fully known. The vital interests of industry in fluoridation will be the focus of the following chapter.

REFERENCES

1. Shaw, J.H., Ed.: Fluoridation as a Public Health Measure. American Association for the Advancement of Science, Washington, D.C., 1954, pp. iv-v.

2. Chronic Illness News Letter, Vol. 5, No. 4, 1954.

3. Maxcy, K.F., Appleton, J.L.T., Bibby, B.G., Dean, H.T., Harvey, A. McG., Heyroth, F.F., Johnson, A.L., Whittaker, H.A., and Wolman, A.: Report of the Ad Hoc Committee on Fluoridation of Water Supplies. Natl. Res. Council-Natl. Acad. Sci. Publ. No. 214, 1952.

4. Ref. 3 above, p. 4.

5. American Medical Association Councils on Pharmacy and Chemistry and Foods and Nutrition: Fluoridation of Water Supplies. J. Am. Med. Assoc., 147:1359, 1951.

6. Farrell, C.L.: Letter to G.L. Waldbott, Oct. 16, 1954.

7. House of Delegates of the American Medical Association: Statement on Fluoridation of Public Water Supplies. Philadelphia, Pa., Dec. 3-6, 1957, p. 14.

8. Ibid., p. 15.

9. Ibid., pp. 14-15.

10. Alesen, L.A.: Letter to George L. Waldbott, Feb. 1, 1958.

11. World Health Organization Report No. 146. Geneva, 1958.

12. Italy's WHO Delegate Opposes Fluoridation: "Must be Cautious." Boston Sunday Herald Traveler, July 10, 1969, Sect. C-7.

13. World Health Organization: Resolution of the World Health Assembly. Fluoridation and Dental Health. WHO Chronicle, 23:512, 1969.

14. Forrest, J.R., Longwell, J., Stones, H.H., and Thomson, A.M.: The Fluoridation of Domestic Water Supplies in North America as a Means of Controlling Dental Caries. H.M. Stationery Office, London, 1953.

15. Executive Board of the American Academy of Allergy: Editorial: A Statement on the Question of Allergy to Fluoride as Used in the Fluoridation of Community Water Supplies. J. Allergy, 47:347-348, 1971.

16. Feltman, R., and Kosel, G.: Prenatal and Postnatal Ingestion of Fluorides—Fourteen Years of Investigation—Final Report. J. Dent. Med., 16:190-199, 1961.

17. Shea, J.J., Gillespie, S.M., and Waldbott, G.L.: Allergy to Fluoride. Ann. Allergy, 25:388-391, 1967.

18. Waldbott, G.L.: Chronic Fluorine Intoxication from Drinking Water. Int. Arch. Allergy Appl. Immunol., 7:70-74, 1955.

19. Waldbott, G.L.: Incipient Chronic Fluorine Intoxication from Drinking Water. Acta Med. Scand., 156:157-168, 1956.

20. Waldbott, G.L: Incipient Chronic Fluorine Intoxication from Drinking Water. II. Distinction Between Allergic Reactions and Drug Intolerance. Int. Arch. Allergy Appl. Immunol., 9:241-249, 1956.

21. Waldbott, G.L.: Tetaniform Convulsions Precipitated by Fluoridated Drinking Water. Confin. Neurol., 17:339-347, 1957.

22. Waldbott, G.L.: Dermatologische Manifestationen bei chronischer Fluor-Vergiftung durch Trinkwasser. Hautarzt, 8:368-370, 1957.

23. Waldbott, G.L.: Allergic Reactions from Fluorides. Int. Arch. Allergy Appl. Immunol., 12:347-355, 1958.

24. Waldbott, G.L.: Urticaria Due to Fluoride. Acta Allergol., 13:456-468, 1959.

25. Waldbott, G.L.: Fluorose, hervorgerufen durch Trinkwasser. Dtsch. Med. Wochenschr., 84:728-730, 1959.

26. Waldbott, G.L.: Fluoride in Clinical Medicine. Int. Arch. Allergy Appl. Immunol., 20, Suppl. 1, 1962.

27. Waldbott, G.L.: Acute Fluoride Intoxication. Acta Med. Scand., 174, Suppl. 400, 1963.

28. Waldbott, G.L.: Allergic Reactions to Fluoride. J. Asthma Res., 2:51-64, 1964; 3:249-251, 1966.

29. Waldbott, G.L.: Hydrofluorosis in the U.S.A. Fluoride, 1:94-102, 1968.

30. Waldbott, G.L., and Cecilioni, V.A.: "Neighborhood" Fluorosis. Clin. Toxicol., 2:387-396, 1969.

31. Public Health Service Grants and Awards, Fiscal Year 1971 Funds, Part I, National Institutes of Health, Research Grants and Research Contracts. U.S. Dept. Health Education and Welfare. Publ. No. (NIH) 72-197, pp. 168, 233, and 366.

32. Federal Grants Criticized. Freedom of Universities at Stake. Pittsburgh (Pa.) Post Gazette, Nov. 21, 1963.

33. Report of the Royal College of Physicians of London: Fluoride, Teeth and Health. 1976, p. 64.

34. Waldbott, G.L.: Letter to the Editor: Fluoridation of Community Water Supplies. J. Allergy Appl. Immunol., 48:253-254, 1971.

35. National Research Council Safe Drinking Water Committee: Drinking Water and Health. 1977, pp. 378 and 396.

36. Am. Dent. Assoc. Newsletter, June 1, 1950. Cf. McNeil, D.R.: The Fight for Fluoridation. 1957, pp. 74 and 80.

37. Kreshover, S.J., Director of the National Institute of Dental Research, as quoted in National Fluoridation News, 21(1):4, October-December 1975.

38. Directory of Dental Consultants and Executive Personnel and Representatives of the American Dental Association to National Agencies and Societies. Bureau of Public Information, Am. Dent. Assoc., Oct. 1, 1955.

39. Polio's Little Brother. Time, Oct. 19, 1959.

40. Rogers, W., Jr.: Surgeon General Predicts Victories in Disease Like Cancer, Heart Trouble. Paterson (N.J.) Evening News, Nov. 6, 1953, p. 40.

CHAPTER 17

INDUSTRY AND FLUORIDATION

INDUSTRY WELCOMED fluoridation with open arms. *Chemical Week,* a publication for the chemical industry, vividly portrayed this fact in 1951 with an enthusiastic news account:

> All over the country, slide rules are getting warm as waterworks engineers figure the cost of adding fluoride to their municipal supplies. They are riding a trend urged upon them by the US Public Health Service, the American Dental Association, the State Dental Health Directors, various state and local health bodies, and vocal women's clubs from coast to coast. . . . it adds up to a nice piece of business on all sides and many firms are cheering the USPHS and similar groups as they plump for increasing adoption of fluoridation.[1]

The beneficiaries named in this article were chemical companies and equipment firms: General Chemical, Harshaw Chemical Co., Blockson Chemical Co., American Agricultural Chemical Co., Aluminum Co. of America (ALCOA), Davison Chemical Corp., and Baugh Chemical Co. *Chemical Week* obviously failed to discuss how many other industries in addition to chemical corporations would eventually gain financially from the unexpected bonanza. Even so, the desire of corporations to sell their products was not the only significant motive for industry to "plump" for the new health measure.

THE PROBLEM

In the early 1930s, ALCOA and other manufacturers of aluminum had a problem so serious that it threatened their very existence. During the smelting and reduction process, when bauxite (aluminum oxide) is dissolved and electrolyzed in molten cryolite, hydrogen fluoride and other volatile fluorides are released into the air, and sodium fluoride remains in the bath.[2] The latter cannot simply be dumped on the ground because it seriously pollutes grass and other forage. Indeed, in 1950 ALCOA's plant in Vancouver, Washington, was fined for dumping fluorides into the Columbia River, and the airborne fluorides heavily contaminated the grass and forage, "which resulted in injury and death to cattle."[3] If it could be established further that human health also suffered from fluoride pollution, the consequences to the company in terms of damage suits would have been immeasurable.

Damage to Animal Life. Many other industries, especially the manufacturers of steel and phosphate fertilizer, shared this problem with ALCOA. On August 25, 1961, W. S. Meader and his wife May, near Pocatello, Idaho, obtained a judgement in the US Court of Appeals, Ninth Circuit, against Food Machinery and Chemical Corp. for the sum of $57,295.80 and against J. R. Simplot Co. for $4,246.41. The factories of these corporations emitted solid and gaseous fluoride compounds which seriously damaged the Meader trout farm and fish hatchery. According to the court record, "eggs were worthless" and did not hatch properly; the fish also exhibited malformations. "During the week after rains, the Meaders were hauling away about a ton of dead fish per day."[4] Fluoride levels in water samples from the Meader hatchery ranged between 0.5 and 4.7 ppm--no different than the fluoride concentrations in food and drinks consumed today by humans in many places. Inevitably, the business of the farm began to deteriorate as "customers were lost."

Damage to fish is not the only source of litigation resulting from environmental fluoride. Ever since the beginning of the industrial revolution, wholesale pollution of air and of the countryside with fluoride fumes and fallout has taken place, and fluoride poisoning has become an important industrial hazard. Early reports of damage came from Great Britain and also from Freiburg, Germany, where by 1893, 880,000 marks (about $200,000) had been paid for current injuries and 644,000 marks for permanent relief. Around the industrial city of Freiburg in Saxony a disease of cattle, endemic for 20 years, was identified in 1907 as fluoride poisoning from the smelters.[5] At about the same time, cattle near copper mines of Anaconda, Montana, were reported to have developed "copper teeth," which were remarkably similar to what

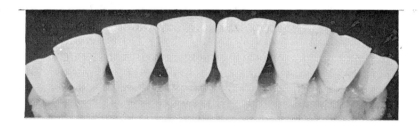

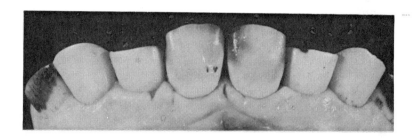

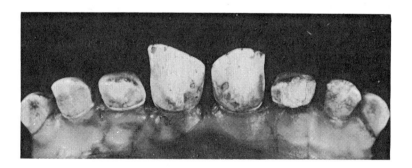

Fig. 17-1. Dental fluorosis in incisor teeth of cattle. Top: normal, 7-year-old.
Middle: moderate effects from intermittent ingestion of fluoride, 4-year-old.
Bottom: severe effects from constant ingestion of fluoride, 4-year-old.
(Courtesy Dr. J. L. Shupe and A. E. Olson,
Utah State University, Logan, Utah.)

was later recognized in humans as "Colorado brown stain" or "mottled teeth" (Fig. 17-1, preceding page).[6]

In the early 1950s American industry was plagued with a virtual epidemic of litigation. In 1950, Mr. and Mrs. Julius Lampert had won their suit against the Reynolds Metals Company's Troutdale aluminum plant for fluoride burns to their gladiolus crops.[7] In Blount County, Tennessee, prior to January 1, 1953, ALCOA had hardly made up the loss of income incurred by 141 farmers and cattle raisers,[8] when another suit charged that fluoride fumes "damaged farmlands, injured registered cattle," making them unmarketable, and caused premature deterioration of teeth, stiffness of joints, knots on ribs, loss of appetite, and general retardation of growth.[9]

Other suits involved the ALCOA plant at Vancouver, Washington, which had to pay cattleman William Fraser $60,000 in 1962 and in the same year, $20,000 to Earl Reeder because of fluoride injury to their cattle on Sauvies Island.[10] In 1961 Fairview Farms, Inc., received $300,000 from the Harvey Aluminum Company's reduction plant in The Dalles, Oregon, because of damage to dairy herds, loss of forage and of milk supply, as well as depreciation of the lands. Orchardist W. J. Meyer and his wife Mary Ann also received $485,000 for "willful damage" to cherry, apricot, and peach crops.[11]

The threat to farming by fluoride pollution can be visualized if we realize that Polk County, which was Florida's leading cattle producer in 1954 with 120,000 head, had some 30,000 fewer cattle by 1965. Fluoride emissions from phosphate plants on local pastures were building up toxic levels as high as 1800 ppm in the grass and other forage. The official maximum allowable concentration for cattle is 40 ppm,[12] but even this level permits significant damage.[13]

Human Health. When human health was at stake, the spectre of these damage suits became even more ominous for the corporations. In the 1955 suit Paul M. Martin and his wife Verla vs. Reynolds Metals, it was proved for the first time in the United States that fumes from an aluminum reduction plant had caused illness to humans.[14] The significance of this litigation is underscored by the fact that seven other aluminum, metal, and chemical companies joined Reynolds Metals as "friends of the court" to obtain a reversal of the judgement against their fellow corporation. Fred Yerke, a Reynolds attorney, "contended that, if allowed to stand, the verdict would become a ruling case, making every aluminum and chemical plant liable to damage claims merely by operating."[15] The verdict did stand: in June 1958, the U.S. Court of Appeals upheld the decision against Reynolds by a five to one vote.[16] Finally, in 1968, the company settled the case by buying the Martin ranch — a solution to the problem that has been followed by other corporations.

Another suit involving human health threatened the Rocky Mountain phosphate plant in Garrison, Montana, when residents complained constantly of "strep" throats, burning eyes, and asthmatic symptoms which they associated with fumes emanating from the plant. Classes of the Garrison school were interrupted 35 times during the first year of the plant's operation (1963-1964) because of fluoride fumes. That fluoride was the chief culprit became evident when ranchers observed: their cows suffered from mottled teeth (Fig. 17–1, page 297) and legs so stiff and painful that they had to graze on their knees (Fig. 17–2, next page). Samples of vegetation near the stack fallout showed fluoride concentrations several thousand times the usual levels.[17] In spite of the installation of pollution control equipment, the plant had to be shut down repeatedly. Finally, the factory discontinued operation altogether for reasons unrelated to the pollution problem.

In another part of the country, a jury decided on March 13, 1972, in favor of P. G. and P. N. Barci, father and son, in the suit of Barci vs. Intalco Aluminum Company of Ferndale, Washington, because of damage to cattle, trees, and to human health. A lung specialist from Spokane testified that P. G. Barci suffered from pulmonary fibrosis, a permanent lung disease which had completely disabled him.[18] About two years later, the same aluminum company lost a $130,500 fluoride emission suit to Ray and Helen Freeman, who resided a mile away from the plant on Lake Terrell.[19]

THE SOLUTION

These are but a few of the numerous law suits highlighting the magnitude of environmental damage by fluoride. Ironically, the expenditures I have discussed are small compared to the cost of installing effective air-cleaning equipment. For instance, by 1957

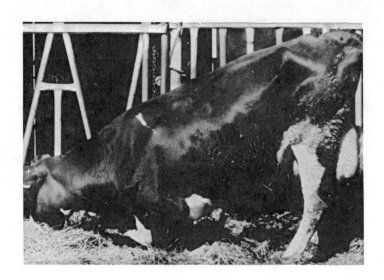

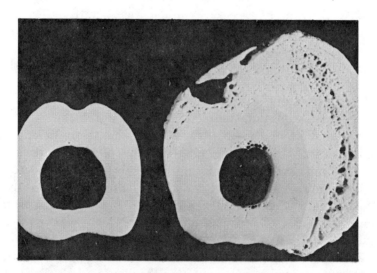

Fig. 17-2. Top: crippling fluoride-induced lameness in mature Holstein cow,
confirmed by definite dental and bone lesions.
Bottom: cross section of metatarsal bones from cows of same breed, size, and
age showing normal appearance (left) and severe osteofluorosis (right).
(Courtesy Drs. J.L. Shupe and A.E. Olson,
Utah State University, Logan, Utah.)

the United States Steel Corporation's Columbia-Geneva Division's plant in Provo, Utah, had spent $9 million to install electrostatic precipitators and other anti-pollution devices. The same company had previously been faced with nearly 900 damage claims totalling approximately $4.5 million.[20] Unfortunately, even high-priced air-cleaning equipment does not solve the problem, since fluoride scrubbed from chimneys does not disappear; it has to be washed onto the land or into rivers and lakes and eventually creates further difficulties.

Dismayed by the prospect of continuous litigation and fearful of recognition of widespread damage to human health, corporations initiated extensive research programs to convince communities and the courts that small amounts of fluorine are not harmful to man. They collaborated with scientists at leading universities and at industrial research laboratories.

One of these temples of learning is the Mellon Institute in Pittsburgh, Pa., founded by Andrew W. and Richard B. Mellon, the former owners of the Aluminum Company of America. LIFE magazine of May 9, 1938, described the Mellon Institute as an "Intellectual holding company and a laboratory for applied science open to the US businessman" where every possible resource and piece of equipment is available to industry. Such varied subjects as shaving, cigarette technology, or insecticides could be studied to improve products or to find new uses for them. LIFE added: "When a manufacturer is in trouble, for example, he finds the market for his goods is shrinking, he goes to the Institute. For $6,000 or more he gets a fellowship entitling him to employ a scientist for a year and use laboratory facilities. When the research is satisfactorily completed, all discoveries are turned over to the manufacturer exclusively."[21] Thus, findings incriminating to the corporations need not be published or presented to the medical and veterinary professions.

Whereas the Mellon Institute was the most logical place to seek aid in their precarious plight, corporations also sought help from other institutions of higher learning, especially the Universities of Tennessee, Cincinnati, and Wisconsin, all of which received large research grants to create a favorable climate of opinion for fluoride. Between 1940 and 1960, a flood of scientific reports issued from these institutions, which acknowledged the receipt of financial support from nine corporations, several of whom had been dumping fluoride into the environment.[22]

One of the scientists engaged in research at the Mellon Institute, Gerald J. Cox, a biochemist, was to play a major role in promoting fluoridation.[23] Some of his research had suggested to him that fluoride "may be specifically required for tooth formation."[24] He therefore recommended that it be added to water supplies as a means of reducing tooth decay.[25] On September 29, 1939, Cox told the Western Pennsylvania Section of the American Water Works Association meeting at Johnstown that "the present trend toward complete removal of fluorine from water and food may need some reversal." Cox's term "reversal" referred to the fact that water works engineers had been recommending 0.1 ppm as the *maximum level of fluoride in drinking water because they felt that at least a tenfold margin of safety should be maintained* (Table 17-1).[26]

Table 17-1

Recommended Maximum Levels of Ions in Water

Used for Drinking and Cooking, 1939[26]

Ion	Max. Level (ppm)
Calcium	30
Magnesium	10
Lithium	5
Iron	0.5
Bicarbonate	150
Carbonate	20
Sulfate	100
Chloride	200
Iodide	0.01
Fluoride	0.1

At that time even the official USPHS regulations stated: "The presence of . . . fluoride in excess of 1 p.p.m. . . . shall constitute ground for rejection of the water supply."[27] Because fluoride had been universally recognized as a toxic agent until then, Cox realized that water works officials might be held liable for poisoning people drinking fluoridated water. He therefore cautioned his audience: "Fluorides are among the most toxic of substances. Mottled enamel results from as little as 0.0001 per cent of fluorine in drinking water [1 ppm]. The results on adults of drinking water containing sufficient fluoride to prevent dental caries in children must be determined."[25] Cox undeniably sensed The Great Dilemma right at the start.

Cox's theory that fluoridated water could protect teeth against decay was based on his own experiments and on evidence provided in 1938 by W. D. Armstrong, professor of biochemistry at the University of Minnesota, and a consultant for the Dental Division of the PHS. In collaboration with P. J. Brekhus, Armstrong had reported more fluoride in enamel of healthy than in decayed teeth.[28] Twenty-five years later, however, his own reinvestigation convinced him that he had misinterpreted his early data, and he realized that the differences in the fluoride content between the sound and the carious teeth in his study were due to differences in the age of the teeth and did not reflect their susceptibility to decay.[29] Thus the basis of Cox's main argument for recommending the addition of fluorides to drinking water was later shown to have been wrong!

In 1943, F. A. Arnold, Jr., of the National Institute of Dental Research in Bethesda, Maryland, took up Cox's suggestion. He advocated fluoridation in the *Journal of the American Dental Association* on the basis of Cox's experiments, Dean's PHS surveys, and the Armstrong-Brekhus fluoride analyses of tooth enamel. Arnold stated: "The cumulative toxic effects on the body from ingestion of fluoride in this concentration is admitted to be a possibility. However, all things considered, such a possibility seems rather remote."[30] Even in 1946 he still maintained in his AAAS report that "such a procedure cannot be recommended for other than research purposes at the present time" and suggested a study which "may take 12-15 years before the final answer is clearly delineated."[31]

In the early 1940s Cox had an excellent opportunity to introduce his idea to scientists when he became a member of the Food and Nutrition Board of the National Research Council[23] and prepared for this illustrious body several pro-fluoridation summaries of the literature on dental caries. Through this organization, with its close link between industry and government, he was able to influence many scientists.

Cox also wielded considerable influence at the political level. In 1962, he was appointed to the Pennsylvania Drug, Device, and

Cosmetics Board to "administer a 1961 legislative act in the registration and regulation of organizations and persons distributing drugs" (including fluoride).[32]   He advised the Pennsylvania State Health Department and guided its policies concerning fluoride.

Cox lost no time in implementing his project. On September 20, 1939, five years before Newburgh and Grand Rapids experiments were initiated, and at the very time when he first suggested the fluoridation idea to the water engineers in Johnstown, he recommended fluoridation for that city;[25]   however, his proposal was rejected. Subsequently he promoted the measure more successfully before chemical and dental organizations, parent-teacher associations, and city councils.

Nevertheless, Cox's research at the Mellon Institute and his political activities fell short of relieving the aluminum industry of its distressing plight. ALCOA also tackled its fluoride pollution problem on another front, namely through the Kettering Laboratory in Cincinnati. This institute was founded in 1930 by gifts of the Ethyl Corporation, General Motors' Frigidaire subsidiary, and the duPont Company to investigate chemical hazards in American industrial operations. Like the Mellon Institute, it has made many valuable scientific contributions. Its 1955 budget of $643,000 was funded by industry (about 90%) and most of the rest by government agencies.[33]   Dr. Robert A. Kehoe, its first chief, one of the nation's leading industrial toxicologists, personified the close link between PHS and industry since he was Medical Director of the Ethyl Corporation and a consultant of the Division of Occupational Medicine of the PHS, the Tennessee Valley Authority, and the Atomic Energy Commission. He and his staff have also been consulted almost routinely by editors of medical journals as to the suitability of articles submitted for publication and have thus given industry a foothold in influencing the medical literature on fluoride. Kehoe and his colleagues at Kettering also played a key role in developing government standards to prevent lead poisoning in industry. These standards have subsequently been criticized severely because they were far too lax.[34]

Since 1931 a considerable portion of the Kettering Laboratory's facilities has been devoted to the study of fluoride, particularly the refrigerant gas Freon 12. Like the Mellon Institute's findings, those of the Kettering Laboratory are made available to the professions and to the public only upon approval of the industrial donor of the grant. Article 8 of one of the contract agreements between the Aluminum Company of America and the Laboratory specified that the University of Cincinnati shall "disseminate for the public good any information obtained. However, before the issuance of public reports or scientific publications, the manuscripts thereof will be submitted to the Donor for criticism and suggestions. Confidential information obtained from the Donor shall not be published without permission of said Donor."[35] The corporations were allowed to interpret the term "confidential information." One can only guess how much valuable research has been lost to the medical profession because of these agreements.

During the mid-20th century, the research that issued from the Kettering Laboratory dominated the medical literature on the toxicology of fluoride. Among its most useful products in the area of fluoride research were the abstracts and an annotated bibliography prepared by Irene R. Campbell covering the literature on fluoride through 1971.[36,37]

Although written mostly by proponents, many scientific articles in Campbell's annotated bibliography reveal serious health hazards of fluoride even in small amounts and at low concentrations. It is impossible to understand, therefore, how Kehoe could state publicly in March 1957 that "the question of the public safety of fluoridation is nonexistent from the viewpoint of medical science."[38]

Kettering Institute scientist E. J. Largent, who subsequently became consultant for Reynolds Metals Company, has written a book entitled *Fluorosis: The Health Aspects of Fluorine Compounds,* which was expressly designed, as indicated on its jacket, to "aid industry in law suits arising from fluoride damage." This book has been used as a reference source by many physicians and health organizations and strongly supports the use of fluoride in drinking water and discounts or minimizes its toxicological effects: "in recent years additional surveys of information have been reported that establish again and again the complete safety of fluoridating drinking water."[39]

TOOTHPASTE MANUFACTURERS

While it is true that many corporations with pollution problems were the driving force in the promotion of fluoridation, the manufacturers of toothpaste also stood to gain from establishing the image of fluoride as a health-promoting, tooth-decay preventive. Their academic center of research has been the Department of Bio-chemistry at the University of Indiana, School of Dentistry, with Professor J. C. Muhler as the senior author of numerous articles on fluoride, particularly under the sponsorship of the Procter and Gamble Company. Although his primary interest has been in fluoride toothpaste, he has also become a strong advocate of fluoridation of drinking water.

On May 22, 1963, a few weeks prior to a vote on fluoridation in Charleston, South Carolina, Muhler referred to fluoridation at a conference on "preventive dentistry" as:

> . . .a revolution in dentistry that will eliminate cavities and enable dentists to do the type of work they prefer and make more money doing it. Gallup polls in 10 large cities in the United States show that dentists who engage in such preventive programs [fluoride application to teeth and fluorida-tion] make more money. These surveys show that dentists who are freed from having to fill cavities have longer vacations and can afford to take trips to Europe, have more children, own bigger houses and buy their wives fur coats.[40]

Although I have great difficulty comprehending how a dentist can make more money by doing less work, it is quite true that Muhler's research dealing with the metabolism of fluorides has yielded an important mass of data. Often directed toward estab-lishing the value of fluoridated toothpaste, Muhler's research culminated in August 1960 with the ADA endorsement of Procter and Gamble's Crest.[41]

As a consequence, Muhler was awarded the title of "Research Professor in Basic Sciences," and received a new laboratory and freedom to work on his chosen projects.[42] ADA officials, on the other hand, were sharply criticized by some of their colleagues at the convention in Los Angeles, October 1960, because it appeared that they had profited from the immediate rise in Procter and Gamble stock following the unprecedented approval of Crest by their Association.[43] After the endorsement was announced, Procter and Gamble stock rose $8 a share,[44] and by May 1961 the sales of Crest had doubled.[45] Crest moved into second place in sales, gaining 25% as its share of the $235 million a year retail tooth-paste market. Colgate's share, still the largest, then dropped from 31% to 27%.[46]

Regardless of his success in the development of Crest, Muhler was obliged to defend the toothpaste industry against another source of competition, the manufacturers of fluoride-containing tablets and fluoride drops. "The effectiveness of a fluoride pill lasts only 20 minutes," Muhler stated in Charleston, South Carolina, "whereas fluoride in the water is spread out over the entire day. To achieve the same benefits with a pill," he added, "you would have to take a fluoride pill every 8 minutes."[40]

The gross error of this contention has been demonstrated by Aasenden and Peebles, who found that fluoride administered in tablet form or in vitamin preparations was more than twice as effective as fluoridated water in preventing cavities.[47] Their figures for 7- to 12-year-old children with caries-free permanent teeth were 54% with the fluoride supplement (tablets and drops) from infancy compared to 23.9% for lifetime exposure to fluoridated water. Actually, a tablet provides an exact dosage of the drug, whereas the amount of fluoride consumed in drinking water cannot be controlled, especially since the early stage of fluoride poisoning induces excessive thirst which calls for greater water intake. Furthermore, tablets and drops can be discontinued at age 10-12 after the tooth enamel is formed or even earlier should ill effects occur.

That simultaneous consumption of fluoride from drugs, tooth-paste, and water created a real risk was suggested by a warning required on the package when fluoride toothpaste was first marketed in 1955. It stated that fluoridated toothpaste should not be used in areas where the water supply is fluoridated.[48] A later decision stipulated that each tube should carry the warning note: "CAUTION: children under 6 should not use CREST" (Fig. 17-3, next page). Both regulations were instituted because the PHS recognized the obvious dangers of an overdose from simultaneous absorption of fluoride from water and from toothpaste. In 1958, however, the two regulations were abandoned, even though no new research was available to prove beyond doubt that the overdose hazard no longer existed.[49] As a matter of fact, subsequent studies by W. S. Weisz raised serious questions about the efficacy

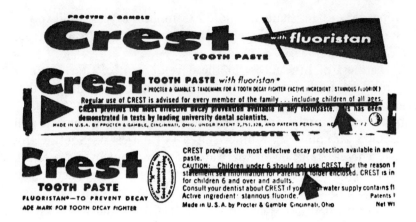

Fig. 17-3. Contradictory recommended-use statements (underlined, arrows) on two different packages of Crest toothpaste sold in the same city at the same time (ca. 1960).

as well as about the safety of toothpastes which contained fluoride.[50]

A conflict also arose between the PHS, which in effect had staked its reputation on fluoridation, and the industries selling fluoride toothpaste. Logically, wide acceptance of fluoride toothpaste and tablets containing fluoride might indicate that there is little or no need for fluoridation. In order to offset such competition, exponents of fluoridation were forced to compromise.

Muhler reversed his original opinion by advocating both: "We don't think that fluoride toothpaste alone or fluoride in drinking water or topically applied alone will prevent cavities. We say that a combination of these together with proper diet and toothbrushing will reduce the number of cavities."[40] Curiously, U.S. fluoride toothpaste advertisements now claim that the only place to get a better fluoride treatment is from your dentist. Only rarely is anything said about fluoridated water.

PHARMACEUTICAL INDUSTRY

There is a parallel between the promotion of Procter and Gamble's stannous fluoride toothpaste, and that of Adeflor, the Upjohn (Kalamazoo, Michigan) Company's fluoride-containing vitamin drops recommended for caries prevention. Neither the toothpaste manufacturers nor the drug companies could have found a ready market for their fluoride products had it not been for the research designed to promote fluoridation of water supplies.

The Upjohn Company provided grants to pediatrician J. S. Walker of Kalamazoo, Michigan, and his associates to determine the daily water consumption of infants and young children up to age "twelve and older" in widely separated areas of the U.S.A.[51] These workers found that generally infants and even older children whose principal source of fluid intake is milk, not water, actually consume less than one pint of water per day, which when fluoridated contains 0.5 mg of fluoride. It is quite clear, therefore, that many children do not receive the recommended dose of fluoride from fluoridated drinking water. Other children, however, run the definite risk of developing dental fluorosis when they consume 1 mg of fluoride in Adeflor drops in addition to the daily 1 mg or more in drinking water plus 0.5 to 1 mg in food.

To cope with this dilemma, the PHS issued a public warning through Professor Philip Jay on November 14, 1962, at the Michigan Annual Pharmacy Lecture at Ann Arbor. "In areas already supplied with fluoridated water," Jay emphasized, "use of added supplements is not only unnecessary but definitely contraindicated."[52] The following year, on September 27, 1963, H. M. Greenleaf, Health Director of Newton, Massachusetts, cautioned against the use of fluorine supplements where water is fluoridated: "Although there is a wide margin of safety, those residents of Newton who have been taking fluoride pills or drops should now discontinue their use concurrently with the start of its [sic] delivery in the water."[53]

The conflict between the pharmaceutical industry and the powerful PHS appears to have been settled when Upjohn released a color film promoting fluoridation of water supplies with Dr. F. J. Stare of Harvard's School of Public Health acting as master of ceremonies.[54] Upjohn simply followed the example of Procter and Gamble's $250,000 hour-long TV show featuring film star Henry Fonda to promote fluoridation during National Children's Health Week.[55] Since these companies are marketing a product competing with fluoridation, their presentations seem to have been a goodwill gesture to mollify the PHS.

SUGAR INTERESTS

The sugar industry stood to profit by fluoridation as much as any other industrial group. If the public were convinced that fluoridation makes teeth resistant to decay, wouldn't mothers be less concerned about their children's consumption of sweets? Wouldn't this help increase the sale of sugar? Ironically, the Sugar Research Foundation, Inc., consisting of about 130 corporations, had long been searching for methods of preventing tooth decay without curtailing sales of their products. The Foundation's 1950 seventh annual report clearly expressed its aim in dental research: "To discover effective means of controlling tooth decay by methods other than restricting carbohydrate [sugar] intake."[56]

Did the sugar industries' goal of preventing tooth decay without decreasing sugar consumption generate large research grants to universities? Two of the institutions most vociferous in the promotion of fluoridation—the Dental Schools of Harvard and of the University of Rochester—have indeed received large grants for fluoride research from the sugar industry. But the grants had strings attached and were sometimes terminated. In January 1958, The Sugar Research Foundation withdrew its support from J. H. Shaw, a biochemist at Harvard's School of Dental Medicine. Dr. Shaw, who had received $57,000 for his research activities, found that all sugars cause tooth decay. His conclusion from his work: "We should cut down on sugar consumption, particularly candy."[57]

OTHER INDUSTRIES

Although the primary financial beneficiaries of fluoridation are steel, aluminum, and other metal manufacturers, the sugar industry, toothpaste producers, pharmaceutical firms, and numerous other corporations also have much to gain from it. Fluoridation equipment, for instance, provides a substantial income to some corporations. In 1967 in the Detroit area alone, the cost for installed fluoridation equipment was estimated by Water Board Manager, G. H. Remus, at $500,000.[58] Detroit is only one of the many large U.S. cities that have spent large sums of money for the installation and maintenance of fluoridation equipment. As early as 1951 USPHS Publication No. 62 named 14 corporations as suppliers of fluoride feeders for communities throughout the U.S.[59]

One personality in the equipment industry stands out among the nation's key promoters – A. P. Black, professor of chemistry at the University of Florida, Gainsville. He was responsible for introducing fluoridation in many Florida cities and for promoting it among members of the American Water Works Association, of which he was a former president. He acknowledged in the *Tampa Sunday Tribune,* December 16, 1951, that members of his family were president and vice-president of a company selling fluoridation equipment.

Other industries such as trucking, railroad, and electric power companies likewise profit from fluoridation, since they serve the companies that gain primarily from the sale of fluoride. Rubber industries also have a stake in fluoridation; they manufacture the rubber lining for tank trucks in which fluosilicic acid is transported to municipalities. In 1966 *Dunlop Dimensions,* the official publication of the DUNLOP Rubber Company of Canada in Toronto, Ontario, clearly demonstrated its own interest and that of the phosphate fertilizer industry. In the past, hydrofluosilicic acid had been "only an incidental by-product of regular phosphoric acid production" at the Electrolytic Reduction Company (ERCO) plants in Port Maitland, Ontario. It was neutralized and thrown away, but now hydrofluosilicic acid liquid is being sold and transported in special rubber-lined tanks.[60]

The acid is so corrosive, *Dunlop Dimensions* stated, "that without the protection afforded by the rubber lining, the steel tank structures would be eaten away in a matter of hours. . . . The future for sales of hydrofluosilicic acid looks extremely good. ERCO, with the growing demand for the acid for use as a fluoridating agent in water supplies, saw a market facing them and built the plant to tap it."[60] ERCO is but one of numerous other phosphate fertilizer companies that have sprung up in recent decades and are now selling the fluoride waste in wash water scrubbed from the chimneys of their factories and collected in settling ponds nearby to fluoridate municipal water supplies of such cities as Detroit, Hamilton, and Toronto.

Interestingly, the corporations that originally sponsored fluoridation rarely promoted their product publicly. In 1950-1951 ALCOA had explicitly advertised sodium fluoride "of a uniform high degree of purity" for addition to water supplies in the

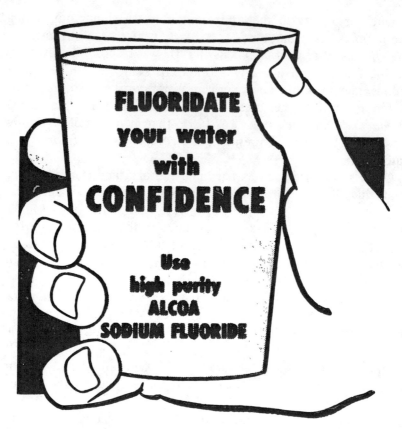

Fig. 17-4. Facsimile of a portion of an ALCOA advertisement in the *Journal of the American Water Works Association,* Vol. 43, No. 6 (1950). The accompanying text states: "ALCOA Sodium Fluoride is particularly suitable for the fluoridation of water supplies. . . . If your community is fluoridating its water supply—or is considering doing so—let us show you how ALCOA Sodium Fluoride can do the job for you. Write to ALUMINUM COMPANY OF AMERICA, CHEMICALS DIVISION, 624 Gulf Building, Pittsburg, Pennsylvania."

Journal of the American Water Works Association[61] (Fig. 17–4, above). On May 22, 1957, however, ALCOA's Chemical Sales Manager, H. P. Bonebrake, stated in a letter to C. A. Barden of Oberlin, Ohio, that his firm was not promoting fluoride for water fluoridation or selling it "directly to any municipality." Nevertheless, Hearings on Fluoridation before the Committee on Interstate and Foreign Commerce, House of Representatives, suggest that ALCOA was the original driving force behind fluoridation:

In 1944 Oscar Ewing was put on the payroll of the Aluminum Company of America, as attorney, at an annual salary of $750,000. This fact was established at a Senate hearing and became a part of the Congressional Record. Since the Aluminum Co. had no big litigation pending at the time, the question might logically be asked, why such a large fee? A few months thereafter Mr. Ewing was made Federal Security Administrator with the announcement that he was taking a big salary cut in order to serve his country.[62]

It was Ewing, as chief of the PHS, who officially gave the green light to fluoridation only five years after the initiation of the 10- to 15-year experiments in Grand Rapids, Michigan, and Newburgh, New York. At that time the permanent teeth of children born under fluoridation had not yet erupted, and therefore no reliable scientific conclusions concerning its benefits could possibly have been reached.

Prior to Ewing's tenure of office in the federal government, Andrew Mellon, the founder of ALCOA, had been the U.S. Treasurer. The PHS was then in the Department of the Treasury. One can only speculate concerning Mr. Mellon's role as protector of his company. Nor can it be ascertained whether or not such scientists as Knutson, Dean, Russell, and their colleagues in the Dental Division of the PHS, were in any way influenced in their desire to please their boss, Oscar Ewing. This thought is bound to occur to anyone who is familiar with governmental agencies; it is also driven home clearly by the Watergate affair. When decisions are made at the top level – be they right or wrong – it is not easy for government employees to report "corruption, waste, or regulatory abuse." The consequences: "Too often they are characterized as troublemakers, then are fired, frozen out of promotions or subjected to personal harassment for the rest of their careers."[63]

Industry's vital role in promoting fluoridation cannot be doubted nor can the leadership of ALCOA be denied in this affair. In carefully orchestrated harmony, industry, science, and the PHS collaborated in a plan that instituted a health procedure touching virtually everyone in America. Enormous research activity produced a mountain of evidence – much positive – that fluoridation was the long-sought answer to our dental health care problems. But what of the serious problems discovered? Why were they obscured, discounted, or simply ignored? If we examine the fluoride literature closely to determine how much of it was supported or generated by industry and/or the PHS, we shall find the answers to our questions. We shall also understand some of the reasons why scientists, physicians, and dentists are generally ignorant of the true consequences of fluoridation.

REFERENCES

1. Water Boom for Fluorides. Chemical Week, July 7, 1951, p. 14.

2. Davenport, S.J., and Morris, G.G.: U.S. Bureau of Mines. Circular 7687, U.S. Dept. of Interior, June 1954, p. 8.

3. Oregon Rancher Asks $200,000 of Aluminum Co. Seattle Times, Dec. 16, 1952.

4. Food Machinery and Chemical Corporation vs. W.S. Meader and May Meader, United States Court of Appeals, Ninth District, Aug. 25, 1961.

5. Ost, H.: Der Kampf gegen schädliche Industriegase. Z. Angew. Chem., 20:1689-1693, 1907.

6. The So-Called Copper Teeth of Cattle. Br. Dent. J., 28:141-142, 1907.

7. Damages Awarded for Crop Burns. Lewiston (Idaho) Morning Tribune, Feb. 6, 1962.

8. Jury Decides Alcoa Liability Ended in 1955. Knoxville (Tenn.) Journal, May 7, 1958.

9. Alcoa Sued for Nearly $3 Million. Knoxville (Tenn.) Journal, July 30, 1955.

10. Sauvies Island. Portland (Oregon) Reporter, June 26, 1962.

11. Harvey Loses Fluoride Case. Hood River (Oregon) News, Oct. 29, 1970.

12. Lewis, H.R.: With Every Breath You Take. Crown Publishers, Inc., New York, 1965, pp. 110-111.

13. Gordon, C.C., and Tourangeau, P.C.: The Impact of Fluoride on the Farmlands of Buckeystown, Maryland, Caused by the Eastalco Aluminum Smelter (cover title). Environmental Studies Laboratory, University of Montana, Missoula, Mont., February, 1977.

14. Three Win in Fume Suit. The Oregonian (Portland), Sept. 17, 1955.

15. Seven Enter Fluoride Case. The Oregonian (Portland), Oct. 15, 1957.

16. Aluminum Firm Loses Appeal in Poison Case. Cleveland (Ohio) Press, June 6, 1958.

17. Smog Battle Ends in Montana Town. New York Times, Sept. 17, 1967.

18. Park, R.: The Intalco Trial. Northwest Passage, Bellingham, Wash., March 20 - April 2, 1972, p. 9.

19. Intalco's Fluoride Emissions Exceed State Standards, Manager Tells Jury. Bellingham (Wash.) Herald, Jan. 17, 1974. Jury Awards Damages from Intalco. Ibid., Jan. 27, 1974.

20. Utah Steel Mill Curbs Pollution. New York Times, Nov. 10, 1957.

21. Science Means Business in This Grecian Temple. LIFE, May 9, 1938, p. 48.

22. Aluminum Co. of America; American Petroleum Institute; E.I. du Pont de Nemours Co.; The Harshaw Chemical Co.; Kaiser Aluminum and Chemical Corp.; Pennsylvania Salt Manufacturing Co.; Reynolds Metals Co.; Tennessee Valley Authority; and Universal Oil Products Co.

23. Institute Hill PTA to Discuss Fluoridation. Butler (Pa.) Eagle, Jan. 28, 1959.

24. Cox, G.J.: Experimental Dental Caries. I. Nutrition in Relation to the Development of Dental Caries. Dental Rays, 13:8-10, 1937.

25. Cox, G.J.: New Knowledge of Fluorine in Relation to Dental Caries. J. Am. Water Works Assoc., 31:1926-1930, 1939.

26. Babbit, H.E., and Doland, J.J.: Quality of Water Supplies in Water Supply Engineering. 3rd Edition, McGraw Hill, New York, 1939, p. 454.

27. USPHS: Public Health Service Drinking Water Standards. Public Health Rep. 58:69-111, 1943 (at p. 80).

28. Armstrong, W.D., and Brekhus, P.J.: Possible Relationship between the Fluorine Content of Enamel and Resistance to Dental Caries. J. Dent. Res., 17:393-399, 1938.

29. Armstrong, W.D., and Singer, L.: Fluoride Contents of Enamel of Sound and Carious Human Teeth: A Reinvestigation. J. Dent. Res., 42:133-136, 1963.

30. Arnold, F.A., Jr.: Role of Fluorides in Preventive Dentistry. J. Am. Dent. Assoc., 30:499-508, 1943.

31. Arnold, F.A., Jr.: The Possibility of Reducing Dental Caries by Increasing Fluoride Ingestion, in F.R. Moulton, Ed.: Dental Caries and Fluorine, 1946, pp. 99-107, and p. 105.

32. Doctor Appointed. Pittsburgh (Pa.) Post Gazette, April 4, 1962.

33. Testimony of Dr. R. Kehoe in Paul Martin Family vs. Reynolds Metals Corp., p. 960.

34. Bryce-Smith, D., and Waldron, H.A.: Lead in Food – Are Today's Regulations Sufficient? Chem. Brit., 10:202-206, 1974.

35. Contract Agreement Between Aluminum Co. of America and U. of Cincinnati, signed by N.P. Auburn, Vice-President and Dean of Administration (April 30. 1947). Testimony McCarthy vs. The Cincinnati Enquirer, 1956.

36. Campbell, I.R., and Widner, E.M.: Annotated Bibliography: The Occurrence and Biological Effects of Fluorine Compounds. The Kettering

Laboratory, Cincinnati, Ohio, 1958.

37. Fluoride Abstracts. Supplement to Annotated Bibliography The Occurrence and Biological Effects of Fluorine Compounds. The Kettering Laboratory, Cincinnati, Ohio, 1955-1971.

38. "Our Children's Teeth," Report to the Mayor and the Board of Estimate of the City of New York by the Committee to Protect Our Children's Teeth, Inc., March 6, 1957, p. 27.

39. Largent, E.J.: Fluorosis: The Health Aspects of Fluorine Compounds. 1961, p. 73.

40. Fluoridation Efforts are Commended. Charleston (S.C.) Evening Post, May 22, 1963.

41. The original endorsement was announced in August 1960. Subsequently, as the result of criticism by dentists and competitive toothpaste manufacturers, ADA officials insisted that they had merely given their "approval" and had "recognized" Crest's value in providing some protection against tooth decay, as reported in the Am. Med. Assoc. News, Jan. 23, 1961.

42. One Toothpaste Wins Dental Society O.K., Detroit Free Press, August 2, 1960, p. 18.

43. Plan to Rescind Toothpaste O.K. Starts Debate Among Dentists. Los Angeles Times, Oct. 19, 1960, p. 4.

44. Toothpaste with Fluoride Endorsed by Dental Group. Tampa (Fla.) Tribune, August 2, 1960.

45. Toothpaste Sales Battle Grows Fiercer; Crest Challenges Front-Runner Colgate. Wall Street Journal, May 4, 1961.

46. Colgate Enters Fluoridated Toothpaste Market, Claims an Improved Ingredient. By Wall Street J. Staff Reporter, Wall Street Journal, Aug. 9, 1961.

47. Aasenden, R., and Peebles, T.C.: Effects of Fluoride Supplementation from Birth on Human Deciduous and Permanent Teeth. Arch. Oral Biol., 19:321-326, 1974.

48. Legal, Sodium Fluoride Label. Chem. Week, July 6, 1957, p. 36.

49. TGA Scientific Section Spotlights Technical Problems Over Wide Area; Names Edman Vice Chairman. More About Fluorides. Drug and Allied Industries, June, 1958, p. 11.

50. Weisz, W.S.: A Comparison of the Relative Effects of Sodium and Stannous Fluoride When Applied Topically. J. Dent. Child., 29:22-35, 1962.

51. Walker, J.S., Margolis, F.J., Teate, H.L., Jr., Weil, M.L., and Wilson, H. L.: Water Intake of Normal Children. Science, 140:890-891, 1963.

52. Jay, P.: Unsupervised Use of Fluoride Items Held Hazardous. Drug News Weekly, Nov. 14, 1962.

53. Fluoridation Advantageous, Greenleaf Says. News-Tribune, Newton, Mass., Sept. 27, 1963.

54. This film was presented by Chester Tossy, D.D.S., of the Michigan State Department of Health at the hearing before the Michigan State House of Representatives Committee on Fluoridation, Cadillac Square Bldg., Detroit, Mich., Oct. 7. 1963.

55. Adams, V.: T.V. Show Given to Dental Group National Unit - Plans Ads on Procter and Gamble Program. New York Times, Aug. 22, 1961.

56. The Problem of Tooth Decay. Seventh Annual Report. Sugar Research Foundation, Inc., 1950.

57. As stated to TIME's reporter, Sweet Tooth, Sour Facts. TIME, Jan. 13, 1958.

58. Remus, G.J.: Personal Communication to the Detroit Common Council, June 11, 1962. Copy in my possession.

59. USPHS Division of Dental Public Health: Better Health for 5 to 14 Cents a Year Through Fluoridated Water. Federal Security Agency, PHS Publ. No. 62, Revised, April 1951.

60. Erco Fluorides Protect Growing Teeth and Dunlop Rubber Protects Erco's Plant. Dunlop Dimensions, March-April-May, 1966, pp. 7-9.

61. High Purity ALCOA Sodium Fluoride for the Fluoridation of Water. J. Am. Water Works Assoc., 42:5, 1950; Fluoridate Your Water With Confidence. Use High Purity ALCOA Sodium Fluoride. Ibid., 43:45, 1951.

62. Hearings before the Committee on Interstate and Foreign Commerce, House of Representatives, Eighty-Third Congress, Second Session on H.R. 2341, May 25, 26, and 27, 1954, p. 51.

63. When Workers Blow Whistle on Federal Waste, Fraud. U.S. News and World Report, Dec. 19, 1977, p. 55.

CHAPTER 18

WHY THE IGNORANCE?

ASK A MEDICAL student, a practicing physician, or the editor of a medical journal what he knows about fluoride, and he will reply that it prevents tooth decay, makes bones stronger, and that too much of it causes mottled teeth and sclerosis of bones. This is usually the sum total of his knowledge on the subject since fluoride is rarely discussed at medical schools or in medical journals. Dr. Elmer Hess, a former AMA president, illuminated the situation in a letter to me dated August 9, 1955: "I think most of us in the American Medical Association feel what we have to depend on the American Dental Association and the United States Public Health Service primarily for scientific facts concerning a situation of this kind, and I am unable to express an opinion as to whether it is safe or not safe."

Even the editors of the AMA *Journal* seem to have trouble finding capable physicians to advise them on the medical aspects of fluoridation and often rely on dentists with no experience in clinical medicine. For instance, in June 1961, D. J. Galagan and J. L. Bernier, whose research had dealt primarily with air temperature and fluoridation and with surgical problems in dentistry, were consulted on a fluoride-related allergic skin disease.[1] Neither had had any clinical background in allergy or skin disease. At a fluoride pollution suit in Oregon, Martin vs. Reynolds Metals Corporation in 1955, the defendant had to retain Dr. Donald Hunter, a British physician, for expert testimony since no one with expertise on fluoride illness was available in the U.S.A. As late as 1974, Dr. E. H. Smith, Jr., a dentist, was asked to write an editorial for the *Journal of the American Medical Association* in which he quoted a politically appointed health officer, the former U.S. Surgeon General Luther Terry, as his authority for claiming that fluoridation "is medically safe for all people of all ages and its benefits last a lifetime."[2]

After three decades of fluoridation, why do physicians and dentists know so little about the hazards of fluoridation? Is this lack of knowledge due to calculated omission of important research from the scientific literature, or have advocates of fluoridation attempted to cover up their Great Dilemma by adroitly side-stepping the adverse health effects?

NEUTRALIZING NEGATIVE FINDINGS

In Chapters 13 and 15 we saw how a USPHS press release attacked Taylor's work on fluoride as a tumor-growth accelerator in an attempt to discredit his original experiments, and how the studies of Rapaport on the relationship of fluoride to Down's syndrome were "neutralized" by an unpublished criticism circulated by a PHS official. The later reports by Taylor and by Rapaport, extending and corroborating their earlier conclusions, are rarely quoted.

Had my own reports of poisoning by fluoridated water been recognized and acknowledged in the mid-1950s, an embarrassing reassessment of fluoridation would have been necessary. The visit to the U.S.A. in 1955 by Dr. Heinrich Hornung, a German health officer and one of Europe's most dedicated advocates of fluoridation, fortunately offered proponents an excellent opportunity to disparage my research. During his so-called "study" tour, Hornung spent considerable time in my Detroit office and home to learn about my cases of fluoride poisoning. To my chagrin, I later discovered that he reviewed my records for the express purpose of detecting any possible flaws that would permit him to downgrade my work, just as Dean and Andervont had visited Taylor's laboratory to undercut his work. Shortly after his return to Germany he addressed a letter to F. S. McKay, who arranged to have it published in the *Journal of the American Dental Association* in September 1956. It immediately became the subject of a widely disseminated news release.

Anyone who reads Hornung's letter will be astonished that such a mélange of hearsay and *ad hominem* argumentation could have been used by the ADA to denigrate my scientific reputation. The strident tone of the letter is set in the opening sentence: "In *The New Leader* of January 2, 1956, I found a *nonsensical* article by James Rorty opposing fluoridation of drinking water." Hornung's entire letter, in fact, abounds with intemperate and biased opinions. Here I have selected only four representative ones: "On the question of fluoridation, his [Waldbott's] reasoning is tarnished constantly by an emotional bias." "Therefore, it can be assumed that the positive answers received to Dr. Waldbott's questionnaire are nothing but the production of suggestion by 'leading' questions. *The 70 cases of chronic poisoning, claimed to be caused by fluoridation, never existed.*" "The American Dental Association and the public health authorities are fully justified in their contention that Dr. Waldbott presented *no proof* to substantiate his belief that chronic poisoning had been caused by water fluoridation, and those organizations, therefore, should proceed with their program." "I feel sorry for the population of those cities where the fluoridation of the water has been rejected on the basis of such unscientific propaganda."[3] (Emphases added.)

One paragraph of Hornung's letter also threw in a reverse form of the "red-herring" technique. He tacitly rejected the theory that fluoridation is a communist plot. Although he did not specifically claim that we even discussed such matters, he clearly tried to associate me with such a view, presumably to embellish his attack on me.

The most perverse aspect of the letter, however, focused on my "70 cases" of chronic fluoride poisoning, the ostensible reason for his communication. Hornung's primary observations, summaries, and conclusions on this vital subject were simply false—and they were known to be false from personal conversations I held with him during his visit. He stated that I did "not find it necessary to investigate these cases scientifically" and that the cases were established on the basis of questionnaires filled with "leading questions." Furthermore, "whenever a single one of these questions was answered positively by one of the recipients of the questionnaire (mostly elderly ladies), this was recorded as proof of poisoning by fluoridation." Claiming to quote these elderly women patients (six of the fourteen he cited were men), he ridiculed and quoted (without permission) out-of-context selected statements from my patients' files.

Upon his return to Germany, Hornung "tried to establish that the symptoms listed in the 70 case histories were irrelevant, and that the questionnaire contained 'leading' (suggestive) questions."

He then translated into German a list of questions apparently based on my own questionnaire, which I had used merely as a screening device, not a primary diagnostic tool. Again, he included fabricated items not in my work: "chronic skin erosion" and "gastritis and atrophy of the liver, especially during summer." He then claimed 50 answers to his questionnaire about chlorine and chlorination (not fluorine and fluoridation). Although he did not publish his claimed responses, he based his accusation that my work was totally false ("never existed") on his own alleged questionnaire, which could have been circulated in a hospital or an insane asylum for all we know.

Never at any time did Hornung mention what I had repeated over and over again: in all cases the symptoms of fluorosis disappeared when the use of fluoridated water was discontinued and reappeared when its use was resumed.[4] Since these scientific facts have been published in my numerous articles already cited, they need not be reiterated here. Hornung was well aware of these facts, yet he never mentioned them.

Had the ADA bothered to contact me before publishing Hornung's curious letter, I could have saved them the embarrassment that history will associate with them for attempting to discredit my scientific work. My immediate reaction was one of dismay and astonishment that a fellow scientist — supposedly sworn to the pursuit of truth — could malign me in such a reckless manner. When I threatened a libel suit against the ADA, they published a letter from me in which I described in some detail the symptoms of chronic fluoride intoxication and the questionnaires that I had "used for preliminary orientation and for screening."[5] I cited a new case of tetaniform convlusions (in a boy) caused by fluoride[6] and concluded the letter by observing: "My research proves that neither a standard concentration of F. in water, nor a standard daily dose of F. in water can be safe for everyone."[5] In a comment at the end of my letter, the editor exclaimed that the ADA did not wish to be confused by scientific facts: "Publication of Dr. Waldbott's letter does not, in any way, alter *The Journal's* opinion that the overwhelming mass of scientific evidence favors fluoridation."

Although the ADA published my letter, they apparently did nothing to counteract the clear fabrications of Hornung's assertions, and the public as well as medical news media propagated the story in many places,[7] which abruptly blocked publication for me in many major American medical journals. And who could blame the editors of these journals if they had not probed deeply into the matter?

On November 4, 1958, when I presented my cases on fluoride poisoning before the Swedish Medical Society in Stockholm through the courtesy of Nobel Laureate Hugo Theorell, Sweden's leading fluoridation advocate, Yngve Ericsson, attempted to discredit me by recounting Hornung's letter.[8] In September 1961 the editor of *Nutrition Reviews* obliquely referred to my work: "The way in which he [Waldbott] had obtained many of the symptoms from questionnaires with leading questions has been described elsewhere."[9] As late as 1970 McClure quoted "Horning" [*sic*] at length to perpetuate the old false impression that by then had been unequivocally refuted.[10] The Hornung affair is one significant reason why dentists and physicians have ignored my reports of fluoride poisoning.

Lest anyone still doubts that the ADA might suppress the truth about adverse effects of fluoride, consider the following evidence. A report in 1958 by the ADA Council on Dental Therapeutics about dietary fluorides claimed that water fluoridation is superior in coverage and cost to individual administration of fluoride supplements.[11] We have already seen that scientific evidence supports the opposite conclusion,[12] and similar evidence was known to the ADA in 1958. As research dentist R. Feltman pointed out to the ADA: "I have been studying the effects of dietary fluorides for approximately the past 10 years. *Your Council knows of this study for they have been in correspondence with me and therefore cannot plead ignorance.*" (Emphasis added.) He concluded his devastating critique concentrating on the many potential hazards to children by observing:

> The statements made, in using fluoride solutions[,] fail to take into consideration the quantity of fluoride that would be ingested when the home fluoridated water supply would be used and therefore causes me to voice again the same objection that I have to community fluoridated water, namely the variations in water intake, and so we find that it is impossible to determine which child will receive the correct quantity, which will receive an excessive amount and which will not receive enough.[13]

Despite this trenchant statement based on extensive research, the ADA continued to promote fluoridation as "safe and effective," without referring to Feltman's explicit contrary findings.

OTHER MEANS OF WITHHOLDING POISONING REPORTS

In 1956 a different approach to deprive physicians of specific information on fluoride poisoning was followed in the Wisconsin town of Wausau. Mrs. J. W. P. had just recovered from a long siege of abdominal spasms and diarrhea upon following the recommendation of her physician that she eliminate fluoridated water for drinking and cooking. On March 24 of that year she was visited by two men, one posing as "the editor" of the nearby Antigo local newspaper, who were able to persuade her to sign her name for release of information about her illness by her physician. Subsequently, the physician was visited by five persons and intimidated to such an extent that he declined to discuss her case with anyone, including his medical colleagues. Later the patient was admitted under my care to a Detroit hospital where, after consultation with several physicians, the diagnosis of fluoride poisoning was fully confirmed.

Other physicians have also had reason to remain silent when they encountered illness caused by fluoridated water. In 1955 Dr. William Wolf, a clinical professor at New York University's School of Dentistry, New York City, also observed four cases of poisoning from drinking water in nearby fluoridated communities. After verifying the diagnosis, he warned his colleagues of fluoridation's danger to health. The following day the dean informed him that his services at the university were no longer needed. When Wolf in turn threatened to give wide publicity to the reason for the proposed action, the dean immediately dropped the matter. Nevertheless, Wolf was discomfited by the whole affair, and refrained from publishing a report of his cases.[14]

In the Indiana town of Tell City near Evansville, another physician had observed poisoning from fluoridated water. In June 1957 in Detroit, I had occasion to study three of Dr. R. J. Miller's cases, Mrs. H. S., Mrs. A.M., and Mrs. S. A. S., and confirmed the diagnosis after careful examination. Symptoms of fluorosis – arthritic changes, especially in the spine, spastic pains and numbness in the arms and legs, gastrointestinal upsets, ulcers in the mouth, blurred vision due to early changes in the retina, and skin eruptions – were promptly alleviated after these patients discontinued drinking Tell City fluoridated water. When Miller attempted to communicate this matter to his colleagues and to sound a public warning through the news media, he was subjected to considerable disparagement and harassment, all of which had such an adverse effect on his standing in the community that he eventually had to abandon his practice in that city and establish himself elsewhere.

Attempts by dental organizations to suppress information about harm from fluoridated water have no doubt followed other avenues, including the following. In 1965 the advertising manager of one of the suburban Detroit newspapers received a form letter signed by the attorney for the Detroit District Dental Society in his capacity as legal adviser to a fluoridation lobbying committee established by the Society. Among the statements in the letter was the following:

> They [opponents of fluoridation] have also made entirely unsupported claims that this public health measure creates hazards and is dangerous, all of which are entirely unwarranted assumptions contrary to well documented basic research.
>
> We anticipate that an attempt will be made to buy advertising in your newspaper in order to utilize your medium to disseminate these statements. . . .
>
> This letter is being written to appeal to you not to participate in any program by publishing these statements, FIGHT WATER POLLUTION, or any similar untrue statements, which can only mislead the public and introduce sensationalism and patent deception into the campaign. We feel that as a responsible member of the community, and as a newspaper man, you recognize the potency of mass communication and the grave responsibility to protect the truth this carries with it.[15]

Who knows what additional pressures – financial and otherwise – have been devised to control the local and national news media? This is but another way to keep knowledge of the health hazards of fluoridation from physicians as well as the public.

PRESSURES ON DENTISTS AND PHYSICIANS

Dental leaders obviously anticipated opposition to fluoridation from their colleagues when they attempted to abridge the consti-

tutional right of freedom of speech by implementing the ADA
Code of Ethics, adopted in November 1950:

> Section 20. Education of the Public. --A dentist may properly participate
> in a program for the education of the public on matters pertaining to
> dentistry provided such a program is in keeping with the dignity of the
> profession and has the approval of the dentists of the community or state
> acting through the appropriate agency of the dental society.

If dentists could not be persuaded by scientific evidence, then the
ADA would legislate approval under pain of censure – in defense
of a Code of Ethics! Opposition by the membership, however, was
widespread, but fear of reprisals suppressed dissent by the rank
and file within the profession. Newspaper correspondent George
Sokolsky exposed this fear in a statement to the ADA *Journal* in
May 1955:

> I find that as many of those whom I interviewed who are members of
> your association are opposed to the process [of fluoridation] as favor it.
> I find also that they live in terror of being quoted. They tell me that they
> may be brought up [before the ethics committee] on charges should I
> quote their names[16]

The published prohibition against dissent was dropped in March
1960, but dentists were admonished not to claim that they represented the majority of dentists when, in fact, their "views were opposed to the society's or to the majority of the dentists in the
community."[17]

As should be anticipated, some dentists vocally opposing fluoridation have felt the wrath of organized dentistry. In 1955, for
example, Dr. R. Pringle and Dr. D. H. Irwin were temporarily suspended from the North Carolina Dental Society for their persistent
public stand against fluoridation.[18] In 1961 Dr. Max Ginns of
Worcester, Massachusetts, was dropped from his state dental society after he refused to discontinue use of a petition, circulated in
1953, which listed 119 dentists and 59 physicians in Worcester
who opposed fluoridation.[19] The petition urged the local dental
society to repeal its pro-fluoridation stand. He was reinstated in
June 1962 after successfully protesting to the Judicial Council of

the ADA,[20] but in November of the same year the ADA House of Delegates voted to uphold the expulsion of Dr. Ginns.[21] In 1969 Dr. I. H. Northfield of Duluth, Minnesota, was suspended from his local dental society for one year for the heresy of opposing fluoridation.[22]

In 1959 Dr. U. L. Monteleone, a dentist in Allentown, Pennsylvania, was forced to appear before the Lehigh Valley Dental Society for his outspoken criticism of fluoridation. When he again successfully opposed fluoridation in 1969, he was subjected to merciless abuse: "Never in my professional life had I ever been subjected to the rude conduct, jeers, laughter, [and] ridicule, which I endured with Dr. Bierman."[23] Such uncivilized tactics were only the beginning; following a narrow defeat of the fluoridation promoters on February 2, 1971, Dr. Monteleone was dismissed from his position at the Cleft Palate Clinic run by the Crippled Children's Society at the Allentown (Pennsylvania) Hospital. Despite the local newspaper's support of fluoridation, it condemned this punitive action of the dentists in a strongly worded editorial: "It is a clear case of vindictive action which should not be tolerated in a democratic society."[24] Dr. Monteleone's "crime"? he had personally examined "24 children from seven different low-income group families" in fluoridated Easton, Pa. Their teeth were badly decayed, and he observed "33 $\frac{1}{3}$% of the children had mottling."[25] As a scientist he had reported his actual findings in a fluoridated community, and the bare truth cost him his position.

How can dentists speak their minds when dental societies and other fluoridation promoters exert such intense pressures? Anyone who has not been brainwashed in the first place will quickly learn that the safest policy is to keep one's mouth shut. No doubt these pressures explain why *no* dentist will speak openly against fluoridation in Wichita, Kansas, where a fierce campaign is being waged as this book is published. Without question the threat of persecution and reprisals is the reason why dentists are equally afraid to speak out against fluoridation in Houston, Texas, where possible fluoridation is also being considered. Loss of group insurance and numerous similar benefits such as hospital privileges and referrals, as well as fear of reprisals, social ostracism, and diminished business–these are tangible reasons why dentists fear to speak out anywhere against fluoridation, even in a democratic republic, where free speech is touted as an inalienable right.

Dentists promoting fluoridation have also repeatedly attempted to persuade local medical societies to adopt the same tactics of harassment and intimidation. For instance, after seven physicians (joined by eight dentists), led by H. F. Koppe, M.D., had petitioned the City Commission of Dayton, Ohio, in July 1955 to postpone adoption of fluoridation, some of them were called before the Executive Committee of the Montgomery County Medical Society for censure at the request of local dentists.[26] The medical committee declined to take any action against the physicians; I can only conjecture about the intense pressures that must have been exerted against the eight dissenting dentists.

In St. Petersburg, Florida, 44 physicians urged the city government to suspend fluoridation until the AMA re-evaluated the matter. Proponents then "succeeded in getting the medical society to pass a resolution to censure all physicians who publicly oppose[d] fluoride." On February 4, 1958, however, the city followed the advice of the physicians and suspended fluoridation until a negative popular vote terminated it on December 15, 1959.[27]

I too have personally experienced similar harassment. Shortly after I had circulated a letter warning physicians about the dangers of fluoridation, the Detroit District Dental Society asked the Council of my medical society to censure me. Two members of the Council told me that Dr. R. Johnson, another Council member, faced the issue squarely: "If one of our members has knowledge on a subject about which we know very little, and if he does not bring it to our attention – *that* would be reason for censuring him." The matter was dropped immediately.

OTHER REPRISALS

Other dissenting physicians, scientists, and health-care professionals, however, have not fared as well as I did. In Calgary, Alberta, Dr. Gordon Bates, the leading Canadian advocate of fluoridation, ordered Dr. W. H. Hill, Medical Officer of Health, to support fluoridation -- "or else." Shortly thereafter, Dr. Hill was removed from the examining board of the Medical School of the University of Alberta, a post he had held for 25 years. A senior engineer with an oil company, C.R. Thomson, who had supported Dr. Hill, was forced to resign after publicly opposing fluoridation, and he was unable to find another job for some time afterwards.[28]

Similar actions against editors of scientific journals pose even more serious threats to the free flow of scientific information. Jonathan Forman, M.D., a well-known allergy specialist in Columbus, Ohio, had been editor of the *Journal of the Ohio State Medical Society* for 25 years. As an outspoken critic of fluoridation, he was subjected to much personal abuse by dentists on both the local and national levels and was eventually asked to submit his resignation as editor in 1958.[29]

Even editors of scientific journals outside medicine and dentistry have been targets of punitive action by the PHS. After John Yiamouyiannis, Ph.D., an associate editor of Chemical Abstracts Service (CAS), a division of the American Chemical Society, repeatedly spoke and wrote against fluoridation, John Small, a public relations employee of the Division of Dental Health, PHS, first telephoned and then sent two communications about Yiamouyiannis to CAS. On August 10, 1970, R. J. Rowlett, Jr., Editor of CAS, wrote to Small: "I have again talked with Dr. Yiamouyiannis and have again made my position as strong and as clear as possible. He will not repeat this kind of performance and remain as an employee of Chemical Abstracts Service."[30] On the following day he again spoke to Yiamouyiannis and issued a memorandum for the latter's personnel files, stating:

> I told him we can no longer tolerate these connections between his beliefs on fluoridation and the CAS organization and its editor. I stated that if I received *one* more such connection between his talks and CAS, I will be obliged to terminate his employment within 30 days. I explained this applied to any talks he makes or any letters or other documents written after 10 August. . . . I stated further that in my opinion he had already connected his name and CAS in too many ways on fluoridation so that he can no longer speak or write on this subject, despite omission of specific reference to CAS, without HEW officials making this connection. . . . he must make the decision as to whether he wishes to continue such public debates or to work for CAS.[31]

To maintain the support of the PHS in Washington, CAS was willing to curtail an employee's freedom of speech, and Yiamouyiannis was harassed until he resigned; litigation followed and is still unresolved.[32]

THE DOSSIERS

Not many scientists who are intimidated or harassed continue very long to oppose fluoridation openly. We have seen some of the things that happen to opponents who dare to persist, but there is much more. Most shocking is the compilation of derogatory dossiers on vocal critics of fluoridation. In cooperation with the Dental Division of the PHS, the public relations arm of the ADA distributed mimeographed copies of selected comments about opponents of fluoridation.[33] This procedure followed the ADA's promotional guidelines of 1953 (see Chapter 15, above).

In 1962 and 1965 these statements were published by the ADA "to furnish information on the background, qualifications and activities of the best known opponents of fluoridation for use by those persons or groups contemplating, planning or engaged in a fluoridation effort on a one-time or continuing basis."[34] Often treading on the knife-edge of libel, the selections reflected an extensive array of unfavorable, empty, and sometimes false statements about many physicians, dentists, and scientists, as well as laymen – almost any effective opponent of fluoridation. The ADA seems to have made no effort to purge clearly false material from the quotations.

A few of the many examples will suffice to demonstrate the ADA's curious attempts to discredit opponents. Dr. Ionel Rapaport's studies on waterborne fluoride and mongolism were discussed at length in Chapter 13, above, and his findings have not been refuted by re-evaluation of the original data. Indeed, Taves has urged, some 20 years later, that a retrospective reinvestigation now be conducted.[35] But the criticisms of Rapaport in the ADA dossier reach far into the depths of "dirty" journalism. They represent the *undocumented* response on May 31, 1963, by Dr. Philip P. Cohen of the University of Wisconsin at Madison to a request by the Health Department of Utica, New York, for a critique of Rapaport and his work:

I have no confidence whatsoever in the significance of the interpretation which Dr. Rapaport has given to his data. In reviewing this matter with him several years ago, he admitted that he had no true knowledge of the actual fluoride exposure of the mothers. Rapaport is not a trained scientist; he has been unable to get his material published in reputable journals and his requests for support from NIH have been consistently rejected.

I regret that Dr. Rapaport's totally unwarranted publication based on erroneous data has reflected on the standards of research at this University. However, I can assure you that his conclusions are totally without basis in fact. . . .[36]

No doubt these unsubstantiated pejorative comments delighted the promoters of fluoridation in Utica, but if any of the charges were true, why did Dr. Cohen not submit them to a scholarly, refereed journal to warn other scientists about Rapaport's "totally unwarranted publication"? The charge that Rapaport's "conclusions are totally without basis in fact" is flatly contradicted by the undeniable truth that the data were matters of *official* record.

If Rapaport was "not a trained scientist," why had he been a lecturer in endocrinology at the École d'Anthropologie in Paris, France? Why had he received a prize in 1950 for his research from the French Academy of Medicine? Why did he receive a Chevalier Award from the Order of Health in 1954? Why, if he was "not a trained scientist," had he been appointed to the position of research Project Associate and later Assistant Professor at the Psychiatric Institute of the University of Wisconsin?

As we have already seen (Chapter 13, above) Rapaport, who earned his medical degree at the University of Paris, published his work on mongolism in "reputable journals" in France – not in the U.S.A. His failure to receive research grants from the National Institute of Health to pursue the positive leads he had uncovered clearly reflected the tight control over the type of fluoride research that the PHS was (and still is) willing to fund. Certainly his findings of a strong association between the occurrence of mongolism and the fluoride content of the mother's drinking water – a subject of vital importance – deserved support for careful and thorough substantiation. All things considered, Dr. Cohen's published statement was an unwarranted, libelous attack on Rapaport.

To neutralize the internationally known Dr. Ludwik Gross, Chief of Cancer Research at the Veterans Administration Hospital in the Bronx, New York, the ADA produced an unpublished *memorandom* from the Dental Division of the PHS. Dr. Gross had stated:

"The plain fact that fluorine is an insidious poison, harmful, toxic and cumulative in its effects, even when injected [ingested] in minimal amounts, will remain unchanged no matter how many times it will be repeated in print that fluoridation of the water supply is safe." The PHS continued:

> He also opposed fluoridation on the grounds that the consumption of water varies greatly, that the margin of safety is narrow and that the engineering problems in large cities are formidable.
>
> The Veteran's Administration which employs Dr. Gross states: "Dr. Gross is free to offer his personal opinion in any relation he may desire. However, Dr. Gross does not speak for the Veteran's Administration of [*sic*] the subject of fluoridation. This agency is not opposed to the fluoridation on [*sic*] public water supplies."[37]

Readers will have to decide what purpose is served by these "trenchant" observations.

Reaching deep into its bag of investigative information, the ADA attacked Dr. V. O. Hurme, a leading dental researcher, by citing an article written in a Missouri medical publication:

> V. O. Hurme, D.D.S., is research director, Forsyth Dental Infirmary, Boston, Mass., in which institution dental service is provided for children. He is the author of a paper entitled "An Examination of the Scientific Basis for Fluoridating Populations" and of a number of public statements questioning the advisability of fluoridation of water supplies. His article produces no evidence that fluoridation is either dangerous or ineffective. A study of his paper leaves the reader with the convictions a) that the author has failed to review the voluminous literature which gives concrete evidence upon points about which he confesses himself to be in doubt and b) that his use of such terms as "mass medication" and "compulsory" procedures reveal an emotional bias which casts doubt on his objectivity.[37]

In rebuttal to Hurme, the commentary from Missouri cited Dr. David Ast, New York State Department of Health, who held different views. The authority of Ast, devoid of any evidence whatsoever, was sufficient in and of itself to despatch Hurme -- so the reader is led to believe!

In my own case, I received an especially long treatment through statements by Dr. J. Roy Doty, two newspaper articles, and a court case. The "critiques" consisted of the customary smears

laced with arrogant innuendo and falsehoods, part of which the
ADA tacitly recognized by publishing my corrections of these
"critiques."[38] The statement attributed to Dr. Doty, however,
must be set in its proper light. In the first place, the passage, although not acknowledged, consists of excerpts written by Cox,
McClure, and Russell,[39] who discussed two points on which I supposedly erred, one of which was that the death of the 22-year-old
soldier reported by Linsman and McMurray "was due to naturally
fluoridated drinking water." As I have already shown in Chapter 9
(page 105, above), these authors were concerned with the patient's
chronic fluoride intoxication that profoundly influenced his
health, and I inferred from the data presented that the patient
died from fluoride in the water he had consumed. Another interpretation quoted by the ADA discussion was that "pyonephrosis
probably followed the local infection at the sternal biopsy site
which provided a portal of entry"—*a highly improbable explanation.*

The other critical point focused on whether an article by F. F.
Heyroth pleaded that patients with nephritis drink nonfluoridated
water. This is merely a semantic quibble, for Heyroth clearly
stated that "it should be possible for physicians who discover such
disease to advise their patients to use nonfluoridated water."[40] The
ADA allows Dr. Doty to describe my statement as a "profound"
error!

FLUORIDATION "NOT DEBATABLE"

There are still other reasons why physicians remain ignorant of
the side effects of fluoridation. Traditionally, when a new discovery is made in medical sciences, its merits and demerits are discussed at medical meetings and in medical journals at the national,
state, and local levels. For instance, when vaccination against
poliomyelitis was introduced first in the 1930s, and again in the
1950s, the subject was covered at numerous medical meetings and
its risk-benefit aspects were freely debated. In contrast, spokesmen
of the ADA and PHS have considered the scientific aspect of fluoridation to be "undebatable" even before long-term studies were
available.

At the 91st annual meeting of the California Dental Association
in San Francisco, April 1961, ADA President Dr. C. H. Patton en-

thusiastically told his dental audience: "I contend [that] the subject [of fluoridation] is not debatable."[41] In 1965, Dr. H. Hillenbrand, Executive Secretary of the ADA, told a press conference at a meeting of the Southern California Dental Association: "Fluoridation of drinking water is no longer a subject that is scientifically debatable."[42] The following year, Dr. M. K. Hine, another president of the ADA, assured his listeners at the National Dental Health Assembly in Arlington, Va.: "Fluoridation is no longer debatable in the scientific community; it should not be debatable in the political community."[43] When McClure was invited to participate in a panel discussion of the scientific aspects of fluoridation held under the auspices of a chapter of the scientific Society of Sigma Xi at the University of Kansas in 1965, he declined on the grounds that he could not "regard water fluoridation as debatable on the basis of its scientific merits."[44]

Naturally, if a subject is "not debatable," anyone with adverse evidence cannot be heard. My scheduled appearance before the District Medical Society in Bismark, North Dakota, was blocked through intervention of the local health officer. The Society had invited me to present my research on fluoride poisoning from drinking water at their meeting on November 5, 1963. On October 18, however, the invitation was withdrawn, because of the "controversial" nature of the subject.[45] Later I was informed by the physician who had originally made the arrangements that the local health officer was responsible for this action. To listen to me apparently would have been an admission that the "not debatable" claim is untrue; historically, such a posture is grossly unscientific. As a leading proponent now concedes: "no scientific question is closed forever."[46]

REJECTION OF ADVERSE FINDINGS

Editors of medical journals have repeatedly rejected research reports unfavorable to fluoridation. Like most physicians, they generally know little about fluoride, and so they turn to the supposedly knowledgeable PHS representatives on their editorial boards. Frequently, then, workers in the Division of Dental Health of the PHS have the final word on the fate of manuscripts dealing with medical as well as with dental aspects of fluoride.

During the more than 25 years that I have been engaged in research on fluoride, I have had extraordinary experiences in this
respect. For instance, the Letters Department editor of the *Journal
of the American Medical Association* had accepted a letter in
which J. J. Shea, an allergist in Dayton, Ohio, S. M. Gillespie, a
Detroit physician, and I had reported on a subject of interest to
every practicing physician: gastrointestinal hemorrhages in five
infants who had been administered fluoride in vitamin drops. That
one of the editors had planned to publish the letter was indicated
by the fact that editorial changes had been made on the manuscript. When the copy edited for the printer reached the desk of
the Editor-in-Chief, J. H. Talbott, however, it was rejected, although the data in it were later published in the *Annals of
Allergy*.[47]

Talbott had written me earlier on August 8, 1961: "I do not pro-
pose, then, to publish another view [on fluorides and fluoridation]
in opposition to that taken by the House of Delegates and the
Council on Foods and Nutrition of the American Medical Association." The editor of another major medical journal, when rejecting
a scholarly review on fluoridation by Dr. D. H. Fogel of Stamford,
Connecticut, used the standard wording September 17, 1964: "To
publish this paper would add further fuel to the fire of heat and
emotion." Scientists at Emory University received a similar reply
from an AMA journal[48] (see Chapter 19, pp. 371-372); one of
them commented that he could not understand how U.S. science
could tolerate such irrational acts.

In 1973 the editor of *Science* rejected another article by V. A.
Cecilioni and me showing harm from fluoridated water. A preliminary report of part of this work had just been awarded first prize
as the best manuscript of the year by *Cutis*, a specialized dermato-
logical journal. Ostensibly, *Science*'s reason for rejection was "because the prototype case, 'Chizzola' maculae [the skin lesions
described above in Chapter 10] has made no impression on American or British dermatologists. At least, it is not described by Rook,
Wilkinson and Ebling, 2nd edition, or in other current books."
This comment is preposterous, since the original research reported
in the article could not have been recorded in any textbook!

One of the most remarkable cases of censorship in science involved the *Journal of the American Dental Association*. During the

mid-1960s, Dr. Albert Schatz had investigated the relationship of artificial fluoridation and increased death rates in Chile. In 1965 he sent in sequence three separate certified letters (return receipt requested) to Dr. Leland C. Hendershot, Editor of the *JADA*, in which he discussed evidence for this frightening consequence of fluoridation. *All three letters were refused and returned to Schatz unopened.* In other words, Hendershot, acting for the ADA, rejected the findings of Schatz, a co-discoverer of streptomycin, without bothering even to open the letters. Scientific censorship is rarely more flagrant than in this example.[49]

MISSING EVIDENCE

Articles that do pass the censors, however, sometimes contain bizarre and revealing information on the subject of fluoridation. In 1965 Dr. D. R. Taves and collaborators, the University of Rochester, N.Y., reported the case of a kidney patient, a nurse 41 years old, who had accumulated in her blood substantial amounts of fluoride resulting from the use of fluoridated municipal water in long-term hemodialysis, a procedure designed to purify the blood.

During repeated treatments over a period of eight months, toxic waste products were removed from the blood, but fluoride also entered the nurse's blood from the dialysate water and collected in her bones, possibly a "beneficial" effect, the authors suggested. At autopsy following her death, the authors discovered an unusually high concentration of fluoride in the bones (5500 ppm) as well as changes typical of chronic fluoride poisoning. They warned: "where no effort can be made to learn more about its possible effects, it would seem prudent to use nonfluoridated dialysate baths for long-term hemodialysis."[50]

My curiosity was aroused about this article, and I wrote Taves two letters about the clinical aspects of the nurse's case. I wondered why the authors had not reported the patient's symptoms in greater detail and what the autopsy data showed, particularly the fluoride levels in soft tissues. Also, the last reference cited in the text was missing.

I was surprised to learn from one of Taves' replies that a detailed clinical account of this case had appeared two years earlier in the *JAMA*,[51] although Taves had not cited the article (where, curiously, the age of the nurse was given as 43, not 41). On the other hand, in his article he acknowledged the cooperation of *Dr. Christine W. Waterhouse,* who was a co-author of the earlier article. The two missing references   the *JAMA* article and the missing footnote – placed an entirely different complexion on the nurse's case.

The reference for the missing footnote reported that excessive accumulation of fluoride occurs in the iliac (hip) bone of patients suffering from kidney disease.[52] The *JAMA* article, however, was an astonishing revelation. "The patient was usually dialyzed for 4 hours. Two longer runs of 6 hours were complicated in the last hour by headaches, confusion, nausea, and, on one occasion, by a grand mal seizure." "Urinary output was depressed for 1 or 2 days after each dialysis secondary to the lowered solute load." "A bizarre neuromuscular irritability characterized by a twitching of the right arm with occasional generalized convulsive seizures developed 5 days after the third dialysis." "Despite the ultrafiltration of 5 to 6 lb of water with each dialysis, the patient remained hypertensive." Furthermore, the patient died a traumatic death: "Within an hour after the fourteenth dialysis the patient convulsed, aspirated, and died suddenly."[51] These graphic details – strikingly characteristic of acute fluoride toxicity – left no doubt in my mind about the contributing role of fluoride in this patient's death.

The Taves report of 1965 then took on new significance. The opening paragraph of the article had observed that "the fluoride concentration in fluoridated water (1 ppm) is normally about six times that in serum." (We now know that the 1-ppm concentration is on the order of 50 to 100 times that of free, ionic fluoride in serum.) "Therefore, when such water is used in the dialysate bath of an artificial kidney, fluoride ions would be expected to move into the patient's blood." Since the patient's blood in this study was subjected to dialysis with 200 to 600 liters of fluoridated water containing a total of 140 to 560 mg of fluoride (0.7 to 0.93 ppm) per treatment, great potential harm was a distinct possibility, clearly borne out by the evidence, as the authors admitted. Yet only a careful reader would discover (at the end of a sentence in the middle of the article) that the patient even died![50]

The macabre clinical details of the nurse's last hours were reported in the 1963 article by Kretchmar *et al.,* but fluoride was not mentioned. In 1965 Taves discussed the role of fluoride but failed to provide even a hint of the patient's gruesome decline, ending in a dramatic convulsion. Most curious, however, is the fact that the 1965 article by Taves *et al.* did *not* cite the earlier article. Why? In April 1965 Taves informed me: "I should have included this reference, but just plain didn't think about it until you asked."[53] In a letter to A. W. Burgstahler 12 years later, Taves wrote: "Yes, the lack of the Kretchmer [*sic*] reference is embarrassing and the reason is that I was ignorant of it until after the paper [by Taves *et al.*] was published. I know that I would have included it had I been aware of it."[54] Yet in the acknowledgement section of his article, Taves thanked *Dr. Christine W. Waterhouse,* a co-author of the 1963 Kretchmar paper, along with Dr. D. F. McDonald and their staffs, for making it possible to study this patient. The evidence forces me to conclude that Taves knew about the article and did not cite it. But why did he later claim that he was not "aware" of it when he wrote his paper?

Did Dr. Waterhouse insist that the 1963 *JAMA* paper not be cited? A possible reason why she might do so is that a potential lawsuit could have developed. This possibility might also explain why the nurse's age was given as 41 in the 1965 article and 43 in the 1963 article. Another possibility is that if the public learned about the dangers of fluoridated water to kidney patients, then promotion of fluoridation might be more difficult. Certainly demands to use fluoride-free water in hemodialysis would be made, as happened recently in Norwalk, Connecticut.[55]

Whatever the true story may be in this case of the missing evidence, the public was denied important information about the true scientific picture of harm to a kidney patient being dialyzed with artificially fluoridated water. As might be anticipated, both articles acknowledged financial support from the Public Health Service.

NATIONAL ACADEMY OF SCIENCES

History often has a way of repeating itself, and sometimes the same character reappears in a similar role. Late in 1977 the

National Academy of Sciences (NAS) published a report of the
National Research Council (NRC) Committee on Safe Drinking
Water. Dr. D. R. Taves, a defender of fluoridation and a frequent
recipient of PHS grants—including support from the Division of
Dental Research in 1977—was selected as the primary author of
the section on fluoride, with no counterbalancing experts to present opposing evidence.

In the 1970s, after growing concern about problems of conflict
of interest and prejudice in its scientific reports, the NRC underwent a general overhaul of its committee operations. Dr. Philip
Handler, President of the NAS, has pointed with pride to his far-
reaching reorganization of the NRC:

> I instituted a rigorous program with respect to potential sources of bias
> and conflict. None of us are good at eating our own words[,] and anyone
> who has taken a position in public will have that position out on the table
> before he or she undertakes service on a committee—whom he or she con-
> sults with, the sources of research funds, the financial connection, posi-
> tions he or she's taken.[56]

In the light of this statement and Dr. Handler's profound concern about environmental health policy, we must ask: why were
only fluoridation proponents and no opponent scientists—to make
a truly bipartisan panel--appointed to the Safe Drinking Water
Subcommittee on Special Ions? More to the point, why was an
internationally known sympathizer chosen to write and make final
judgment about criticisms of the controversial fluoride section of
the report?

Selecting a patently biased Subcommittee on Special Ions was
serious enough, but to turn a deaf ear to numerous fully documented criticisms of the report is inexcusable. After the preliminary
draft of the fluoride section of the report was circulated for comments and the *Summary Report: Drinking Water and Health* appeared, numerous critiques were sent to Dr. Handler's office and
forwarded to the NRC Safe Drinking Water Committee. For example, on July 8, 1977, Dr. A. W. Burgstahler sent a letter more
than five pages long, single-spaced, detailing serious shortcomings
and errors in the fluoride section of the just-released *Summary
Report*. When this critique remained unanswered, he wrote yet
another long letter on August 16, 1977, discussing in five and a

half single-spaced pages a multitude of serious omissions, misinterpretations, and erroneous conclusions in the draft copy of the full report.

On August 22, 1977, I also sent to Dr. Handler a three page, single-spaced communication summarizing the results of more than 400 clinical cases I have treated. I observed: "Your report [draft copy] has cited solely my early (1962) work on illness from fluoridated water and a 1967 paper dealing with allergic reactions from fluoride-containing vitamins and toothpaste." I enclosed a partial list of my fluoride publications from 1962 to 1977 plus an article on the fluoride-cancer question. I emphasized how I had used double-blind tests, as well as laboratory data, and how patients had been relieved of their symptoms merely by changing to fluoride-free water.

I also commented that much other evidence invalidated the report and that the "fluoride section of the report cannot be salvaged" without drastic revision. I further pointed out that the "NRC report in its present form will cast a dark shadow on the reputation of the National Academy of Sciences."

From here and abroad many other strong criticisms based on scientific data were also forwarded to Dr. Handler and reflected similar conclusions.[57]   Neither Handler, Taves, the Safe Drinking Water Committee, nor any neutral outside committee provided any evidence whatever to refute the validity of these critiques. Instead, Dr. Handler finally replied to me on October 16, 1977:

> There are of necessity differences of opinion regarding any scientific problem as complex as that of fluoride effects. The current report reflects the considered and best judgment of a knowledgeable committee and has been released as a report of the National Research Council.

All my adverse scientific evidence was simply dismissed and swept away in a sea of unsubstantiated generalities.

Handler's reply to Burgstahler was far more revealing and fascinating. He remarked that since the "substantive" contents of the report were the responsibility of the NRC Committee, he had forwarded Burgstahler's comments to the Chairman of the Committee. At the same time, however, he recognized their possible significance. Although the official report was in galley proofs,

Handler, in an "unprecedented"[58] move, *delayed release of the final printed version of the report* "until the authoring committee had an opportunity to review your comments."[59] Without question, changes *could have been made before the report was released to the public.* The response, however, was completely negative: "Since there is no disposition on the part of the Committee, after reviewing your comments, to revise the substance of the report, we are proceeding with plans to release the printed document."[59]

The rest of the letter proffered generalities about difficulties in obtaining a consensus on a controversial subject, the review of the literature by the Committee, and the possible adverse effects of fluoride. "Special attention was given to the claims of any adverse effects of fluorides, *since proof of no effect is not possible [sic]."* [Emphasis added.] The report called for more research in such areas as possible fluoride-related congenital abnormalities and cancer incidence and mortality, yet it ignored much of the already existing adverse evidence cited by Burgstahler. Nor did it take any notice of a contradictory report of the Canadian National Research Council[60] that had been sent for review to Dr. Edward Groth of the Environmental Studies Board of the NRC in the summer of 1977. Again, Dr. Handler's letter concluded: "The current report reflects the considered and best judgment of a knowledgeable Committee. . . ."[59] Dr. Handler had an opportunity to discard or revise the highly criticized fluoride section of the report, whose specific and general defects had been emphasized by numerous scientists. Instead, he decided to accept the opinion of a committee – primarily that of one of its members -- which was unchecked by outside objective resources.

Although this is not the place to enumerate all the serious defects of the fluoride section of the report, I must comment briefly on a clear attempt to omit available pertinent evidence and therefore to deprive the public of information vital to the health of everyone in the country.

The author of the fluoride section was fully apprised both in writing and orally (by telephone and in person) of data that negated his conclusion that no harm would result from drinking fluoridated water. Although much of this evidence dealt with general considerations – ranging from cancer, chromosome damage, and mongolism to general intolerance, gastrointestinal symptoms and reversible ill effects – one particular point was emphasized from an early date, namely undeniable fluoride damage to kidneys. On January 28, 1977, Burgstahler wrote Taves and referred to the forthcoming AAAS Symposium in Denver on "Continuing Evaluation of the Use of Fluorides." He asked "why the panel did not include participants with pertinent new data such as S. L. Manocha" of the Yerkes Primate Research Center and others.

When Taves visited Lawrence, Kansas, on March 8, 1977, Dr. H. L. McKinney, in company with Burgstahler, asked him specifically to explain why Manocha's work demonstrating kidney damage in squirrel monkeys drinking fluoridated water (1 and 5 ppm F)[61] should not be accepted at face value, especially because of its implications for humans. Although Taves admitted he had not yet read the paper, he offered the opinion that the experiments were probably flawed, possibly because the air temperatures were higher near the cages of the fluoridated squirrel monkeys, causing them to drink more water.

In his letter of August 16, 1977, to Handler, Burgstahler referred to the Manocha report and on September 12, 1977, he again wrote Taves specifically about it:

In the final 10 months of the 18-month study, "water consumption was considerably higher in the animals [squirrel monkeys] on higher [1 and 5 ppm] fluoride intake" than those with no fluoride in the drinking water. Moreover the kidneys "showed significant cytochemical changes, especially in the animals on 5 ppm fluoride in the water." Changes in enzyme activity were also noted. [Brackets in original.]

Many other matters previously discussed during the visit on March 8, 1977, were touched on in the fluoride section of the final NRC report. On November 14, 1977, Taves claimed that each monkey in the Manocha study should have been housed in a separate cage rather than having only three cages for the three groups of monkeys. How this could have affected kidney function was not made clear, but then Taves was not clear about the details of Manocha's work even at this late date.[62]

Despite these lengthy discussions on kidney damage, especially as described in the unrefuted paper by Manocha et al., the final NRC report suggested under the heading "Research Recommendations," point no. 8, that "The nonhuman–primate study of Manocha *et al.* (1975) should be repeated with 5 ppm water and better controls, to check the reported renal enzyme changes."[35] Why were the *already published results* of Manocha's work[61] not included in the report's discussion of the effects of fluoride on kidney function?

In short, why did the NRC report consciously omit much evidence damaging to fluoridation, very important evidence specifically brought to the attention of the author of the fluoride section of the report? Why were reversible effects of chronic fluoride poisoning downplayed and rejected, despite an intense discussion of the subject with Taves on March 8, 1977, in which Burgstahler and McKinney presented personal knowledge of cases of this type? Numerous requests to Taves for rational alternative explanations of these cases have remained unanswered. Remembering the example of the Rochester nurse, I am led to conclude that the missing evidence provides a case study of history repeating itself.

The broader implications of this entire episode should be thought provoking. In violation of its own code designed to prevent bias, the National Academy of Sciences permitted the appointment of a one-sided subcommittee of the NRC Safe Drinking Water Committee to report on the safety of fluoride; the report was written by D. R. Taves, a leading supporter of fluoridation who minimized the known harm caused by fluoride and omitted vital evidence from the report. In numerous scientific critiques, researchers cognizant of this evidence notified both Taves and the Academy. Critics made every effort to seek a balanced report that presented an accurate statement of the evidence – all to no avail. If the most august scientific body in the United States is unable to prepare an objective report of all important data about the effects of fluoridation, is it any wonder that scientists remain uninformed about the matter?

OTHER ATTEMPTS TO MINIMIZE HARM

The manner in which the case of the Rochester nurse and the fluoride section of the Safe Drinking Water Committee report were presented underscores a basic reason why the medical profession generally sees no hazard in fluoridation: statements by authors minimizing harm from fluoridated water. For instance, in

1967 M. C. Latham and P. Grech reported a high incidence of severe dental fluorosis, extensive nail abnormalities, goiter, and skeletal fluorosis in areas of Tanzania with as little as 1 to 3 ppm fluoride in the drinking water. Their article in a U.S. public health journal, however, was accompanied by a 25-line disclaimer of any negative implications for fluoridation as well as the suggestion that "the osteosclerosis found in subjects in the survey does perhaps add support to the view that, in lesser amounts, fluoride consumed over many years may be beneficial to older subjects by reducing the incidence of osteoporosis."[63]

In 1965 when J. W. Morris described 20 cases of advanced skeletal fluorosis in Arizona Indians drinking natural fluoride water, he claimed that skeletal fluorosis produces "no demonstrable physiologic adversities"—a statement that contradicts the plain data in his own article, as well as in many others, of spontaneous fractures and advanced skeletal changes.[64] In 1972 physicians at the Mayo Clinic in Minnesota reported two teen-age cases of systemic fluorosis and impaired renal function associated with fluoride in drinking water; in one case the concentration was 0.4 to 2.6 ppm and in the other 1.7 ppm.[65] Instead of dwelling on the significance of these findings for individuals whose kidneys are not functioning normally in fluoridated areas, the authors opened their article with the irrelevant and misleading comment: "It is generally agreed that water fluoridation is safe for persons with normal kidneys." The article, of course, discussed two patients whose kidneys were *mal*functioning.

An even more striking contradiction appears in the account by the National Center for Disease Control of an incident of nonfatal fluoride poisoning at a rural school in Stanly County, N.C. On April 16, 1974, 201 pupils and 12 adults whose orange juice had been prepared with over-fluoridated drinking water, became ill with nausea and vomiting (see Chapter 7 above, page 93). While conceding that illness was produced by the equipment malfunction, the report failed to stress the seriousness of the harm that could arise under such circumstances.

At a Norwegian poisoning center, 34 cases of illness from fluoride tablets and topical application of fluoride were dismissed as being unrelated to fluoride on the basis of dubious provocative tests in two of the cases, although the cause was clearly established by the clinical data.[66] These examples show that observations unfavorable to fluoridation are frequently couched in language deprecating any harm to human health. How can physicians be expected to extract the truth from such contradictory and confusing statements?

REPETITION OF EXPERIMENTS

The fluoride research literature reveals still another peculiar and striking feature. On several occasions authors have been induced to repeat their investigations evidently for the purpose of countering their own research — since their subsequent conclusions were usually diametrically opposite to their original results. For example, in 1957, Ramseyer, Smith, and McCay published a report on the effects of lifetime exposure of laboratory animals to fluoride and concluded: "In old age missing teeth and periodontal disease were frequent in rats which had received sodium fluoride supplementation, especially at the higher levels" (5 and 10 ppm F). "Hypertrophy and hyperplasia of the kidney tubules were found in rats receiving fluoride [1, 5, and 10 ppm in the drinking water] but were not observed in the unsupplemented animals."[67] Such results clearly do not help the fluoridation hypothesis, and the study was repeated by McCay and E. B. Bosworth. This time they reported finding no significant cumulative effects of fluoride on the kidneys: "A wide range of changes were found in the kidneys. It is our interpretation that these changes may be expected in any series of rats of this age."[68]

In a similar manner, after Herman initially had found large amounts of fluoride in kidney stones,[69] he received a PHS grant and two collaborators to carry out new research on the basis of which the medical profession and the public were assured that such high fluoride levels cause no harm.[70] How do scientists determine which investigation to believe? Is "latest" always "best" or "most accurate?"

INTERNATIONAL SOCIETY FOR FLUORIDE RESEARCH

By 1960, many physicians and scientists here and abroad recognized the need for meetings and free discussion on fluoride research. Therefore, Professor A. Gordonoff, Pharmacology Department, University of Bern (Switzerland), and Professors A.

Benagiano and S. Fiorentini, Eastman Dental Institute in Rome, and I organized an international scientific conference. We invited many outstanding scientists irrespective of their stand on fluoridation. Everyone contacted expressed keen interest in the meeting, which was to be held at the George Eastman Dental School in Rome, one of the foremost European institutions of dental research. Unfortunately, a few weeks before the scheduled date, the Italian scientists cancelled the meeting. No reason was given. I was also compelled to cancel an alternative plan for holding the meeting in Holland.

Through last-minute efforts by Professor Gordonoff, we were able to hold the conference in Bern, October 15–17, 1962. Most of those attending had carried out original research on fluoride, and every one of the 60 participants expressed great satisfaction for an unfettered opportunity to exchange information and views with other leaders in the field. The papers and discussions were scheduled for publication in July 1963. In fact, they were in galleys when the publisher was threatened with a boycott of future business. Professor Gordonoff, who edited the book with my assistance, explained that "certain individuals, whose names were not given to me, have approached the publisher and threatened to boycott him if he publishes the volume. He informed me that he has withdrawn his commitment to publish it."[71] Money also changed hands.[72] Another European firm, however, published the book the following year.[73]

The success of the Bern conference led to the founding of the International Society for Fluoride Research (ISFR). In 1966 the forerunner of the ISFR, called the American Society for Fluoride Research, held a meeting in Detroit that included participants from Europe and Asia as well as North America. Although the meeting was strictly scientific, PHS and ADA officials immediately saw it as a threat to their promotion of fluoridation in Detroit. On the eve of the conference the ADA issued a highly critical press release without having seen or heard any of the program.[74] A news writer in *Science* even questioned by implication whether the fledgling organization had a right to call itself a "scientific society" until it became affiliated with the AAAS.[75]

Despite these scurrilous attacks on its predecessor, the ISFR has been meeting regularly about once a year since 1968. Through its conferences and its journal *Fluoride,* it has been contributing materially to the advancement of research on fluoride, especially on matters biological and medical. At no time has the Society been involved in the politics of fluoridation. Its members hold widely differing views on the subject and on the role of fluoride in air and water pollution. Biochemists, physicians, dentists, veterinary scientists, botanists, physicists, chemists, and engineers from many parts of the globe have participated in its meetings.

Nevertheless, promoters of fluoridation have interfered with this worthwhile congregation of researchers. For instance, several U.S. scientists who had at one time contributed papers to the conferences or to the *Fluoride* journal have suddenly withdrawn without giving any reasons, despite strong previous interest. One scientist, who had been engaged in basic research on fluoride for six years, shed some light on this matter when he informed me that he was no longer permitted to pursue research on fluoride at his institution, which relied on PHS research grants. He inquired whether the Society could assist him in finding a new position where he could continue his fluoride studies. Another, who was scheduled to participate in the program of one of the conferences, candidly acknowledged that the PHS, which was supporting his research, would not give him permission to attend.

Fluoride, the official journal of the Society, is a veritable encyclopedia covering all aspects of fluoride research. Nevertheless, *Index Medicus,* published by the PHS' National Library of Medicine and a major source of references to fluoride-related health topics, has repeatedly declined to include *Fluoride* in its list of journals indexed. On the other hand, *Excerpta Medica, Biological Abstracts, Chemical Abstracts, Pollution Abstracts, Oceanic Abstracts, Current Contents,* and *Science Citation Index,* all include *Fluoride* in their coverage. Since this journal is the only one in the world devoted exclusively to fluoride research, why does the National Library of Medicine consistently decide "not to include *Fluoride* in *Index Medicus,*"[76] although many other journals far less important to human health, such as purely chemical journals, are included?

The foremost effect of banning *Fluoride* is that various public health figures–doctors, dentists, etc.–are deprived of access to information about the numerous effects of fluorides on humans, animals, and plants. The following example speaks for itself. On May 3, 1978, Dr. James B. Lucas, Deputy Director, Environmental Protection Agency, Cincinnati, Ohio, wrote me about cases of airborne fluoride poisoning in Ohio that I have been investigating and closed his letter by requesting a copy of *Fluoride* because he clearly had not seen it: "the local library is not receiving it."

In the swine flu vaccination campaign the PHS made every effort to mobilize all the "troops" at the national, state, and local level. When lives are supposedly at stake, our federal health officials can disseminate information with blinding speed. Why have they, then, recently closed the door for two more years on the indexing of an international journal containing vital information that every physician, dentist, and public health official should have at his or her finger tips. Why, in the name of health, does the PHS promote this ignorance?

*

Why do most scientists and laymen remain ignorant of the dangers of fluoridation? Some of the answers have been presented in this chapter. No single reason by itself sufficiently explains the general state of mind regarding fluoridation, but one point is clear: scientists and the public are not ignorant because the many opponents of fluoridation have been silent. Quite the contrary, from the very beginning they have cried out with loud voices, enumerating the scientific, logical, and moral reasons for not adding an unnecessary cumulative toxic substance to public water supplies. What has been their reward? — harassment, intimidation, persecution, loss of precious reputation, research grants, and employment. The sad conclusion is that had the Public Health Service taken another posture, fluoridation would now be on the historians' shelves with other mistakes of the past.

REFERENCES

1. Fluoridated Water. J. Am. Med. Assoc., 175:1062, 1961.

2. Smith, E.H., Jr.: Editorial: Fluoridation of Water Supply. J. Am. Med. Assoc., 230:1569, 1974.

3. Hornung, H.: Fluoridation: Observations of a German Professor and Public Health Officer. J. Am. Dental Assoc., 53:325-326, 1956.

4. Waldbott, G.L.: Incipient Fluorine Intoxication from Drinking Water. Acta Med. Scand., 156:157-168, 1956.

5. Waldbott, G.L.: The Reader Comments: Waldbott Presents His Views on Fluoridation. J. Am. Dent. Assoc., 55:873, 1957.

6. Waldbott, G.L. Tetaniform Convulsions Precipitated by Fluoridated Drinking Water. Confin. Neurol. 17:339-347, 1957.

7. Waldbott, G.L.: A Struggle With Titans. 1965, pp. 232-233.

8. Swedish Medical Society Transactions, Stockholm, Nov. 4, 1958.

9. Metabolism of Fluorides. Nutr. Rev., 19:259-262, 1961. For reply, see Waldbott, G.L.: Letter to the Editor: The Physiologic and Hygienic Aspects of the Absorption of Inorganic Fluorides. Arch. Environ. Health, 4:459, 1962.

10. McClure, F.J.: Water Fluoridation: The Search and the Victory. 1970, pp. 264-265.

11. ADA Council on Dental Therapeutics: Prescribing Supplements of Dietary Fluorides. J. Am. Dent. Assoc., 56:589-591, 1958.

12. Aasenden, R., and Peebles, T.C.: Effects of Fluoride Supplementation from Birth on Human Deciduous and Permanent Teeth. Arch. Oral. Biol, 19: 321-326, 1974.

13. Feltman, R.: The Reader Comments: Dietary Fluorides. J. Am. Dent. Assoc., 57:104, 1958.

14. Wolf, W.: Letter to G.L. Waldbott, June 18, 1955.

15. Butler, H.W., Legal Adviser, Metropolitan Detroit Committee to Retain Fluoridation: Letter to Advertising Manager of Mellus Newspapers, Oct. 22, 1965.

16. Sokolsky, G.: The Reader Comments: Mr. G. Sokolsky Replies. J. Am. Dent. Assoc., 50:567, 1955.

17. Conway, B.J.: An Introduction to the Principles of Ethics. J. Am. Dent. Assoc., 60:307, 1960.

18. Ethics Committee: J. North Carolina Dent. Soc., 38:144, 1955.

19. Drop Dentist in Fluoride Row. Boston Daily Record, Sept. 28, 1961.

20. Fluoridation Adversary Reinstated. The Evening Gazette, Worcester, Mass., June 23, 1962.

21. Gordon, N.: Dental Assn. Upholds Ouster of Fluoridation Foe. The Boston Herald, Nov. 21, 1962, p. 10 B.

22. Northfield, I.H., D.D.S.: Notarized Statement, Duluth, Minn., Aug. 5, 1969.

23. Monteleone, U.L.: Victory in Allentown. National Fluoridation News, 17(1):4, Jan.-Feb. 1971.

24. Editorial. Allentown (Pa.) Morning Call, Nov. 5, 1971. See also ibid., Oct. 11, 1970.

25. Monteleone (in Ref. 23, above): "A story of these findings was published in the [Allentown] Sunday Call-Chronicle, Jan. 31, 1971."

26. Shea, J.J.: Letter to G.L. Waldbott, July 27, 1955. See National Fluoridation News, 1(8):3, September 1955.

27. St. Petersburg Discontinues F. National Fluoridation News, 4(2):2, Feb.-March 1958. For list of the 44 physicians, see ad in St. Petersburg (Fla.) Independent, June 29, 1957.

28. Thomson, C.R.: Letter to Mrs. G.L. Waldbott, Feb. 11, 1959. Copy in my possession. Cf. The Albertan, June 7, 1957; North Hill (Alberta) News, June 19, 1958.

29. Dr. Forman Quits OSMJ Editorship. The Columbus (Ohio) Citizen, Nov. 13, 1958.

30. Rowlett, R.J., Jr.: Letter to John Small, 10 August 1970. Copy in my possession.

31. John Yiamouyiannis v. Chemical Abstracts Service et al., Plaintiff's Exhibit R-9: Confidential Memorandum, Personnel Files, written by Russell J. Rowlett, Jr., Editor of CAS, regarding John Yiamouyiannis - Anti-fluoridation Talks, 11 August 1970. Copy in my possession.

32. Editor Files $3.8 Million Federal Suit in Job Loss. Columbus (Ohio) Citizen-Journal, Nov. 8, 1972, p. 3.

33. Nader Interview. National Fluoridation News, 16(5):1, Nov.-Dec. 1970. Cf. Greenberg (in Ref. 75, below).

34. Bureau of Public Information, American Dental Association: Comments on the Opponents of Fluoridation. J. Am. Dent. Assoc., 71:1155-1183, 1965. Cf. ibid., 65::694-710, 1962.

35. Taves, D.R.: Fluoride: Research Recommendations, in Drinking Water and Health. Safe Drinking Water Committee, National Research Council — National Academy of Sciences, Washington, D.C., 1977, p. 399.

36. Ref. 34 above, pp. 1176-1177.

37. Ref. 34 above, p. 1171.

38. Ref. 34 above, pp. 1180-1183. See also Waldbott, Ref. 5 above.

39. McClure, F.J.: Letter to P. Jay, Sept. 29, 1954; Russell, A.L.: Letter to P. Jay, Sept. 28, 1954; An Analysis by G.J. Cox of Medical Evidence Against Fluoridation of Public Water Supplies by G.L. Waldbott, undated. Copy in my possession.

40. Heyroth, F.F.: Toxicological Evidence for the Safety of the Fluoridation of Public Water Supplies. Am. J. Public Health, 42:1568-1575, 1952.

41. ADA Head Says Fluoridation Not Debatable. San Francisco Examiner, April 17, 1961, p. 3.

42. Fluoridation Foes: 'Emotional Primitives.' Los Angeles Times, May 11, 1965.

43. 1966 National Dental Health Assembly. Emphasis: Fluoridation. Sponsored by the U.S. Public Health Service and the American Dental Association, Feb. 6-8, 1966, Arlington, Va. Public Health Service Publication No. 1552, p. 1.

44. McClure, F.J.: Letter to J.E. Fox, Sept. 17, 1965. Copy in my possession.

45. Pierson, R.W., Secretary-Treasurer of the 6th District Medical Society, Bismark, N.D.: Letter to G.L. Waldbott, Oct. 18, 1963.

46. H.C. Hodge, as quoted in Glenchur, P.: Fluoridation: Local Water's Safety Queried. The Daily Californian, Berkeley, Calif., May 2, 1978, p. 8.

47. Shea, J., Gillespie, S.M., and Waldbott, G.L.: Allergy to Fluoride. Ann. Allergy, 25:388-391, 1967.

48. Seabrook, C.: Anti-Fluoridation Forces Outnumbered. The Atlanta (Ga.) Journal and Constitution, June 29, 1975, p. 2A.

49. Franklin, J.: Censorship Suppresses Information Unfavorable to Fluoridation. National Fluoridation News, 20(3):3-4, July-Sept. 1974. Photos of the three envelopes appear on p. 4 in this article. Cf. Schatz, A.: Fluoridation and Censorship. Prevention, June 1965.

50. Taves, D.R., Terry, R., Smith, F.A., and Gardner, D.E.: Use of Fluoridated Water in Long-Term Hemodialysis. Arch. Intern. Med., 115:167-172, 1965.

51. Kretchmar, L.H., Greene, W.M., Waterhouse, C.W., and Parry, W.L.: Repeated Hemodialysis in Chronic Uremia. J. Am. Med. Assoc., 184:1030-1031, 1963.

52. Blayney, J.R., Bowers, R.C., and Zimmerman, M.: Evanston Dental Caries Study. 22. A Study of Fluoride Deposition in Bone. J. Dent. Res., 41:1037-1044, 1962.

53. Taves, D.R.: Letter to G.L. Waldbott, April 16, 1965.

54. Taves, D.R.: Letter to A.W. Burgstahler, March 25, 1977. Copy in my possession.

55. Wassung, J.: Letter to A.W. Burgstahler, May 8, 1978. Copy in my possession.

56. Lepkowski, W.: Handler Reflects on NAS, Science Issues. Chem. & Eng. News, 56(7):20-21, Feb. 13, 1978.

57. I am aware of communications from Prof. A.H. Mohamed, Dr. H.C. Moolenburgh (Holland), Dr. Dean Burk, Dr. J. Yiamouyiannis, Lord Douglas of Barloch (England), and Mrs. Alfred Taylor.

58. Interview, A.W. Burgstahler at the National Academy of Sciences with P.L. Sitton, Assistant to the President of the NAS, Oct. 12, 1977.

59. Handler, P., President of the National Academy of Sciences: Letter to A.W. Burgstahler, Oct. 26, 1977. Copy in my possession.

60. Rose, D., and Marier, J.R.: Environmental Fluoride 1977. National Research Council Canada, Report No. 16081 [July 1978].

61. Manocha, S.L., Warner, H., and Olkowski, Z.L.: Cytochemical Response of Kidney, Liver and Nervous System to Fluoride Ions in Drinking Water. Histochem. J., 7:343-355, 1975. This paper cites pertinent fluoride research by Dr. Handler (1945), who "observed significant accumulation of

lactic acid and hexose-6-phosphate in liver and muscle of the animals which ingested large doses of fluoride in their drinking water."

62. Telephone conversation, D.R. Taves with A.W. Burgstahler, Nov. 14, 1977.

63. Latham, M.C., and Grech, P.: The Effects of Excessive Fluoride Intake. Am. J. Public Health, 57:651-660, 1967.

64. Morris, J.W.: Skeletal Fluorosis Among Indians of the American Southwest. Am. J. Roentgenol. Radium Ther. Nucl. Med., 94:608-615, 1965.

65. Juncos, L.I., and Donadio, J.V., Jr.: Renal Failure and Fluorosis. J. Am. Med. Assoc., 222:783-785, 1972.

66. Løkken, P., and Borchgrevink, C.F.: Reported Adverse Effects in Caries Preventive Use of Fluorides in Norway. Norw. Tannlaegeforen Tidskr., 87:248-254, 1977. (Abstracted in Fluoride, 11:100-101, 1978; cf. Editorial: Reliability of the Double-Blind Test in Fluoride Poisoning, ibid., 11:43-45, 1978.)

67. Ramseyer, W.F., Smith, C.A.H., and McCay, C.M.: Effect of Sodium Fluoride Administration on Body Changes in Old Rats. J. Gerontol., 12:14-19, 1957.

68. Bosworth, E.B., and McCay, C.M.: Pathologic Studies on Rat Kidneys: Absence of Effects Ascribed to Fluoride Following Long-Term Ingestion of Drinking Water Containing Fluoride. J. Dent. Res., 41:949-960, 1962. Cf. Lovelace, F., Black, R.E., Kunz, Y., Smith, C.A.H., Bosworth, E.B., Wang, C.N., Austria, L., Park, R.L., and McCay, C.M.: Metabolism of Fluoride in Old Rats and Hamsters. J. Appl. Nutr., 12:142-151, 1959.

69. Herman, J.R.: Fluorine in Urinary Tract Calculi. Proc. Soc. Exp. Biol. Med., 91:189-191, 1956.

70. Herman, J.R., Mason, B., and Light, I.: Fluorine in Urinary Tract Calculi. J. Urol., 80:263-268, 1958. Cf. Herman, J.R., and Papadakis, L.: The Relationship of Sodium Fluoride to Nephrolithiasis in Rats. J. Urol. 83:799-800, 1960.

71. Gordonoff, T.: Letter to G.L. Waldbott, Sept. 2, 1963. For a further account, see Waldbott (in Ref. 7 above), pp. 275-285.

72. Interview, A. Schatz with T. Gordonoff and Ch. Leimgruber. See Schatz, A.: Some Comments on Two Books Dealing with the Toxicology of Fluorine Compounds. Pakistan Dent. Rev., 15:68ff., 1965. Also, telephone conversation, A.W. Burgstahler and H.L. McKinney with A. Schatz, May 14, 1978. The amount of money involved was 10,000 Swiss francs.

73. Gordonoff, T., Ed.: The Toxicology of Fluorine. Symposium, Bern, 15-17 October 1962. Schwabe & Co., Basel/Stuttgart, 1964.

74. Editorial: The Richmond (Va.) News Leader, Sept. 30, 1966. Cf. Detroit Sunday News, Sept. 25, 1966.

75. Greenberg, D.S.: Fluoridation: A Meeting in Detroit Raises Some Questions. Science, 153:1499-1500, 1966. For comment, see Burgstahler,

A.W.: Letter to the Editor: Detroit Fluoride Conference, ibid., 154:590, 1966.

76. Vasta, B.M., Chief of Bibliographic Services Division, National Library of Medicine: Letter to A.W. Burgstahler, April 26, 1978. Copy in my possession.

CHAPTER 19

CONCLUSION

Controlled fluoridation is one of the four great, mass preventive health measures of all time. The "four horsemen" of health are: the pasteurization of milk, the purification of water, immunization against disease, and controlled fluoridation of water.[1]

* * * * *

The evidence has been examined, critically and repeatedly, and the specific allegations of injury and of hazard have been carefully evaluated. The conclusion in every instance, from every body of investigators with recognized competence in toxicology, epidemiology, and medicine has been the same: *Fluoridation of public water supplies is safe.*[2]

* * * * *

We are told, for example, that the effects of fluorine on some organ or tissue can be controlled by controlling the concentration of fluorine in drinking water, without regard to how much water is consumed, or how much fluorine is consumed in food or inhaled in air, and without regard to how much of the fluorine taken in is absorbed, or how much of that gets to the place where the effect is produced. The whole idea is so absurd on its face that it is hard to see how any sane person could give it the slightest credence. Yet this preposterous idea permeates almost everything written about the effects of fluoride; thousands of "experts" have accepted it as gospel; millions of laymen believe it because the experts say so even when their own common sense tells them it can't be true.[3]

* * * * *

NO OTHER PROCEDURE in the history of medicine has been praised so highly nor at the same time condemned so thoroughly. Few other examples exist where healthbringers have ignored so much unequivocal scientific evidence of human harm – actual as well as potential – in order to implement a controversial health measure. Fluoridation, a program of almost inescapable mass medication, has no parallel in the experience of man.

In the early 1950s when the PHS, ADA, and AMA openly endorsed fluoridation, scientists really knew very little about the possible consequences of adding fluoride to the drinking water. As dental researcher V. O. Hurme observed in 1952: "So far medical researchers have paid relatively little attention to the problem of chronic fluorine toxicosis." "One can summarize the situation by asserting that medical approval of fluoridation, based on thorough long-term investigations, is still needed." "Since the big problem in fluoridation is the ruling out of subclinical injury, or the existence of a health hazard to persons who are not completely healthy, one is entitled to ask about the quantity and quality of animal experimentation that has been done in relation to fluoride consumption." "Apparently animal experimentation has not placed us in a strong position for recommending immediate adoption of universal fluoridation where the natural fluoride content of water supplies is low."[4]

Although I was unaware of this prescient review when I began to publish my findings on illness from artificially fluoridated water, my discoveries showed good reason why Hurme should have been seriously concerned.

WATER CONSUMPTION AND FLUORIDE INTAKE

The fundamental structural weaknesses of fluoridation have increased with time until the very heart of the program has suffered a massive coronary. In 1939, when Cox proposed adding industrial-waste fluorides to drinking water for the prevention of tooth decay, water engineers were recommending at least a 10-fold factor of safety for fluoride in domestic water supplies. Recognizing that unattractive dental mottling was found wherever drinking water contained as much as 1 ppm fluoride, they had suggested that 0.1 ppm be the *maximum* desirable concentration of fluoride in a public water supply; 1.0 ppm in the water source was sufficient reason for rejection.[5]

Scientists in the USPHS had other views, however, for by 1942 they believed, on the basis of Dean's research, that a concentration at about 1-ppm fluoride in the drinking water afforded optimal protection against tooth decay with minimal risk of dental fluorosis and no other known "public health hazard." Consequently, they set the maximum permissible fluoride level in public water supplies at 1.0 ppm instead of 0.1 ppm.[6] Four years later they raised it again, to 1.5 ppm,[7] apparently on the strength of PHS investigator McClure's research on five healthy young men: "drinking water containing 1.8 to 1.9 p.p.m. fluorine[,] or any drinking water which contributes an average of not more than 3.0 to 4.0 mg. fluorine daily to the ingesta, is not liable to create endemic cumulative toxic fluorosis."[8] The same report also stated that 4.0 to 5.0 milligrams "may be the limits of fluorine which may be ingested daily without an appreciable hazard of body storage of fluorine."

McClure's estimates in the 1940s of water consumption and the average daily intake of fluoride from food and drinking water are given in Table 19-1.[9-14] (See next page.) The current 0.7-1.2 ppm fluoridation standards established in the U.S. in 1961 are based on these figures plus the effect of temperature. According to the USPHS they provide a two-fold margin of safety, since the *maximum permissible level is set at 1.4-2.4 ppm.*[15] In this concentration range, however, even Dean encountered excessive dental fluorosis.[16] Moreover, with a fluoride intake as low as 0.5 mg/day from food and 3.6 mg/day from drinking 1.5 liters/day of 2.4-ppm fluoride water,[17] the total daily ingestion of fluoride easily reaches the lower end of McClure's "appreciable hazard of body storage of fluorine."

Since the 1940s, when McClure published his estimates, the fluoride content of food has risen significantly. Foods and beverages processed or prepared with fluoridated water show a 2- to 5-fold increase in fluoride level, so that today the fluoride intake of an adult *from food alone* in a fluoridated community is not 0.2 to 0.3 mg/day but about 1.0 to 3.4 mg/day (see again, Table 19-1 on the next page). Moreover, in the recent NRC report *Drinking Water and Health,* the average amount of drinking water (in all forms) consumed per healthy person (adult) was taken as 2 liters/day, not 1.0-1.5 liters/day.[18] Thus the *average* total fluoride intake even in a community with 1-ppm fluoride in the drinking water now *easily exceeds McClure's 5 mg/day limit.* The AMA

Table 19-1

Estimates of Average Daily Fluoride Intake with Fluoridation[a]

Year of report	Fluoride from food water (mg)[b]	Volume of water (liters)	Fluoride from water (mg)[b]	Total F intake (mg)	First author (Ref.)
1943[c]	0.03-0.56	0.4-1.2	0.4-1.2	0.4-1.7	McClure[9]
1949	0.2-0.3	1.0-1.5	1.0-1.5	1.2-1.8	McClure[10]
1965	0.5-1.5	1.0	1.0	1.5-2.5	Hodge[11]
1966	1.0-2.0	1.0-3.0	1.0-3.0	2.0-5.0	Marier[12]
1971	0.8-0.9	1.0-1.5	1.0-1.5	1.8-2.4	San Filippo[13]
1974	1.7-3.4	1.0-2.0	1.0-2.0	2.7-5.4	Kramer[14]

[a] For critical commentary, see C.S. Farkas: Total Fluoride Intake and Fluoride Content of Common Foods: A Review. *Fluoride,* 8:98-105, 1975.

[b] Based on a concentration of 1 mg/liter (1 ppm) fluoride in the water. Fluoride intakes increase or decrease according to the fluoride concentration and the volume of water consumed.

[c] For children 1 to 12 years old. All the other estimates are for healthy adults.

recognizes that this is true but denies the possibility of any hazard at this level of intake[19] — *contrary to the original findings of the PHS on which fluoridation was premised!*

Balance studies also show that over 80% of the fluoride present in food and over 90% of the fluoride in drinking water is absorbed by the body.[20] When regional and occupational variations are also considered, even higher intakes are not mere possibilities but realities. Under adverse environments or in diseases like diabetes or nephritis, fluoride burdens of 10-20 mg/day are not at all unlikely. The potential for physical harm is therefore extremely serious, even in a community raising the fluoride content of the water to only 1 ppm, for the total intake from food and water *is now in the range of 5 mg/day.* Are the possible benefits to teeth worth the lurking dangers?

TEETH

In fact, how reliable are reports of the impressive decay reductions credited to fluoridation? What role do concurrent procedures –improved oral hygiene, use of dental floss, interdental stimulators, regular tooth brushing, better nutrition, removal of candy machines from schools, regular dental check-ups, topical applications, etc.–have on the total dental picture? How many consumers in a fluoridated community drink low-fluoride bottled water? What effect does bias have on the data and conclusions? As Hurme observed: "Statistical generalizations are never better than the seemingly little individual units upon which they are based. The procedures of examining teeth are very difficult to standardize and the influence of personal bias on the part of the examiners equally difficult to eliminate."[4]

In the ninth year of fluoridation in Newburgh, N.Y., school examinations disclosed a significantly greater need for dental work than in the nearby nonfluoridated control city of Kingston.[21] In fluoridated Easton, Pa., dentist U. L. Monteleone found that the teeth of the economically deprived children were in no better condition than those in nonfluoridated Allentown, Pa.[22] In Illinois and Indiana, dental researchers showed there is little difference in dental practice and income between fluoridated and nonfluoridated communities; moreover, in the fluoridated cities restorations in primary teeth and orthodontic work accounted for a larger proportion of dental services.[23]

In any risk-benefit situation there must be at least *some* benefit for all if the procedure is to be justified. As we have just seen, fluoridation does not always seem to work: when we speak of *average* benefits we really mean that some persons are NOT receiving any benefits at all. Furthermore, when dental fluorosis (mottling) occurs, as it does in 10 to 20% of the exposed population, the recipients can be worse off than without fluoridation. Disfiguring mottling is a source of great psychological as well as physical trauma for the individual. The AMA has called it "the most delicate criterion of harm from fluoride ingestion,"[24] which is true only with *some* children, not others; adults, of course, do not develop dental fluorosis and can be harmed without showing mottling.

Are there other illusory aspects of fluoridation statistics? How much effect does delay in the eruption of teeth have on the validity of comparisons if the rate of decay is about the same after caries begins? If patient work loads, the number of fillings made, and dentists' incomes and practices are not appreciably different in fluoridated and nonfluoridated communities,[23] how can there be much real cost saving with fluoridation? But since dental researchers "have told the public it works," how can they report anything but benefits from fluoridation?

GENERAL HEALTH EFFECTS

Dental fluorosis, unfortunately, is only the tip of a gigantic iceberg of fluoride damage. In India various forms of arthritis-producing skeletal fluorosis result from 1-2 ppm-fluoride water.[25] Debilitating skeletal fluorosis has been observed in Spain with only 1.2 ppm fluoride in the water.[26] In South Africa young children in economically deprived areas suffered serious ill effects—bone deformities, depressed thyroid function, gastrointestinal disorders, etc.—where the water contained 3.6 ppm fluoride. The report concluded: "it is clear that the drinking water containing as little *as 1 to 2 parts of fluorine per million parts* [italics in original] may in certain circumstances cause serious disturbances of general health and especially in normal thyroid function and in the normal processes of calcium-phosphorus metabolism."[27]

The persistence of free ionized fluoride in the bloodstream, even at very low concentrations (about 0.01 ppm), and its ability to penetrate cell membranes and to interfere with enzyme function and mineral balance throughout the body help explain many disorders and pathological conditions arising from fluoridation. No other electrolyte in the human body is so reactive chemically as is fluoride. Bones and teeth are therefore only two of its many targets. The former belief that soft tissues contain little or no fluoride is no more than a fairy tale.

What mischief can the omnipresent fluoride ion cause in the body? Mutagenesis, birth defects, and cancer are three serious associations of the first order.[28] Confirmations are multiplying constantly, such as Klein's findings on the deleterious effects of fluoride on DNA repair.[29] No longer can these results be brushed aside with the magic words "not confirmed," or by misrepresentation of the actual scientific evidence. Roholm identified a variety of ailments with skeletal fluorosis, and my clinical investigations, confirmed by other clinicians, have elaborated the preskeletal phase. The wide range of symptoms induced by fluoride may provide important clues about the origin of many common disorders for which adequate explanations have not been found.

For example, do not the following cases indicate that fluoride is involved in gastric ulcer? In a group of 60 retired aluminum workers with signs of skeletal fluorosis, 30 (or 50%) of them had gastritis and dyspepsia, and 7 (or 12%) had gastric or duodenal ulcers.[30] A nine-year-old boy was twice subjected to surgery for gastric hemorrhages before physicians recognized that the damage was caused by fluoride tablets.[31] Even infants have developed gastrointestinal bleeding, as seen by blood in their stools, from daily ingestion of vitamins containing 0.5 mg of fluoride.[32]

Other evidence also strengthens this link. The fact that acid urine increases the formation of undissociated HF which penetrates bladder tissue[33] provides a reasonable basis for understanding the adverse reaction of fluoride with acid gastric juice. To what extent this mechanism plays a role in cystitis, pyelitis, and urethritis requires further investigation. I have repeatedly observed complete, seemingly miraculous, cures of such disorders simply by putting the patient on a low-fluoride regimen.

Some cases of arterial sclerosis also indicate fluoride involvement. Two persons, who had lived less than 20 years in fluoridated Grand Rapids, attained fluoride levels as high as 8400 ppm in their aortas. Another individual living in a *non*fluoridated city had as much as 2340 ppm in his aorta.[34] In Ames, Iowa, the aorta of a premature infant had 59 ppm fluoride.[35] Pericapillary toxic inflammation, the hallmark of Chizzola maculae — an early symptom of chronic fluoride toxicosis — is also caused by fluoride.[36]

Consistent with these findings are certain trends in changes reported for mortality due to heart disease. Although the differences were not large, age-adjusted death rates due to heart disease during the period 1950-1970 showed a greater decrease in nonfluoridated cities of 25,000 to 200,000 population than in comparable fluoridated cities.[37] On the other hand, larger cities had just the opposite pattern, a result confirmed by Taves for the 20 largest fluoridated and 15 largest nonfluoridated U.S. cities. Taves has postulated that "intermediate levels of fluoride inhibit soft-tissue calcification *in vitro* and are associated with less aortic calcification *in vivo*."[38] This interpretation is questionable, however, since the fluoride levels needed to inhibit apatite formation in the *in vitro* study[39] were about 5 to 10 times the ionic fluoride levels found in the blood with fluoridation. An even more telling criticism is that the *in vivo* study was based on erroneous data.[40] In the last analysis, then, the discrepancy between the results from the larger and smaller cities may have other, entirely different origins, such as the growth and population structure of the two sets of cities since 1950.

The frequent occurrence of arthritis in the preskeletal phase of fluorosis strongly suggests that certain kinds of arthritis, especially in the spine (spondylitis), may often be due to fluoride. Pinet and Pinet have given a striking account of their X-ray findings in 148 cases of endemic skeletal fluorosis in the Sahara[41] that I believe closely resemble the spinal changes frequently found elsewhere but which are usually attributed merely to aging. Increased accumulation of fluoride with age is well established, as is the increase of arthritis with age. The subject clearly merits more research.

Another widespread problem of great interest to practically everyone is the connection of fluoride with headaches. In my medical practice I have found that severe, migraine-like headaches have often been relieved dramatically by the simple expedient of having patients stop drinking fluoridated water. This occurred even when the illness had been of long duration and had been completely refractory to numerous other treatments. Other clinicians have observed similar disappearance of headaches when their patients were taken off fluoridated water.[42] Related neurological disorders are now also being linked to fluoride, particularly certain kinds of retinitis[43] and possibly certain forms of demyelinizing diseases.[44]

The kidneys are another prime target for damage from fluoridated water. Several of my patients with serious kidney impairment have had their kidney function restored simply by changing to nonfluoridated water for all drinking and cooking. We also know that persons with nephritis store excessive amounts of fluoride in the body and are more susceptible to skeletal fluorosis than persons with healthy kidneys. Moreover, young children with nephrogenic or pituitary diabetes who drink excessive amounts of water containing 1 ppm[45] or even 0.5 ppm[46] fluoride can develop disfiguring dental fluorosis. In one of these studies the authors advised that "a portion of the ingested water that these children consume should be supplied from a nonfluoridated source."[45]

Although the National Kidney Foundation is reported to believe that fluoride does not harm the kidneys, many studies in the scientific literature emphatically refute such a claim. In 1957, Ramseyer *et al.* demonstrated (with accompanying photomicrographs) that rats drinking fluoridated (1, 5, and 10 ppm) water for 520 days sustained clearly discernible hypertrophy of their kidneys, whereas controls on fluoride-free water did not.[47] After nine months on 1-ppm fluoridated drinking water, golden hamsters underwent a 48% reduction in activity of the enzyme succinic dehydrogenase in the kidney compared to controls on fluoride-free water.[48] In 1975, Manocha *et al.* showed that the kidneys of squirrel monkeys drinking 1 and 5 ppm-fluoridated water "showed significant cytochemical changes [increased activity], especially in the animals on 5 ppm fluoride in their drinking water." In the final 10 months of this study, monkeys drinking fluoridated water consumed more water than those drinking distilled water. Humans suffering from fluoride poisoning also consume much more water, and the reason, as in the case of the monkeys, is probably "a result of functional changes in the kidneys."[49] Without question, fluoride harms the kidneys.

The significance of fluoride toxicity for kidney patients undergoing long-term hemodialysis is equally clear. In this procedure the amount of fluoride transferred to the patient from a 1-ppm fluoridated dialysate bath can easily amount to 50 mg or more per week. As pointed out in a Canadian–U.S. study, abnormal bone formation and other deleterious effects are excessive when fluoridated water is employed in hemodialysis: "patients maintained on long-term hemodialysis using fluoridated water for periods of years will encounter an unacceptable frequency and degree of osteomalacia."[50]

Fluoride also affects plants as well as animals and man. Gladiolus and rose cuttings, for example, exhibit flower and stem damage after they are placed in fluoridated water compared to controls in fluoride-free water; gladiolus leaf-tip burn is also caused by 1-ppm fluoride in water.[51] Likewise, cuttings of a popular indoor foliage plant called "baby doll" (*Cordyline terminalis*), used extensively in dish gardens because of its attractive red coloration, often exhibit leaf "tip necrosis in the propagation bed. This necrosis is caused by fluoride found in the soil-water solution."[52] Ponderosa pine, apricot, and peach trees are also extremely susceptible to airborne fluoride, but fluoride-induced damage has been well documented in many other kinds of plants as well.[53] Study of the botanical effects of fluoride offers much promise for further investigation.

The adverse health effects of fluoridated water are extensive, serious, and insidious; they offset any possible benefit to teeth, no matter how great. If individuals most susceptible to harm in a population are to be protected, as the NRC Safe Drinking Water Committee report states, then anyone demonstrably intolerant to fluoride, as many of my patients have been, must be protected from fluoridated water. This goal may be achieved by furnishing these individuals with distilled or other fluoride-free water, or simply by ceasing to fluoridate water supplies. *Never* should physicians attribute to psychosomatic origins an intractable case where the symptoms coincide with those listed in this book.

My two collaborators in this enterprise have themselves suffered the reality of reversible chronic fluoride toxicosis from artificially fluoridated water, and I have treated close to 500 similar patients who displayed what should now be called the **Chronic Fluoride Toxicity Syndrome.** Many other physicians have also treated this disease, and various clinicians have written about it. If caught in time, the disease can be diagnosed and arrested with ease, for the symptoms can be reversed merely by switching to distilled (preferably) or other low-fluoride water and by eliminating as much fluoride from the diet and environment as possible. If the symptoms do not disappear or diminish within two weeks, however, a physician should be consulted at once to determine possible alternative causes and solutions. I shall elaborate on my numerous clinical cases in another work to appear in the near future.

FLUORIDATION AND GOVERNMENT

Considering the demonstrable harm fluoride does to humans, animals, plants, and the environment,[54] why has our government become deaf and blind on a matter of such vital concern? Whenever adverse findings appear, health officials or scientists immediately deny the facts or conclusions, criticize key aspects of the work, sometimes before they have examined it, or urge retraction of the conclusions. Occasionally, outright suppression of the work is attempted. The previous chapter enumerated many of these machinations, but there are far more than can be recounted here.

John Small, a top troubleshooter with the National Fluoridation Information Service of the USPHS, has been involved in many skirmishes that could present difficulties for any dispassionate discussion of fluoridation. Frequently he has intervened by letter, telephone, or in person when any threatening cloud appears on the horizon. For example, the following passage from a review article published in 1970 drew certain "unpleasant" conclusions about the effects of fluoride air pollution on animals:

> Whenever domestic animals exhibited fluorosis, several cases of human fluorosis were reported, the symptoms of which were one or more of the following: dental mottling, respiratory distress, stiffness in the knees or elbows or both, a skin lesion, or high levels of F in teeth or urine [six references cited]. Man is much more sensitive than domestic animals to F intoxication [ref.].[55]

In late summer 1971 Small telephoned the agency of the U.S. Department of Agriculture where the author worked and "expressed concern" about the serious implications of the above-quoted statement.[56] In an apologetic letter of September 7, 1971, the author responded to the Director of the Division of Dental Health that the first word of the offending statement should be changed to "In some cases when."[57] Small's "search and destroy" activities are as well known as they are effective, and among anti-fluoridationists the phrase "Small strikes again!" seems to have a double meaning.

This example points to the manner in which governmental agencies — particularly the Dental Division of the PHS — attempt to control information on fluoride toxicity. Often favorable statements on fluoridation are solicited by the PHS to answer or anticipate problems. For example, the American Academy of Allergy, responding to a request by the PHS, issued a statement that there was "no evidence" of hypersensitivity or intolerance to fluoride.

The National Kidney Foundation, apparently responding to another PHS request, has denied there are any problems caused by fluoridation for kidney patients, although even the PHS has backed off from recommending the use of fluoridated water for hemodialysis. The National Cancer Institute has fed data to foreign scientists and then categorically denied any association of cancer with fluoridation on the basis of "independent" analyses of the data by these same scientists.[58]

During the last few years the Environmental Protection Agency (EPA) has taken over from the PHS much of the primary activity for promoting fluoridation, although the 1974 Safe Drinking Water Act expressly forbids the federal government or any agency thereof from attempting to require fluoridation anywhere.[59] The EPA has based its support of fluoridation solely on the one-sided propaganda information published by the PHS and its allies. Who can therefore truthfully assert that the EPA is protecting the American public from a harmful procedure?

The EPA position was originally defined in its fluoridation manual by E. Bellack, a chemist of the Fluoridation Laboratory, USPHS Division of Dental Public Health. In April 1970, while still with the PHS, however, Bellack had co-authored another revealing article with R. J. Baker, Technical Director for the Wallace and Tiernan Division of the Pennwalt Corporation, a leading supplier of fluoridation equipment and of fluoride chemicals. Their paper conceded that in the manufacture of phosphate fertilizer the practice of scrubbing the particulate and gaseous fluoride wastes from the surface of the chimneys created a new problem to his corporation: "In many cases, the water from the scrubbers was merely disposed of in the nearest stream thus contributing to water pollution."[60]

Bellack and Baker suggested that fluoridation of water might become a market for the waste hydrofluorosilicic acid collected in storage ponds from phosphate fertilizer plants. These wastes were more desirable for fluoridation than was sodium fluoride, "both from the cost standpoint and also because of the simplicity and convenience of feeding a material which was already in solution . . . ." It was a simple matter to deliver it by tank truck to a nearby water works and also obtain a good price for it. In concentrated form, however, this grade of hydrofluorosilicic acid is even more toxic than sodium fluoride: other contaminants are lead, antimony, and arsenic. Thorough analysis of these waste solutions would no doubt produce many other surprises of an unpleasant kind.

Many who read this book will scoff at the idea that government would deliberately act in a manner detrimental to our well-being, but examples here and abroad prove otherwise. Science is almost always profoundly influenced by government. In Nazi Germany, for example, Adolf Hitler believed that Germans were a biologically superior race; Jews, on the other hand, were labeled inferior – not on the basis of scientific evidence, but solely for political and ideological reasons. The catastrophic impact of this Nazi "idealism" has been thoroughly exposed and justly condemned, and we must never forget the incredible ideological impact that government-sponsored ideas have had on the development of human biology.

Soviet science has also experienced its moments of disrepute. From the late 1930s until the early 1960s, especially in the late 1940s, certain biological (agrobiological) subjects were strongly influenced or controlled by T. D. Lysenko and his coterie. These areas of thought, emphasizing the ability of scientists to manipulate inheritance through environmental alterations (conditioning), fit nicely with Marxist beliefs that the state could mold the individual into certain configurations; hence, Joseph Stalin adopted Lysenko's premises, and anyone holding opposing views – Mendelian concepts about particulate inheritance, for example – was dealt with harshly. Lysenko's followers published innumerable articles, reports, and books discussing their Lamarckian "facts" and conclusions. Advanced scientific degrees and professional reputations were established on an enormous, but ludicrous, mass of "data," now admitted to be essentially incorrect.[61] The dictatorial control of science dangerously impeded the objective pursuit of truth based on facts – facts issuing from the laws of nature, which cannot be changed by government or man.

Democracies do not have the omnipotent control over science that totalitarian governments have. But they do exercise power, and they have sometimes made dramatic mistakes that have adversely affected many lives. The U.S. Department of Agriculture, for example, has from time to time embarked on disastrous programs to eradicate the fire ant and the gypsy moth. Although well-intentioned, these DDT spraying programs have destroyed millions of birds, animals, fish, and other wildlife, not to speak of the great harm done to domesticated animals and humans as well. Ironically, the fire ant and gypsy moth are still with us, despite the millions of dollars spent plus an equal number of good intentions.[62] The harm remains.There is an uncanny parallel with fluoridation.

Another example of how government controls and manipulates science provides an even closer, astonishing parallel with the fluoridation affair. In 1963 the Atomic Energy Commission (AEC) assigned Drs. John Gofman and Arthur Tamplin, Lawrence Radiation Laboratory, Livermore, California, the task of examining the effect of low-level radiation on cancer and especially leukemia. They issued a report in 1969 charging that the government's maximum permissible dose of radiation was allowing perhaps 32,000 extra cancer deaths each year. They recommended "An immediate reduction of permissible maximum radiation to no more than one-tenth the present limit [170 millirads/year]." They believed that there is no "threshold" "below which radiation is harmless." In fact, Gofman exclaimed: "It is an outrageous lie that only high doses of radiation are harmful."[63]

The AEC promptly responded by issuing an immediate rebuttal and soliciting a group of 29 scientists to denounce "the alarmist views of a tiny minority of experts." Every effort was made to discredit and harass Gofman and Tamplin mercilessly, by drastically reducing their staffs and funding, and by other tactics as well. Indeed, they claimed that "AEC representatives and other atomic technologists have attempted to intimidate them and censor their research since it is not favourable to the nuclear-power lobby."[64]

Radiation scientist Dr. Irwin Bross has also concluded on the basis of original research (diagnostic X-rays) that "exposures to radiation in the one-rad range [100–1,000 millirads] are hazardous to health," and much more so than he originally thought.

> There is no longer any scientific question that radiologists and other physicians who claim these low levels of radiation are 'harmless' (and who use them indiscriminately) are killing their patients. I don't believe it absolves these professionals to say they are hurting their patients with the best of intentions.[65]

Dr. Bross feels that the AEC (now Nuclear Regulatory Commission), its industrial counterparts, and scientists in related fields have been "lying" for 25 years to the public about the hazards of low-level ionizing radiation. Increased cancer and leukemia rates are inevitable consequences.

What has been the government's response to Bross and his conclusions? The NCI terminated its contract with him after eight years of support. He received an on-site visit from an "angry radiologist." *Science,* specifically Philip Abelson, the editor, rejected publication of his findings. He has also experienced various attacks on his work by the profession and other harassments.[65] In short, Bross has been treated exactly as if he had been a scientific opponent of fluoridation. Even if Tamplin, Gofman, Bross, and others are absolutely wrong on every point, which seems unlikely, they have legitimately asked: are governmental agencies justified in suppressing opposing points of view?

Two-time Nobel Prize Laureate Linus Pauling also knows what happens when scientists oppose "Big Science" controlled by government. For many years Pauling has advocated vitamin C as a valuable asset in promoting health and well-being among mankind. Since 1971 extensive experimental and clinical studies have been conducted on vitamin C as a cancer-control agent. The results have been very promising – in some cases remarkably good. Nevertheless, the NCI has recently rejected Pauling's request for a mere $50,000 to pursue this promising line of research. Considering its lackluster track record in the last 20 years while spending *billions* of dollars, we must wonder why the NCI has refused to support a recognized scientific leader in a potentially life-saving project? We must also question why, in the light of much contrary evidence, the NCI has decided to commit $300,000 to see if vitamin C *causes or promotes cancer!*[66]

Without question, ideas contrary to orthodoxy – as determined by the NCI, PHS, or any other governmental agency – can be opposed very effectively by cutting off funds and supporting the opposite views. Support for vitamin C and opposition to fluoridation may seem like strange bedfellows, but they are bedfellows nevertheless, and the same strategies have been employed against both positions. It is no coincidence that Dr. F. J. Stare, a leading advocate of fluoridation, is at the same time a leading opponent of Pauling and his views on vitamin C.

Scientists may find it extremely difficult to believe that respected governmental agencies like the USPHS or the U.S. Department of Agriculture, which have wrought so much good, could have a darker side of their characters. The admirable contributions public health officials have made I freely admit and applaud, but we cannot deny that in the area of fluoridation, the PHS, EPA, NCI, and other federal agencies have often acted contrary to the best interests of the public they are sworn to serve. Indeed, government officials often have ruthlessly attempted to suppress views contrary to their own; they have maintained, in the face of much clearly adverse evidence, an entrenched and self-serving policy that was misguided and unsubstantiated from its inception. Hiding our heads in the sand about these nefarious actions will not cancel them, any more than erasing tape recordings or pleading innocence before the public could have made the Watergate scandal belatedly disappear.

SUPPRESSION OF EVIDENCE: SCIENCE'S WATERGATE

How can scientific evidence be suppressed in the free world? Easily. Anyone who has read this far has irrefutable evidence on this point, and what has already been discussed represents only the foothills of a gigantic mountain chain that would dwarf the Himalayas. Tragically, suppression of reputable data extends into almost every proponent argument.

Why, for example, did the AMA fail to cite scientific work on poisoning reports when the following words appeared in September 1975?

> There have been no adequately documented reports based on controlled research of any adverse systemic effects from fluoride ingestion at recommended levels used in public water supplies for the prevention of dental caries.[19]

My work alone had by then described hundreds of cases resulting from artificially fluoridated water, and yet the AMA *did not cite one single paper of mine on this topic,* nor any of the many works by other authors with similar information. Paradoxically, one of the seven footnotes to the passage quoted above was by F. B. Exner, M.D., who did describe extensive harm.[67] The ordinary scientific or lay reader, however, could hardly know this since the publication cited is rare and very difficult to find.

Suppression of information on this point is scarcely unique in this part of the AMA document, for throughout the work there are other serious omissions, as well as false statements and excessive interquotes of proponent literature. Furthermore, approximately 25% of the references were published before 1960 during the early push for fluoridation. The ADA statement on fluoridation in 1974 also committed similar errors of omission[68] and the *JADA* issue for February 1977 carried an article that falsely concluded: "There is no evidence that water containing optimal concentrations (0.7–1.2 ppm) of fluoride impairs general health."[69] My well-known work was not cited, presumably on the accepted tradition that whatever the friends of fluoridation do not believe simply is not knowledge.

Proponents of fluoridation have exported these same tactics of suppression of evidence. The British Dental Association, for example, issued a statement on fluoridation in 1976 which cited only my early works of 1958 and 1959 plus my 1967 article with Drs. Shea and Gillespie discussing intolerance/allergy to fluoridated toothpaste.[70] Also in 1976 the Royal College of Physicians (RCP) of London implied in their report on fluoridation[71] that I was the only physician to discover and describe reversible ill effects from fluoridated water. They cited *only* my articles before 1964 and nothing since then.

Omission of pertinent scientific data is at best a demonstration of poor scholarship; when the health of millions is at stake, however, it is intolerable. The reader can judge from the following example whether or not the RCP has acted responsibly. According to H. A. Cook, London, England, the RCP committee contacted him on June 30, 1975, requesting that he and/or the Scientific Committee for the Study of Fluoridation Hazards (of which he was secretary) submit any evidence to assist in the RCP deliberations for the report. He asked when the evidence was due, and learned from the Committee on July 28, 1975, that the deadline was the following day. Cook immediately informed the Honorable Secretary of the Committee that he needed two more weeks to assemble material. He then learned that Dr. Hugh Sinclair, Oxford University, had been told that the report *was already in print.*

On August 7, 1975, when Cook's report "was nearly finished," he discovered from the mouth of the Secretary himself that the RCP "report was indeed finished and *had been even before they had contacted him.*" [Emphasis added.] The Secretary claimed, however, "that it was not yet in print, and they were prepared to consider my data and amend their report in proof if necessary!"[72]   Except for citing two references to Cook's work on fluoride in tea,[73]   the committee did not do so, of course, and the clear implication is that the RCP snubbed the "U.K. and the international community in their report on fluoridation by taking no evidence from them until their report was completed."[72]   The report glowingly recommended fluoridation at the 1-ppm level and in effect suppressed many reports of harm.

This devious approach of omitting or suppressing evidence is one of the clearest and most disturbing parts of the history of fluoridation. Careful examination of fluoridation literature proves this beyond doubt. As the Editor-in-Chief of the *University of Ottawa Medical Journal* commented as early as 1965:

> It is true that the reports of adverse effects of fluorides on man are relatively few. Physicians by and large are unaware of the existence of such problems. It [chronic fluorosis] is hardly mentioned in the textbooks or in the medical literature. Of equal significance is the fact that rarely does one find reference in the proponent literature to the publications reporting damage to animals and humans from fluoridated drinking water at or near the so-called safe concentration.[74]

The instances of this procedure of ignoring any contrary findings are incredibly numerous. When asked to comment on the work of Rogot *et al.* on fluoridation and urban mortality, Dr. Dean Burk wrote:

> The article is an excellent example, currently and commonly developing even at intermediate levels of scientific activity, of clearly deliberate omission of due reference to extensive contrary reports and conclusions in the widely available literature that are contrary to the cited conclusion in the article, and of failure of the publishing journal to correct this obviously glaring omission.[75]

Rogot's conclusion was the standard denial that "no relationship was found between fluoridation and cancer death rate trends."[37] Failure to cite the Burk-Yiamouyiannis study cannot be attributed to incompetence on the part of the four authors as well as the journal; as Burk reemphasized: "The omissions were deliberate."[75]

In the case of the recent NRC report, we also know that many omissions were deliberate. Once again, no work of mine beyond 1962 was cited. Although Dr. I. Rapaport published important articles on mongolism in 1956, 1957, 1959, 1960, 1961, and 1963,[28] Taves cited only the 1959 report. The article by Manocha, Warner, and Olkowski (1975) on kidney function[49] was not discussed in the text of the fluoride report; it appeared only in the section on "Research Recommendations," with the customary implication that it was somehow defective.[76]

The research by Manocha et al. is of course a source of great embarrassment for the supporters of fluoridation because the controls were very tight, and the investigators were capable and experienced. If this book has accurately portrayed the difficulties experienced by authors attempting to publish adverse data on fluoridation, then the article by Manocha et al. should have encountered problems. In fact, it did — the article was rejected by the AMA *Archives of Environmental Health.* One of the consultants remarked:

> I would recommend that this paper not be accepted for publication at this time for the following reasons: 1.) This is a sensitive subject and any publication in this area is subject to interpretation by anti-fluoridation groups. Therefore, any detrimental fluoride effect has to be conclusively proven. . . . 3.) The key question is whether these cytochemical changes are reversible (an adaptation) or irreversible (leading to pathology). This key question is not answered.[77]

In other words, because the authors had shown adverse cytochemical changes in primate kidneys from fluoridated water (1 and 5 ppm), their work should be suppressed! If a detrimental fluoride effect was not conclusively proven, why block publication of the paper? Whether or not the changes were reversible was irrelevant, for persons drinking fluoridated water all their lives would not easily find out if their kidney problems were reversible. Another of the AMA consultants expressed similar views that

scientific evidence must be subsidiary to preconceived conclusions:

> The safety of the 1 ppm level in the drinking水has been exhaustively and
> repeatedly demonstrated for more than 70 million residents of the USA
> and one wonders whether anything is gained by 'beating on a dead horse'
> or reviving an issue that has already been resolved. In short, the work tends
> to merely raise the question and cast doubt through monkey studies that
> appear to have no basis for man. Moreover, the questions regarding the
> safety of the 1 ppm fluoride level are based on rather tenuous
> cytochemical studies.[78]

For anyone to maintain that primate studies on monkeys have
no relevance for humans does not merit further comment.
Cytochemical studies of course provide fundamental information
about the effect of fluoride on man.

Ironically, Manocha *et al.* anticipated many potential objections
and instituted numerous extra precautions in their experimental
procedures. For example, the cages were moved periodically by
Warner to cancel any possible effects from any unobserved draft.
Special care was also directed to the dietary regimen, and "all
animals were maintained on an optimum diet." But the *pièce de
résistance* is that the histochemical procedures *were repeated twice
on the kidneys and confirmed!*[78]

The investigators spent an extraordinary amount of time and
effort collecting their data, and every precaution was taken to
cancel potential bias. There is no justification whatsoever for
rejecting their findings essentially for nonscientific reasons. Had
Taves really been interested in unearthing faulty controls in the
experiments, he could have telephoned the authors at the Yerkes
Primate Research Center, as he telephoned Dr. A. H. Mohamed when
attempting to discredit Mohamed's work.[79] Instead, Taves
criticized the primate study *before he had even read it* and later
recommended that the experiments be *repeated,* a request the
Yerkes scientists would be pleased to fill if the USPHS will fund
additional work.[78]

Editors of scientific journals frequently participate in suppression of information. In December 1974, E. H. Smith, Jr., Assistant
Surgeon General for Dental Services of the U.S. Army, wrote a
guest editorial for the *JAMA* in which he claimed: "Extensive research, conducted over a period of 35 years, has established be-

yond question the benefits of 1.0 or 1.5 ppm of fluoride in communal drinking water in reducing tooth decay. These same studies have also proven unequivocally the safety of fluoridation for those who drink the treated water."[80]

Both statements are false, but they are the usual claims proponents make. What should really shock all of us, however, is the fact that only a few months later, during most of March 1975, the editor of the *JAMA* had in his possession a report, dated February 25, 1975, from H. T. Petraborg, M.D., who discussed 22 cases of fluoride poisoning from artificially fluoridated water in the Milwaukee, Wisconsin, area. These cases completely refuted Smith's sweeping claims of no harm from fluoridated water. Instead of correcting the misleading editorial by publishing Petraborg's communication, the *JAMA* Senior Editor wrote him that "we find that we are unable to put it [the report] effectively to good use for publication."[81] There is no rational excuse for this act of suppression. We might also ask: what happened to another critique of Smith's editorial by P. E. Zanfagna, M.D.?[82]

Increased corrosion of water pipes is another problem categorically denied by proponents, including the EPA. Nevertheless, corrosion is a well-documented result of fluoridation, especially in areas with soft, nonalkaline water supplies. Waterworks engineers have encountered demonstrably accelerated corrosion after fluoridation began in Concord, N.H.; Wilmington, Massachusetts; Schenectady, New York; Seattle, Washington, and elsewhere.[83] Even the EPA concedes: "Under special conditions of water quality, a small increase in the corrosivity of potable water that is *already* corrosive may be observed after treatment with alum, chlorine, fluorosilicic acid, or sodium silicofluoride."[84] Solid evidence shows much wider damage, and so we are told another lie by the defenders of fluoridation.

Can the problem of suppression of evidence – a very serious component of The Great Dilemma – be solved? Not until journal editors rely on *bipartisan* panels of referees and honestly judge work on the basis of intrinsic merit, rather than "saving the appearances." Not until the heads of our scientific organizations have the courage to reject shoddy reports whose errors have been brought to their attention; perhaps not until a new generation of independent thinkers invade our centers of learning.

SCIENCE'S DILEMMA

The decay of scientific inquiry is not confined to fluoridation; it has spread like a cancer into many areas. P. M. Boffey, AAAS science writer, has documented an astonishing variety of scientific problems issuing from an illicit merger of governmental/industrial interests. Six major areas were identified: radioactive waste disposal, the supersonic transport, defoliation, the safety of food additives, persistent pesticides, and airborne lead – to which we must add the fluoride problem. The National Academy of Sciences, according to Boffey, has not handled these six problems responsibly. For example, the NAS Food Protection Committee has apparently been influenced by industry, which supplied 40% of its budget in 1972. The Committee has not been overly concerned about the hazards of food additives. Boffey has warned: "Be cautious about accepting the Academy's pronouncements as the Unchallengeable Word from On High."[85] The importance of this caveat is obvious from the questionable way in which NAS President Philip Handler dealt with the serious shortcomings in the fluoride section of the NRC report *Drinking Water and Health* (1977).

Because much scientific research is conducted in industrial laboratories and industry-supported institutions, scientists often fail to speak out about health hazards for fear of losing their jobs: "Industrial scientists who fail to challenge conspiracies of silence within their firms are not rebuked: rather they are often quietly rewarded for their loyalty."[86] On the other hand, scientists who blow the whistle usually lose their jobs. W. H. Rodgers, Jr., has documented at some length the enormous control certain industries, especially those connected with fluoride,[87] have on our nation's scientific enterprises, and there are many other examples of this corruption of science.[88]

This book has presented the story of an intense struggle within the scientific community over a controversial subject, which has never won universal approval. Failure to overcome opposition has led proponents to resort to nonscientific tactics, and so the story is now primarily one of political intrigues, harassment, intimidation, suppression of evidence, control of the media, propaganda, and questionable scientific work. Proponents claim to be guided by the light of objectivity and truth, but a recent statement in *Science* may appropriately be applied here out of its original context: "Unconscious or dimly perceived finagling is probably endemic in science, since scientists are human beings rooted in cultural contexts, not automatons directed toward external truth."[89]

The irony of this conclusion in a publication of the AAAS is perhaps best seen in the statement on "The Integrity of Science" by the AAAS Committee on Science in the Promotion of Human Welfare:

> Free dissemination of information and open discussion is an essential part of the scientific process. Each separate study of nature yields an approximate result and inevitably contains some errors and omissions. Science gets at the truth by a continuous process of self-examination which remedies omissions and corrects errors. This process requires free disclosure of results, general dissemination of findings, interpretations, conclusion, and widespread verification and criticism of results and conclusions.[90]

Fluoridation poses a remarkable dilemma for science; it is science "run amok." Until scientists stop marching in mindless lock-step fashion to the authorities' siren music of endorsements, and begin *reading the original research literature for themselves* to check the claims made by proponents *and* opponents, The Great Dilemma cannot be resolved. All the negative evidence in the world cannot penetrate an ossified mind that refuses to be "confused by the facts."

THE PATIENT'S DILEMMA

The Great Dilemma of physicians, dentists, and scientists pales beside a far more pressing question: after untold personal suffering, how can millions throughout the world who are sensitive or intolerant to fluoride be restored to health? Especially vulnerable are nephritic and diabetic patients who drink more than the average amounts of water, and allergic patients whose tolerance to drugs is often impaired. Their personal dilemma is a pragmatic one of what to eat and drink without aggravating their illness. Because in the early stage of fluorosis many organs of the body can be affected, and because specific unequivocal laboratory tests for chronic fluoride poisoning are not yet available, most physicians do not recognize the disease. As with many other undiagnosed disorders, they often attribute the ailments to "nerves." In my experience, the resulting widespread use of pain killers has repeatedly added new problems to the victim of fluorosis.

Some laboratory tests, however, may at least provide clues. For example, minor changes in the serum calcium, serum phosphorus, and alkaline and acid phosphatase are sometimes helpful, but these indicators are not a constant feature of the disease. Slight abnormalities in liver, kidney, and thyroid function may also be revealing, but urinary and even blood fluoride levels are not reliable indexes of fluoride illness. Twenty years ago the double-blind test was a sound method for confirming the diagnosis, but the unforeseen increase in the fluoride content of food effectively precludes complete elimination of fluoride and often jeopardizes the reliability of such tests. The greatest aid in the diagnosis, therefore, is a thorough case history--as in most other toxicological situations. Physicians also must carefully rule out other possible illnesses with mimicking symptoms before they consider the possibility of poisoning from fluoridated water.

Certain definite physical signs, characteristic of nonskeletal fluorosis, do exist. In the early stages in women and children, for example, the skin lesion called "Chizzola maculae" provides a useful, clearly visible clue to the diagnosis.[91] The simultaneous occurrence of symptoms suggestive of stomach ulcer, arthritis (especially in the spine), and diarrhea, particularly when accompanied by headaches, muscular pains, and paresthesias, is almost always indicative of chronic fluoride poisoning. Excessive thirst, increased urination, and sudden episodes of acute abdominal pains often diagnosed as "intestinal flu" also point to fluoride intoxication. Temporary improvement during the patient's absence from a fluoridated community is another tell-tale sign. Progressive exhaustion associated with increasing general debility, even to the point of being completely bed-ridden, furnishes additional evidence for the diagnosis.

With respect to treatment, let me emphasize that the best remedy for chronic fluorosis is strict avoidance of fluoride in water, foods, beverages, drugs, dentifrices, and air. It is impossible, however, to eliminate the halogen completely from food, particularly in vegetables and fruits. The fluoride content of these foods is highly erratic, depending on where they were grown, how they were prepared, and to what extent they were fertilized and sprayed or exposed to atmospheric contamination. Furthermore, some foods like tea, ocean fish (especially with bones), chicken skin, chocolate (prepared in fluoridated water), prepared cereals, gelatin, and any item soaked or processed in fluoridated water are likely to have elevated levels of fluoride. Probably the foods most consistently low in fluoride are milk, eggs, red meats (excluding organs), produce having a protective rind (such as watermelon, lemons, bananas, and coconuts), fruits packed in their own juices (pineapples), and foods canned abroad in nonfluoridated, low-fluoride countries. In general, canned foods vary greatly in their fluoride content depending on many different factors. Persons intolerant to fluoride should watch their diet carefully and switch to other brands if symptoms occur after consuming a particular food.

Since fluoridated toothpaste has precipitated temporary recurrence of systemic symptoms in several of my patients, its use should be strictly avoided by afflicted persons. Drugs containing fluoride should not be used, particularly fluoride-containing anesthetics, such as Halothane and Enflurane. Sensitive persons should also stay away from areas having industrial air pollution, and they should *never* ingest large amounts of fluoride as a treatment for osteoporosis.

Some studies on the effect of certain vitamins, especially pyridoxine (B_6) and ascorbic acid (C), suggest that they may be of some assistance in countering fluoride toxicity. The use of calcium and magnesium salts has also been recommended in order to decrease fluoride absorption from the stomach and thus assist in eliminating the halogen through the bowels. None of these measures, however, has proved to be as effective as strict avoidance of ingested, imbibed, and inhaled fluoride, an approach that always requires careful attention by patients.

If symptoms do not disappear or diminish markedly within two weeks, patients should consult their physicians for diagnosis of other possible causes. Patients who improve, on the other hand, may periodically suffer temporary setbacks when inadvertently subjected to small intakes of fluoride. Severely affected individuals may require several months or even longer for complete recovery.

DENTAL CARIES: ALTERNATIVE SOLUTIONS

Are there safe, effective ways to prevent tooth decay? Although dental caries is not a fluoride-deficiency disease, many dental researchers have been so mesmerized by the favorable and enthusiastic early reports of the anti-caries effects of fluoridated water that they have neglected to follow up other, far more impressive findings. For example, even before fluoridation, W. A. Price, D.D.S., and others demonstrated the very low incidence of dental caries among populations throughout the world that have retained sound, unrefined native diets compared with those that have adopted modern, refined foods. Later, in his clinic in Cleveland during the depression of the 1930s, Price showed that just "one reinforced meal at noon for six days a week . . . completely controlled the dental caries of each member of the group" of children who attended. What were the magical ingredients?

> The nutrition provided these children in this one meal included the following foods. About four ounces of tomato juice or orange juice and a teaspoonful of a mixture of equal parts of a very high vitamin natural cod liver oil and an especially high vitamin butter was given at the beginning of the meal. They then received a bowl containing approximately a pint of a very rich vegetable and meat stew, made largely from bone marrow and fine cuts of tender meat: the meat was usually broiled separately to retain its juice and then chopped very fine and added to the bone marrow and meat soup which always contained finely chopped vegetables and plenty of very yellow carrots; for the next course they had cooked fruit, with very little sweetening, and rolls made from freshly gound whole wheat, which were spread with the high-vitamin butter. The wheat for the rolls was ground fresh every day in a motor driven coffee mill. Each child was also given two glasses of fresh whole milk. The menu was varied from day to day by substituting for the meat stew, fish chowder or organs of animals. . . . analysis showed that these meals provided approximately 1.48 grams of calcium and 1.28 grams of phosphorus in a single helping of each course. Since many of the children doubled up on the course, their intake of these minerals was much higher.[92]

During both world wars, increased use of wholegrain bread products and unprocessed foods, together with a greatly reduced consumption of refined carbohydrates, markedly diminished the incidence of tooth decay. A related pilot study of "wholemeal bread" families in England by a medical officer of health and a dental surgeon revealed that over 50% of the test children aged 5 to 7 drinking nonfluoridated water and eating only wholemeal instead of white or refined flour products from infancy were completely free of caries, whereas fewer than 20% of comparable children in the official British fluoridation studies were caries-free.[93]

This view that tooth decay is fundamentally a dietary-mineral deficiency disease led A. Åslander to develop the concept of "complete tooth nutrition" for the prevention of dental caries. He found that well-formed, completely caries-free teeth resulted from the daily ingestion of a broad-spectrum mineral supplement (uncalcined bone meal) from infancy through adolescence. These studies were begun in 1940 in a region of Sweden where tooth decay was universal; today the same subjects have teeth that are entirely free of cavities or fillings – with no adverse effects.[94] Dental researcher P. H. Laplaud of France has hailed this approach as a sound, practical, and economical way to eliminate tooth decay among the general public.[95]

Laboratory and epidemiological studies also confirm that dietary factors other than fluoride are extremely important for the prevention of dental caries. Besides the major tooth-building minerals calcium and phosphorus, other elements such as magnesium, strontium, molybdenum, vanadium, and zinc evidently can play a significant role in caries resistance. On the other hand, too much selenium, copper, manganese, or cadmium may make the teeth more susceptible to decay.[96] Higher chewing loads from coarse, unrefined foods exercise the jaw and teeth more and probably are also important in the caries-immunity of people having little or no fluoride in their drinking water.[97] Furthermore, restoration of heat-labile organic nutrients like lysine, thiamine, and pyridoxine to refined food diets decreases dental caries in man as well as in animals.[98]

Certain studies, using electron microscopy, indicate that tooth decay usually begins with an internal breakdown of protein in the enamel.[98] Well-nourished teeth are therefore much less subject to this initial phase of caries. In the second stage, bacterial attack produces cavities, as demonstrated by the failure of animals in germ-free environments to develop cavities until they are inoculated with cavity-producing bacteria like *Streptococcus mutans*.[99] Impressive results from the vaccination of monkeys fed refined food diets suggest that immunization of children and even adults against cavity-producing bacteria may soon be possible.[100] Meanwhile, to counter today's cariogenic, refined food diets, improved nutrition and good oral hygiene are vital to good dental health.

Considering the outstanding success that other public health measures have achieved in controlling such dreadful afflictions as smallpox, typhoid, diphtheria, poliomyelitis, measles, cholera, and

tuberculosis, it is surprising that a procedure claiming to produce
only "partial prevention" of a major civilization disease —
tooth decay—continues to be so vigorously promoted, especially in view of the availability of far more effective alter-
natives.

₀ Parents who still insist on fluorides for their children's teeth can
dispense fluoride tablets or vitamins, supervise the use of fluoridated mouth rinses, or have their dentist apply topical fluoride
treatments. But I must add a word of CAUTION: these procedures
—like fluoridation— can be dangerous to a child who is sensitive
or intolerant to fluorides. Even in the hands of the most responsible parent or competent professional, disastrous results can occur,
as shown by the following example. In New York City during
1976, a three-year-old child, in good health, received a prophylactic fluoride treatment. The dental technician had applied a "mixture of 4% stannous fluoride solution and pumice" to the boy's
teeth. During the treatment, while still under professional supervision, the child accidentally swallowed ½ Lily cup of 4% stannous
fluoride solution, and within five minutes vomited and suffered a
convulsive seizure. Three hours later he died from cardio-respiratory
arrest during another seizure.[101] Good nutrition does not cause
children to die dramatically, and good eating habits promote other
life-long benefits in addition to better teeth.

WILL THE GREAT DILEMMA END?

Is there any cogent reason why millions of fluoride-sensitive
persons should suffer from a perplexing illness so that others can
enjoy the illusion of better teeth? Prophetic words spoken by dentists, doctors, scientists, and others in the 1940s and 1950s fore-
told most of the problems we have encountered since fluoridation
began. The simple truth is that The Great Dilemma should have
been avoided in the first place. Where did the defenders of public
health take the wrong turns and why?

For nearly a decade after 1931, the PHS sought to *remove* excessive fluoride from water supplies because of endemic mottled
teeth. But after 1940 the balance began to tilt in the opposite direction—to *augment* water supplies with fluoride. On the basis of
studies on a very small number of healthy young men, plus limited
surveys of health effects in natural fluoride areas, PHS scientists

concluded that fluoride had no significant adverse effect on health, except for occasional mild mottling. Even that minor problem, so they thought, could probably be controlled in time.

Morbidity and mortality data apparently also reinforced the PHS optimism, for fluoridated and nonfluoridated areas seemed to have the same rates. On May 18, 1978, to a loud fanfare by the news media, still another reconfirmation by Dr. J. D. Erickson has appeared: "There was no evidence of a harmful effect, including cancer, attributable to fluoridation."[102] Does Erickson's evidence corroborate his conclusion, or does it again, as in the case of his mongolism data,[103] actually support an opposing argument? Since the details of the analysis are not included in his paper, I shall refrain from an extensive critique at this time, but the evidence in the article shows "plainly" that the "age-race-sex-adjusted [death] rates" during 1969-1971 in the 24 fluoridated cities are about 5% *greater* than in the 22 nonfluoridated cities: 1,156.0 (F) vs. 1,102.4 (non–F) per 100,000 population. Only after *additional adjustment* by analysis of covariance for city population density and median education do the figures barely reverse. Thoughtful readers will wonder why *only two* additional adjustments (one of which was itself already adjusted) were applied, when many others could also have been made   for low-income levels, climate, hospitals in the area, air conditioning in the houses, types of housing (multi-unit structures, etc.), length of residency, and water hardness, to name only a few – especially since the author himself admits that *exactly the opposite results might have been achieved had different covariance factors been selected for analysis.*[104] Without analysis for covariance the age-race-sex-adjusted data show: *higher rates* for overall mortality (5%) as well as for cancer-malignant neoplasms (about 4%), and cardiovascular causes (about 8%). With analysis for covariance of factors other than the two selected by the author, the results may accentuate the already marked disadvantage of the fluoridated cities.

These results should be remembered as still other questions arise. Why was the indirect method used when the direct method – using actual age-race-sex-specific figures and not calculated hypothetical rates   presents a statistically more accurate determination? Why was 1965 selected as an arbitrary cut-off date for fluoridation, thus excluding several major fluoridated cities? Why was

Houston not included at least partially as a nonfluoridated city? Why were cities approximately the same size and population density not compared directly, rather than by comparing watermelons with oranges? Lack of time-trend data is still another serious shortcoming, which freezes and obscures trends. In summary, then, this article hardly inspires any confidence in the safety of fluoridation, statistical manipulations notwithstanding.[105]

As a practicing allergist, I am less concerned with unrevealing averages cited in statistics than I am with the individual responses of patients. I constantly assess their reactions to suspected intoxicants, and I often remove suspected agents from their environments. Early in my medical career, I treated a patient sensitive to iodized salt, whose symptoms were reversible simply by switching to plain salt;[106] in 1934 I had the good fortune to hear a paper about a patient who suffered from "asthma and so-called functional colitis" largely caused by chlorine in drinking water. These symptoms disappeared when the patient drank only distilled water and reappeared with chlorinated water.[107]

It was only natural for me, in the 1950s, to begin testing for sensitivity to another halogen in water—fluoride—by having patients in fluoridated areas switch to nonfluoridated water for all drinking and cooking. As we have seen, the results were dramatic, and persons who had vainly sought relief from their manifold ailments suddenly found themselves well again simply by avoiding fluoridated water and high-fluoride food. Other physicians of course have fully confirmed these findings. The stark reality of ill effects from fluoridated water can no longer be denied.

Had the Public Health Service undertaken appropriate screening and testing—as should have been done in the swine-flu inoculation program—it would have discovered, long before endorsing and promoting fluoridation, that there are persons who are sensitive to 1-ppm fluoridated water. PHS scientists would also have found that these individuals became well when they changed to nonfluoridated water. If this approach had been tried in natural fluoride areas with persons suffering from otherwise undiagnosed symptoms of the type caused by fluoride, the PHS itself would have discovered exactly what I have found—many cases of reversible chronic fluoride poisoning.

We are told, however, that nothing out of the ordinary was uncovered. Why not? With all its vast resources and manpower, the

PHS certainly should have been able to discover what others have encountered here and abroad. Possibly the answer is that public health physicians are not oriented toward the study of the individual but the public at large. By not seeking out persons with *reversible* illness and subjecting them to appropriate diagnostic tests of the type I have described, health officials completely overlooked the very effects they concluded were not occurring! It is shocking and deeply ironic that the sophisticated methods of modern epidemiology — so successful in other areas — should have uncovered nothing more serious than mottled enamel as a toxic effect of fluoridated water.

What can be done to throw off the shackles of the past? Despite all its previous "unqualified" endorsements of fluoridation, the Public Health Service can immediately stop playing ostrich, forget what certain industries will say, and begin to publicize the symptoms and causes of reversible chronic fluoride illness. The PHS does not hesitate to warn the public about the hazards of air pollution, lead poisoning, drug abuse, alcoholism, cigarette smoking, etc., so why should it not be willing to do so about fluoride, an equally clear danger to health? Fluoride should no longer enjoy immunity as a "protected pollutant,"[108] and state and local health officials should be exhorted to make honest investigations of illness from fluoridated water and report their findings to the public. Physicians and dentists especially should be allowed to cooperate in this endeavor without fear of reprisals.

Water works engineers, too, can start exercising their traditional responsibility and insist that only safe, potable water be supplied to the public. Consumers should be warned if fluorides are present in the water and what consequences follow from consuming fluoridated water. Failure to do any less is an abdication of responsibility by engineers to make the water as safe as possible.

The Environmental Protection Agency can also cease pretending to "see no evil" about fluoridation. Just because it is a Federal agency does not compel it to go along with everything claimed by the Dental Health Division of the PHS. Under the Safe Drinking Water Act of 1974 the EPA is charged with setting national drinking water standards that provide maximum possible protection to the most sensitive members of the community, not just to persons who enjoy good health. This principle is also enunciated in the NRC report *Drinking Water and Health*, but unfortunately it is completely ignored in the case of fluoride.

If the EPA, PHS, and water engineers do not act, will the present impasse continue? Probably not for very much longer, for more and more scientists and physicians throughout the world are learning about the nondental toxic effects of fluoride in drinking water. They see all too clearly what is happening with fluoridation. As in any struggle for the ascendancy of truth, it is only a matter of time before mistaken views are exposed and discarded; time always sides with the truth.

Meanwhile, officials of the PHS, EPA, NAS–NRC, AAAS, WHO, RCP, AMA, and ADA should ask themselves how they will appear in the ultimate judgment of history for suppressing the very findings they are sworn to reveal. Although they could have "blown the whistle" years ago, when adverse effects were first reported, they failed to do so. And their culpability is constantly increasing as more and more evidence of harm from fluoridation comes to light; all their efforts to contain the bad news will ultimately collapse like the bursting of a dam as the floodwaters of public indignation are unleashed. Their loss of prestige will be inescapable, and science's golden image will be more severely tarnished than it has ever been in the past.

* * * * *

As I enter the twilight of my long and active medical career, I know that the path I chose long ago, though strewn with many obstacles, is the only one I could have taken. No more satisfying nor humane goal can be attained than the truth which alleviates the suffering of mankind. When medical practitioners everywhere also recognize the severity of the problems of chronic fluoride toxicosis, and laws mandating truly safe drinking water are sincerely enforced, the health of millions will dramatically improve. Only then will fluoridation cease to be The Great Dilemma.

REFERENCES

1. Terry, L.L.: The Fourth Great Preventive Measure, in Summary and Recommendations, 1966 National Dental Health Assembly. Emphasis: Fluoridation. Feb. 6-8, 1966, Arlington, Va. USPHS Publ. No. 1552, p. 4.

2. Sterner, J.H.: Is It Safe! Is It Sound! Terry (in Ref. 1, above), p. 4.

3. Exner, F.B.: Affidavit. Seattle, Wash., ca. 1967.

4. Hurme, V.O.: An Examination of the Scientific Basis for Fluoridating Populations. Dent. Items of Interest, 74:518-534, 1952.

5. Babbit, H.E., and Doland, J.J.: Quality of Water Supplies in Water Supply Engineering. 3rd Edition. 1939, p. 454.

6. U.S. Public Health Service Drinking Water Standards, Adopted September 25, 1942. Public Health Rep., 58:69, 1943. Section 4.21 reads: "The presence of . . . fluoride in excess of 1.0 p.p.m. shall constitute ground for rejection of the [water] supply."

7. U.S. Public Health Service Drinking Water Standards, 1946. Public Health Rep., 61:371-384, 1946.

8. McClure, F.J., Mitchell, H.H., Hamilton, T.S., and Kinser, C.A.: Balances of Fluorine Ingested from Various Sources in Food and Water by Five Young Men. Excretion of Fluorine Through the Skin. J. Ind. Hyg. Toxicol., 27:159-170, 1945. (Reprinted in Fluoride Drinking Waters, 1962, pp. 377-384.)

9. McClure, F.J.: Ingestion of Fluoride and Dental Caries. Quantitative Relations Based on Food and Water Requirements of Children One to Twelve years Old. Am. J. Dis. Child., 66:362-369, 1943. (Reprinted in Fluoride Drinking Waters, 1962, pp. 283-286.)

10. McClure, F.J.: Fluorine in Foods. Survey of Recent Data. Public Health Rep., 64:1061-1074, 1949. (Reprinted in Fluoride Drinking Waters, 1962, pp. 287-294.)

11. Hodge, H.C., and Smith, F.A.: Metabolism of Inorganic Fluoride, in J.H. Simons, Ed.: Fluorine Chemistry, Vol. IV. 1965, p. 171.

12. Marier, J.R., and Rose, D.: The Fluoride Content of Some Foods and Beverages—a Brief Survey Using a Modified Zr-SPADNS Method. J. Food Sci., 31:941-946, 1966.

13. San Filippo, F.A., and Battistone, G.C.: The Fluoride Content of a Representative Diet of the Young Adult Male. Clin. Chim. Acta, 31:453-457, 1971.

14. Kramer, L., Osis, D., Wiatrowski, and Spencer, H.: Dietary Fluoride in Different Areas in the United States. Am. J. Clin. Nutr., 27:590-594, 1974. Cf. Prival, M.J., and Fisher, F.: Adding Fluorides to the Diet. Environment (St. Louis), 16(5):29-33, June 1974; also, Rose, D., and Marier, J.R.: Environmental Fluoride 1977. CNRC Report No. 16081, 1978.

15. USPHS Drinking Water Standards. 1961 Revision. Public Health Rep., 76:782, 1961. Republished in Drinking Water Standards Revised 1962. PHS Publ. No. 956, Washington, D.C., 1962.

16. Dean, H.T.: Chronic Endemic Dental Fluorosis (Mottled Enamel). J. Am. Med. Assoc., 107:1269-1272, 1936.

17. According to the NRC Safe Drinking Water Committee report

Drinking Water and Health (1977, p. 370), a 1970 USPHS survey showed that "Nearly 1 million people in 524 communities [in the U.S.] were receiving water with more than 2 mg/liter of naturally occurring fluoride."

18. Ref. 17, above, p. 11.

19. Report prepared by J.L. Shupe, N.J. Leone, and D.C. Fletcher: Efficacy and Safety of Fluoridation. Am. Med. Assoc., Chicago, Ill., Sept. 1975. Cf. Ref. 24, below, pp. 14-15.

20. Spencer, H., Lewin, I., Wiatrowski, and Samachson, J.: Fluoride Metabolism in Man. Am. J. Med., 49:807-813, 1970. Cf. Prival and Fisher (in Ref. 14, above).

21. Forst, J.A., M.D., Division of Pupil Personnel Services, The University of the State of New York, The State Education Department, Albany, N.Y.: Letter to Dr. J.D. Kerwin, Oct. 26, 1954. Cf. J. Rorty, in The American Fluoridation Experiment, Revised Edition. 1961, p. 18.

22. Monteleone, U.L.: Victory in Allentown. National Fluoridation News, 17(1):1-4, Jan.-Feb. 1971.

23. Douglas, B.L., Wallace, D.A., Lerner, M., and Coppersmith, S.B.: The Impact of Fluoridation on Patterns of Dental Treatment. J. Public Health Dent., 31:275-281, 1971. For comment on initial report, see Lear, J.: Fluoridation and the Dentist. Saturday Review, Aug. 2, 1969, p. 50.

24. House of Delegates, Am. Med. Assoc.: Statement on Fluoridation of Public Water Supplies. Philadelphia, Dec. 3-6, 1957, p. 15.

25. Jolly, S.S., Prasad, S., Sharma, R., and Rai, B.: Human Fluoride Intoxication in Punjab. Fluoride, 4:64-79, 1971.

26. Rodríguez, I.A.: Estudio Médico del Fluoro. Univ. Salamanca, 1955.

27. Steyn, D.G.: Chronic Fluorine Poisoning Caused by the Drinking of Subterranean Waters Containing Excessive Quantities of Fluorine, in T. Gordonoff, Ed.: The Toxicology of Fluorine. 1964, pp. 53-57.

28. For references, see Chapter 13, above.

29. Klein, W., Kocsis, F., and Wottawa, A.: DNA Repair and Environmental Substances. Ber. Osterr. Studienges. Atomenenerg. (SGAE Ber.), No. 2613 (1976). See also: Klein, W., Kocsis, F., and Altmann, H., ibid., No. 2355 (1974).

30. Czerwinski, E., and Lankosz, W.: Fluoride-Induced Changes in 60 Retired Aluminum Workers. Fluoride, 10:125-136, 1977.

31. Waldbott, G.L.: Editorial: Gastric Ulcer and Fluoride. Fluoride, 10: 149-151, 1977.

32. Shea, J.J., Gillespie, S.M., and Waldbott, G.L.: Allergy to Fluoride. Ann. Allergy, 25:388-391, 1967.

33. Whitford, G.M., Pashley, D.H., and Stringer, G.I.: Fluoride Renal Clearance: A pH-Dependent Event. Am. J. Physiol. 230:527-532, 1976.

34. Geever, E.F., McCann, H.G., McClure, F.J., Lee, W.A., and Schiffmann, E.: Fluoridated Water, Skeletal Structure, and Chemistry. Health Serv.

Mental Health Admin. Health Rep., 86:820-828, 1971.

35. Bacon, J.F.: Arterial Calcification in Infancy. J. Am. Med. Assoc., 188: 933-935, 1964. For further discussion, see Chapter 8, above, p. 106.

36. Cristofolini, M., and Largaiolli, D.: Su di una probabile tossidermia da fluoro. Revista Med. Trentina, 4:1-5, 1966.

37. Rogot, E., Sharrett, A.R., Feinleib, M., and Fabsitz, R.R.: Trends in Urban Mortality in Relation to Fluoridation Status. Am. J. Epidemiol., 107: 104-112, 1978.

38. Taves, D.R.: Fluoridation and Mortality Due to Heart Disease. Nature (Lond.), 272:361-362, 1978.

39. Taves, D.R., and Neuman, W.F.: Factors Controlling Calcification in Vitro: Fluoride and Magnesium. Arch. Biochem. Biophys., 108:390-397, 1964.

40. Nordin, B.E.C., in British Medical Research Council Report, Medical News (London), Sept. 26, 1969. Exner, F.B.: Open Letter to J. Talbott, Editor, J. Am. Med. Assoc., Nov. 11, 1966. Copy in my possession.

41. Pinet, A., and Pinet, F.: Endemic Fluorosis in the Sahara. Fluoride, 1:86-93, 1968.

42. Petraborg, H.T.: Chronic Fluoride Intoxication from Drinking Water (Preliminary Report). Fluoride, 7:47-52, 1974; Grimbergen, G.W.: A Double Blind Test for Determination of Intolerance to Fluoridated Water (Preliminary Report), ibid., 7:146-152, 1974; Petraborg, H.T.: Hydrofluorosis in the Milwaukee Area. Ibid., 10:165-169, 1977.

43. Geall, M.G., and Beilin, L.J.: Sodium Fluoride and Optic Neuritis. Br. Med. J., 2:355-356, 1964.

44. Franke, J., Rath, F., Runge, H., Fengler, F., Auermann, E., and Lenart, G.: Industrial Fluorosis. Fluoride, 8:61-85, 1975.

45. Greenberg, L.W., Nelson, C.E., and Kramer, N.: Nephrogenic Diabetes Insipidus with Fluorosis. Pediatrics, 54:320-322, 1974.

46. Klein, H.: Dental Fluorosis Associated with Hereditary Diabetes Insipidus. Oral Surg., 40:736-741, 1975.

47. Ramseyer, W.F., Smith, C.A.H., and McCay, C.M.: Effect of Sodium Fluoride Administration on Body Changes in Old Rats. J. Gerontol., 12:14-19, 1957.

48. Sullivan, W.D.: The In Vitro and In Vivo Effects of Fluoride on Succinic Dehydrogenase Activity. Fluoride, 2:168-175, 1969.

49. Manocha, S.L., Warner, H., and Olkowski, Z.L.: Cytochemical Response of Kidney, Liver and Nervous System to Fluoride Ions In Drinking Water. Histochem. J., 7:343-355, 1975.

50. Cordy, P.E., Gagnon, R., Taves, D.R., and Kaye, M.: Bone Disease in Hemodialysis Patients with Particular Reference to the Effect of Fluoride. Can. Med. Assoc. J., 110:1349-1353, 1974.

51. Waters, W.E.: Relationship of Water Salinity and Fluorides to Keeping

Quality of Chrysanthemum and Gladiolus Cut-Flowers. Proc. Am. Soc. Hortic. Sci., 92:633-640, 1968; Influence of Well Water Salinity and Fluorides on Keeping Quality of "Tropicana" Roses. Proc. Fla. State Hortic. Soc., 81:355-359, 1968. Also, Spierings, F.: Injury to Gladiolus by Fluoridated Water. Fluoride, 3:66-71, 1970. These findings have been cited in New Scientist (46: 143, 1970) as "irrefutable evidence of the harmful effects of fluorine [at the 1-ppm concentration] in water supplies."

52. Poole, R.T., and Conover, C.A.: Influence of Propagation Media and Amendments on Fluoride Toxicity of *Cordyline Terminalis* 'Baby Doll'. Fluoride, 8:85-92, 1975.

53. Cf. Marier, J.R., and Rose, D.: Environmental Fluoride. Can. Natl. Res. Council Publ. No. 12,226, Ottawa [1971], pp. 15-18.

54. Groth, E., III: An Evaluation of the Potential for Ecological Damage by Chronic Low-Level Environmental Pollution by Fluoride. Fluoride, 8:224-240, 1975. See also Refs. 1-4, Chapter 3, above.

55. Lillie, R.J.: Air Pollutants Affecting the Performance of Domestic Animals. A Literature Review. Agricultural Research Service, U.S. Dept. Agric. Handbook No. 380, Washington, D.C., August 1970.

56. For a similar telephone call by J. Small, see Chapter 18, above, p. 328.

57. Lillie, R.J.: Letter to Director, Division of Dental Health, NIH, Sept. 7, 1971. Copy in my possession.

58. The National Cancer Program (Part 2. Fluoridation of Public Drinking Water): Hearings before the Intergovernmental Relations and Human Resources Subcommittee of the Committee on Government Operations, House of Representatives, Ninety-fifth Congress, First Session, Sept. 21 and Oct. 12, 1977. Washington, D.C., 1977, pp. 11-12; 63-67; 81-82; 205-218; 263-270.

59. Public Law 93-523, signed into effect by President Gerald Ford Dec. 16, 1974: "No national primary drinking water regulation may require the addition of any substance for preventive health care purposes unrelated to contamination of drinking water." Par. (6), Sec. 1412(b). For details and comment, see National Fluoridation News, 21(1):1-2, Jan.-March 1975.

60. Bellack, E., and Baker, R.J.: Fluoridation Chemicals – The Supply Picture. J. Am. Water Works Assoc., 62:223-224, 1970.

61. Medvedev, Z.A.: The Rise and Fall of T. D. Lysenko, trans. by I.M. Lerner. Columbia Univ. Press, New York, 1969. Cf. Joravsky, D.: The Lysenko Affair. Harvard Univ. Press, Cambridge, Mass., 1970.

62. Carson, R.: Silent Spring. Houghton Mifflin, Boston, 1962, Ch. 10. Cf. Hinckley, A.D.: The Gypsy Moth. Environment (St. Louis), 14(2):41-47, March 1972.

63. Lawson, H.G.: Nuclear Split. Argument Breaks Out Over the Health Impact of Peaceful Atom Uses. Wall Street Journal, May 20, 1970, pp. 1,23.

64. Wick, G.: They Won't Shut Up. New Scientist and Science Journal, 50:532-533, 1971.

65. Bross, I.D.J.: Low-Level Ionizing Radiation is Hazardous to Health: A Coverup and Its Consequences. Testimony presented before U.S. House of Representatives Subcommittee on Health and Environment, Feb. 8, 1978. (Full text in National Health Federation Bulletin, 24(5):2-7, May 1978. See also Ref. 105, below.)

66. Salaman, M.: Linus Pauling Can't Get Money, NCI Spends $300 Thousand To Prove Him Wrong. Public Scrutiny, 1(3):6, April 1, 1978. Cf. NCI Explains Vitamin 'C' Study Taxpayers Hit for $300 Thousand. Ibid., 1(4):16, May 1, 1978. See also, Pauling, L., and Robinson, A.B.: The Linus Pauling Institute – A Reply. New Scientist, 77:98-101, 1978.

67. Exner, F.B.: The "Margin of Safety" in Fluoride Treatment in a Fluorine-Polluted Environment. Seattle, Washington, April, 1970. Cf. Exner, F.B.: Fluorine Pollution of Air, Water and Soil (Sources and Effects on Plants Animals and People). Presented at the Second Meeting of the International Society for Fluoride Research, Barcelona, Spain, Jan. 27-29, 1969.

68. Am. Dent. Assoc.: Fluoridation Facts: Answers to Questions About Fluoridation. Chicago, Ill., 1974.

69. Newbrun, E.: The Safety of Fluoridation. J. Am. Dent. Assoc., 94: 301-304, 1977.

70. Br. Dent. Assoc.: Fluoridation of Water Supplies: Questions and Answers. Br. Dent. Assoc., The Fluoridation Society, and The Health Education Council, London, Jan. 1976.

71. Report of the Royal College of Physicians of London: Fluoride, Teeth and Health. 1976.

72. Cook, H.A.: Letter to A. W. Burgstahler, Aug. 13, 1975. Copy in my possession.

73. Cited on p. 22 (No's. 16 and 17) of Ref. 71, above.

74. Brodsky, L.: A Criticism of Fluoridation. Univ. Ottawa Med. J., 10(1): 4-10, Sept.-Nov. 1965, at p. 8.

75. Burk, D.: Letter to Mrs. D. E. Winkler, Orinda, Calif., April 12, 1978. Copy in my possession.

76. Taves, D.R.: Fluoride, in Drinking Water and Health. 1977, p. 399.

77. Manocha, S.L.: Letter to A.W. Burgstahler, Nov. 18, 1975. Copy in my possession. Amplified by Ref. 78 below.

78. Telephone conference: A. W. Burgstahler and H. L. McKinney with S. L. Manocha and H. Warner, May 26, 1978. Manocha, S.L.: Letter and personal communication to A.W. Burgstahler, June 2, 1978. Telephone call, H.L. McKinney to H. Warner, June 6, 1978.

79. Taves (in Ref. 76, above), p. 391.

80. Smith, E.H.: Fluoridation of Water Supply. J. Am. Med. Assoc., 230: 1569, 1974.

81. Archer, J.D., Senior Editor, J. Am. Med. Assoc.: Letter to H. T. Petraborg, March 27, 1975. Copy in my possession.

82. Crosby, W.H., Coordinator of When Friends or Patients Ask About. . .: Letter to P. E. Zanfagna, Dec. 27, 1974. Copy in my possession.

83. For accounts, see National Fluoridation News, 2(4):3, April 1956; 2(7):1-2, July-August 1956; 2(8):2, Sept. 1956; 3(4):3, April 1957; 9(1):4, Jan.–Feb. 1963; 21(3):1-2, July-Sept. 1975. For discussion, cf. Gotzsche, A. L.: The Fluoride Question: Poison or Panacea? 1975, pp. 130-134.

84. Dangel, R.A., Fluoridation Engineer, U.S. Environmental [Protection?] Agency, Boston, Mass.: Letter to Division of Dentistry, USPHS, Oct. 10, 1975. Quoted in USPHS Memo FL-89, August 1976.

85. Boffey, P.M.: The Brain Bank of America: An Inquiry Into the Politics of Science. McGraw-Hill, New York, 1975.

86. Professional Bulletin No. 2 of the Federation of American Scientists, Nov. 1974.

87. Rodgers, W.H., Jr.: Corporate Country. Rodale Press, Emmaus, Pa., 1973.

88. Edsall, J.T.: Scientific Freedom and Responsibility. Report of the AAAS Committee on Scientific Freedom and Responsibility. Science, 188: 687-693, 1975. Cf. St. James-Roberts, I.: Are Researchers Trustworthy? New Scientist, 71:481-483, 1976.

89. Gould, S.J.: Morton's Ranking of Races by Cranial Capacity. Science, 200:503-509, 1978.

90. AAAS Committee on Science in the Promotion of Human Welfare: The Integrity of Science. Am. Sci., 53:174-198, 1965.

91. See Chapter 10, above, pp. 141-144.

92. Price, W.A.: Nutrition and Physical Degeneration. A Comparison of Primitive and Modern Diets and Their Effects. Am. Acad. Appl. Nutr., Los Angeles, 1948, pp. 288-290.

93. Turner, E., and Vickery, K.O.A.: The Wholemeal Bread Family – A Pilot Study. Vitalst. Zivilisationskr., 11:99-102, 1966.

94. Åslander, A.: Correlation Between Tooth Nutrition and Dental Caries According to the Laws of Nature. Odontol. Tidskr., 73:595-612, 1965; The Technique of Complete Tooth Nutrition, Pakistan Dent. Rev., 18(4):2-9, Oct. 1968.

95. Laplaud, P.H.: Prévention Sociale de la Carie Dentaire. Thèse pour le doctorat en chirurgie dentaire, Dactylo-Sorbonne, Paris, 1969, pp. 125-126.

96. Cf. Dalderup, L.M.: Nutrition and Caries. World Rev. Nutr. Diet., 7:72 -137, 1967; Ludwig, T.G.; Adkins, B.L., and Losee, F.L.: Relationship of Concentrations of Eleven Elements in Water Supplies to Caries Prevalence in American School Children. Aust. Dent. J., 15:126-132, 1970. Cf. Curzon, M. E.J., and Losee, F.L.: Dental Caries and Trace Element Composition of Whole Human Enamel: Western United States. J. Am. Dent. Assoc., 96:819-822, 1978.

97. Neumann, H.H., and DiSalvo, N.A.: Caries Absence Among "Primitives." New York J. Dent., 35:355-358, 1965.

98. Sharpenak, A.E.: The Etiology and Prevention of Dental Caries. N.Y. State Dent. J., 33:592-600, 1967.

99. Cf. Dalderup (in Ref. 96, above), p. 122. Also see Ref. 100, below.

100. Lehner, T.: A Vaccine Against Dental Decay. New Scientist, 78:216-218, 1978.

101. Church, L.E.: Fluorides – Use With Caution. J. Maryland State Dent. Assoc., 19:106, Aug. 1976. Is there a parallel in the manner of death of this child and that of the nurse described in Chapter 18, above, pp. 336-337?

102. Erickson, J.D.: Mortality in Selected Cities with Fluoridated and Non-Fluoridated Water Supplies. N. Engl. J. Med., 298:1112-1116, 1978.

103. See Chapter 13, above, pp. 214-215 and 218-219.

104. Telephone call, A.W. Burgstahler and H.L. McKinney with J. D. Erickson, June 2, 1978.

105. Statistics can be manipulated to support almost any reasonable hypothesis and can also be used to obscure important differences between opposing interpretations. Analysts must always move beyond numbers if they are to achieve any substance of truth. Bross has remarked: "As a professional biostatistician for 25 years, I am well aware that it is hard for most people, and most scientists, to appreciate the distinction between a good statistical analysis and a bad one." Irwin D. J. Bross, Ph.D., Director of Biostatistics, Roswell Park Memorial Institute, Buffalo, N.Y.: Hazards to Persons Exposed to Ionizing Radiation (and to Their Children) from Dosages Currently Permitted by the Nuclear Regulatory Commission. Revised for presentation to the Nucl. Regul. Comm., Washington, D.C., April 7, 1978.

106. Waldbott, G.L.: Discussion of paper cited in Ref. 107, below, p. 201.

107. Watson, S.H., and Kibler, S.K.: Drinking Water as a Cause of Asthma. J. Allergy, 5:197-198, 1934.

108. Jerard, E., Ed.: The Case of the Protected Pollutant [New York, 1969].

LIST OF MAJOR SYMPTOMS:

CHRONIC FLUORIDE TOXICITY SYNDROME

MOST OF THE FOLLOWING reversible ill effects caused by fluoride were first recognized among aluminum workers in the 1930s by the Danish health officer Dr. Kaj Roholm. Not all the symptoms are necessarily present at the same time. Their severity and duration (often episodic) depend on a person's age, nutritional status, environment, kidney function, amount of fluoride ingested, genetic background, tendency to allergies, and other factors.

To test for fluoride intoxication, *the following procedures must be rigorously followed.* Avoid all fluoridated water (substitute distilled or other nonfluoridated, low-fluoride water), fluoridated beverages, fluoride-rich foods (tea, ocean fish, gelatin, skin of chicken, etc.), fluoridated toothpastes, and any other source of environmental fluoride, including cigarette smoke and industrial pollution (see Chapter 19, pages 376-377, above). If symptoms are in fact caused by fluoride, they should diminish markedly within a week and largely disappear within several weeks. If symptoms persist, consult a physician for possible alternative problems. *True fluoride toxicosis* can be reproduced by re-exposure to fluorides from whatever source.

CAVEAT: *The following list contains symptoms that can have other origins even in someone suffering from chronic fluoride poisoning:*

Chronic fatigue not relieved by extra sleep or rest
Headaches
Dryness of the throat and excessive water consumption
Frequent need to urinate
Urinary tract irritation
Aches and stiffness in muscles/bones (arthritic-like pain)
    In lower back   In neck area
    In jaws   In arms, shoulders, legs
Muscular weakness
Muscle spasms (involuntary twitching)
Tingling sensations in fingers (especially) and feet
Gastrointestinal disturbances
    Abdominal pains   Blood in stools
    Diarrhea   Bloated feeling (gas)
    Constipation   Tenderness in stomach area
Feeling of nausea (flu-like symptoms)
Pinkish-red or bluish-red spots (like bruises, but round or oval) on
    the skin that fade and clear up in 7-10 days.
Skin rash or itching, especially after showers or bathing.
Mouth sores (also from fluoridated toothpaste)
Loss of mental acuity and ability to concentrate
Depression
Excessive nervousness
Dizziness
Tendency to lose balance
Visual disturbances
    Temporary blind spots in field of vision
    Diminished ability to focus (possible retinal damage)

ADDITIONAL READING

Blount, P.C.: *Compulsory Mass Medication*. The Clair Press, London, 1964.

Buck, R.M.: *The Grim Truth About Fluoridation*. G.P. Putnam's Sons, New York. 1964.

Caldwell, G., and Zanfagna, P.E.: *Fluoridation and Truth Decay*. Top-Ecol Press, 3025 Highridge Road, LaCrescenta, Calif. 91214. 1974.

Campbell, I.R., Widner, E.M., and Kukainis, I.P.: *Annotated Bibliography: The Occurence and Biologic Effects of Fluorine Compounds*. Vol. 1. *The Inorganic Compounds*. The Kettering Laboratory, University of Cincinnati, Cincinnati, Ohio. 1958. Supplement: *Fluoride Abstracts: 1955-1971*. The Kettering Laboratory. 1967-1971.

Cannell, W.A.: *Medical and Dental Aspects of Fluoridation*. H.K. Lewis & Co., Ltd., London. 1960.

Committee on Biologic Effects of Atmospheric Pollutants, National Research Council: *Fluorides*. National Academy of Sciences, Washington, D.C. 1971.

Eagers, R.Y.: *Toxic Properties of Inorganic Fluorine Compounds*. Elsevier, Amsterdam-London-New York. 1969.

Fluoridation of Water: *Hearings before the Committee on Interstate and Foreign Commerce*. U.S. House of Representatives, Eighty-Third Congress, Second Session, on H.R. 2341. May 25, 26, and 27, 1954. U.S. Government Printing Office, Washington, D.C. 1954.

Exner, F.B., Waldbott, G.L., and Rorty, J.: *The American Fluoridation Experiment*. Revised Edition. Devin-Adair Co., New York. 1961.

Gordonoff, T., Ed.: *The Toxicology of Fluorine* (Symposium, Bern, Switzerland, October 15-17, 1962). Schwabe & Co., Basel/Stuttgart. 1964.

Gotzsche, A.L.: *The Fluoride Question: Panacea or Poison?* Stein and Day, New York. 1975.

Hodge, H.C., and Smith, F.A.: *Fluorine Chemistry.* Vol. IV. J.H. Simons, Ed. Academic Press, New York and London. 1965.

McClure, F.J., Ed.: *Fluoride Drinking Waters.* U.S. Dept. Health, Education, and Welfare, Public Health Service, Institute of Dental Research, Bethesda, Md. 1962.

McClure, F.J.: *Water Fluoridation: The Search and the Victory.* U.S. Dept. Health, Education, and Welfare, Public Health Service, Institute of Dental Research, Bethesda, Md. 1970.

McNeil, D.R.: *The Fight for Fluoridation.* Oxford University Press, New York. 1957.

Moulton, F.R., Ed.: *Fluorine and Dental Health.* American Association for the Advancement of Science, Washington, D.C. 1942.

Moulton, F.R., Ed.: *Dental Caries and Fluorine.* American Association for the Advancement of Science, Washington, D.C. 1946.

The National Cancer Program (Part 2.–Fluoridation of Public Drinking Water): *Hearings before the Subcommittee on Intergovernmental Relations and Human Resources of the Committee on Government Operations.* U.S. House of Representatives, Ninety-fifth Congress. Sept. 21 and Oct. 12, 1977. U.S. Government Printing Office, Washington, D.C. 1977.

Newbrun, E., Ed.: *Fluorides and Dental Caries.* Second Edition. Charles C. Thomas, Springfield, Ill., 1975.

Polya, J.: *Are We Safe? A Layman's Guide to Controversy in Public Health.* F.W. Cheshire Pty., Ltd., Melbourne, Australia. 1964.

Proceedings of the Symposium on Fluorosis -- October 1974. Indian Academy of Geoscience, Osmania University, Hyderabad, India, 1977.

Roholm, K.: *Fluorine Intoxication: A Clinical-Hygienic Study with a Review of the Literature and Some Experimental Investigations.* NYT Nordisk Forlag, Arnold Busck, Copenhagen, and H.K. Lewis & Co., London. 1937.

Rose, D., and Marier, J.R.: *Environmental Fluoride 1977.* National Research Council Canada. Report No. 16081. Ottawa, Ont., Can. [July 1978].

Royal College of Physicians of London: *Fluoride, Teeth and Health.* Pitman Medical Publishing, Ltd., London. 1976.

Safe Drinking Water Committee, National Research Council: *Drinking Water and Health.* National Academy of Sciences. Washington, D.C. 1977.

Shaw, J.H., Ed.: *Fluoridation as a Public Health Measure.* American Association for the Advancement of Science, Washington, D.C. 1954.

Smith, F.A., Ed.: *Pharmacology of Fluorides,* in *Handbook of Experimental Pharmacology,* Vol. 20, Parts 1 and 2. Springer-Verlag, Berlin-Heidelberg-New York. 1966, 1970.

Steyn, D.G.: *The Problem of Dental Caries and The Fluoridation of Public Water Supplies.* Voortrekkerpers Beperk, Johannesburg. 1958.

Sutton, P.R.N.: *Fluoridation: Errors and Omissions in Experimental Trails.* Second Edition. Melbourne Univ. Press, Melbourne, Australia. 1960.

Vischer, T.L.: *Fluoride in Medicine.* Hans Huber, Bern, Switzerland. 1969.

Waldbott, G.L.: *Fluoride in Clinical Medicine.* S. Karger, Basel-New York. 1962. (Suppl. 1, Vol. 20, *International Archives of Allergy and Applied Immunology).*

Waldbott, G.L.: *Health Effects of Environmental Pollutants.* Second Edition. C.V. Mosby Co., St. Louis, Mo. 1978.

Waldbott, G.L.: *A Struggle With Titans.* Carlton Press, New York. 1965.

WHO Monograph No. 59: *Fluorides and Human Health.* World Health Organization, Geneva. 1970.

OTHER SOURCES

American Dental Association, 211 East Superior Ave., Chicago, Ill. 60611.

International Society for Fluoride Research, P.O. Box 692, Warren, Mich. 48090.

National Fluoridation News, Route One, Gravette, Ark. 72736.

National Pure Water Association, 223 Newtown Road, Worcester WR5 1JB, England.

U.S. Public Health Service, National Center for Disease Control, Atlanta, Ga. 30333; also USPHS, Division of Dental Health, Rockville Pike, Bethesda, Md. 20014.

INDEX

Note: Daggers (†) designate pages on which literature and sources are cited. All persons named in the text are indexed; otherwise only first-named and principal authors in the references are listed.

ABOUT THE AUTHORS

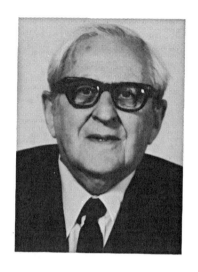

GEORGE L. WALDBOTT was graduated from medical school at the University of Heidelberg in 1921 and interned at Henry Ford Hospital, Detroit, Michigan during 1923-24. He is one of the first allergy specialists in the United States and has enjoyed an active and successful career in that discipline. In 1927 he carried out the first pollen survey in the State of Michigan; ten years later, he conducted the first comprehensive air survey for fungi in the United States. He first advocated bronchoscopic lavage as an emergency lifesaving treatment for asthma patients; he also reported the first sudden anaphylactic fatality from penicillin. Another first in his career was his description of a lung disease, caused by smoking, which leads to emphysema (*not* Loeffler's Disease). He initially drew attention to the significance of the thymus gland in allergies. He is the world's leading medical expert on the clinical aspects of chronic fluoride toxicity, as well as a widely consulted authority on the health effects of environmental contaminants.

Dr. Waldbott has written many books, monographs, and articles. The best known longer works are: *Contact Dermatitis* (Charles C. Thomas, Springfield, Ill., 1953); *A Struggle With Titans* (Carlton Press, New York, 1965); *Health Effects of Environmental Pollutants* (The C.V. Mosby Company, St. Louis, 1973; Second edition, 1978); "The Physiologic and Hygienic Aspects of the Absorption of Inorganic Fluorides," *AMA Archives of Environmental Health*, 2:155-167, 1961; 4:450, 1962; "Fluoride in Clinical Medicine," *International Archives of Allergy and Applied Immunology*, Suppl. 1 to Vol. 20:1-60, 1962; "Acute Fluoride Intoxication," *Acta Medica Scandinavica*, Suppl. 400 to Vol. 174:1-44, 1963; and hundreds of other publications.

His professional affiliations and honors are far too numerous to list in detail. They include among others: co-founder and former president of the Michigan Allergy Society; Fellow of the American Academy of Allergy; Fellow of the American College of Physicians; Fellow of the American College of Chest Physicians; Honorary Member of the Spanish and French Allergy Societies; Affiliate Member of the Royal Society of Medicine, London, England; founder and chief of four allergy clinics in Detroit; founder and Secretary of the International Society for Fluoride Research and editor of the journal *Fluoride*.

Dr. Waldbott has studied cases of fluorosis at many locations in the United States as well as in Canada, Switzerland, Italy, Germany, Sweden, Belgium, and Spain. He has treated more than 500 cases of fluoride toxicity and practices medicine in Warren, Michigan.

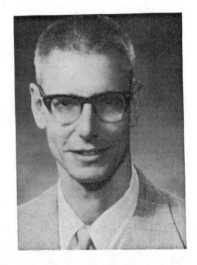

ALBERT W. BURGSTAHLER received his B.S. degree in chemistry (Magna cum Laude) from the University of Notre Dame (1949) and his M.A. (1950) and Ph.D. (1953) degrees in organic chemistry from Harvard University. After post-doctoral studies at the University of London, a year as an instructor at Notre Dame, and further post-doctoral research at the University of Wisconsin, Madison, he joined the faculty at the University of Kansas in 1956, where he is now a professor of chemistry.

Prof. Burgstahler maintains active research in organic synthesis and the chemistry and chiroptical properties of natural products; he has authored or coauthored over 50 scientific publications in these areas. His interest in fluoride research began in the early 1960s with work on the synthesis and biological properties of fluorinated amino acids. He then enlarged this focus to the overall literature of fluoridation, recently emphasizing the connection of fluoride with Down's syndrome (mongolism).

He is a past president of the International Society for Fluoride Research and a co-editor of its journal *Fluoride*. From 1961 to 1964 he was an Alfred P. Sloan Research Fellow and in 1965 received a Notre Dame Centennial of Science Award.

H. LEWIS McKINNEY was graduated with Distinction from the University of Oklahoma before continuing his advanced studies at Cornell University, where he received his Ph.D. in History of Science (1967). He has taught the history of biology and medicine as a faculty member at Yale University, School of Medicine, and he was subsequently a Public Health Service Special Postdoctoral Fellow at Yale before joining the faculty at The University of Kansas. He is now Professor of the History of Science, specializing in biology and medicine. He is particularly interested in scientific innovation and the interaction between science and society.

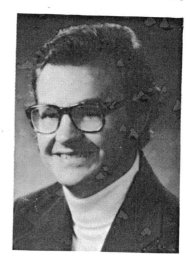

Professor McKinney has published many articles and books, including *Lamarck to Darwin: Contributions to Evolutionary Biology, 1809-1859* (Coronado Press, Lawrence, Ks., 1971; Fourth printing 1977) and *Wallace and Natural Selection* (Yale University Press, New Haven, Conn., 1972). His articles have appeared in *The Journal of the History of Medicine and Allied Sciences, The Dictionary of Scientific Biography,* the *Encyclopedia of American Biography, Isis,* and elsewhere.

His *Wallace and Natural Selection* (1972) was a finalist for the National Book Award (Sciences category) in 1973.